TESTIMONIALS

RE: Permanent Diabetes Control (book)   www.mydiabetescontrol.com

Dr. Konduru is an intelligent and committed scientist who has learned to manage his diabetes and cardiovascular risk factors. This book represents a comprehensive and readable review that could help many people with diabetes.

Dr. Marshall Dahl
BSc, MD, PhD, FRCPC, Certified Endocrinologist
Faculty of Medicine
University of British Columbia
Vancouver, British Columbia, Canada

RE: Dr. Rao Konduru's Publications   www.mydiabetescontrol.com

1. Permanent Diabetes Control
2. The Secret to Controlling Type 2 Diabetes
3. Reversing Obesity
4. Reversing Sleep Apnea
5. Reversing Insomnia
6. Drinking Water Guide (www.DrinkingWaterGuide.com)

TO WHOM IT MAY CONCERN
Dr. Rao Konduru, PhD is a patient of mine who has suffered from chronic diabetes for most of his life; He also suffered from uncontrollable obesity, sleep apnea and chronic insomnia for the past 3 to 4 years. He has managed to reverse all of these conditions by taking non-pharmacological and science-based natural measures with great success. He has created 6 how-to user guides/books with regard to how he achieved this, and I recommend these books for anyone suffering from these conditions.

Sincerely,
Dr. Ali Ghahary, MD
Brentwood Medical Clinic
4567 Lougheed Hwy
Burnaby, British Columbia, Canada

RE: Permanent Diabetes Control (book)   www.mydiabetescontrol.com

Headline: Excellent Guide Regarding Diabetes
Dr. Rao Konduru's book, Permanent Diabetes Control, is a very useful guide and roadmap for anyone wishing to manage their diabetes well. It is an easy read and will be of great benefit. I intend to recommend this book to my diabetic patients.

Dr. Gary Almas, DPM-Podiatrist
4170 Fraser Street
Vancouver, British Columbia, Canada

RE: Permanent Diabetes Control (book)   www.mydiabetescontrol.com

We all know that food raises blood sugars, especially those big meals. We also know that exercise may reduce blood sugars. But Dr. Konduru teaches us how to put one and one together.

This book provides us with a method to accomplish a healthy lifestyle. Dr. Konduru learned it the hard way. After experiencing complications he decided to find the way his body likes to be treated. We, on the other hand, should learn from his experience and start implementing perfect blood sugar controls right now! Thank you, Dr. Rao Konduru, for providing the diabetic community with such a comprehensive book, on everything related to blood sugar control, including all up-to-date technology. I would recommend this book to every newly diagnosed and veteran diabetic!

Rabbi Hirsch Meisels
Moderator, FriendsWithDiabetes.Org
Spring Valley, New York, USA

RE: Permanent Diabetes Control (book)   www.mydiabetescontrol.com

Dr. Rao Konduru, in his book Permanent Diabetes Control, has made an outstanding contribution to the field of diabetes management. This is a book that will inspire its readers, whether diabetic or not, to make changes that will improve the quality of their lives forever. Through his own innovative experiments, Dr. Konduru has succeeded in developing a method of diabetes control that has allowed him, incredibly, to reduce his insulin dose by 60%, to reverse critical heart disease, thus avoiding bypass surgery, and to stabilize his blood glucose levels. In Permanent Diabetes Control, Dr. Konduru has carefully explained this method so that others may benefit from his revolutionary discovery. Join him in controlling your diabetes!

Ms. Ricki Ewings, BA, TT
Professional Freelance Writer and Editor
Member, Editors' Association of Canada
Hotline Co-Chair, EAC-BC
Vancouver, British Columbia, Canada

RE: Reversing Sleep Apnea (book)   www.reversingsleepapnea.com

Dear Rao,
I read your book this weekend and it is an impressively comprehensive and extremely well-documented review of the broad spectrum of therapies available to treat and help relieve sleep apnea. You are to be heartily congratulated on a finely-researched and very practical work that will be accessible and useful to a wide audience of readers. I wish you every success.

Best regards,
Mr. Martin R. Hoke
President
RhinoSystems, Inc.
Brooklyn Heights, OHIO-44131, USA

REVIEWS: Permanent Diabetes Control (book)

Please do not ignore reviews. Please read all reviews thoroughly.
You can learn a lot by reading through the reviews below:

Lyndsie
5.0 out of 5 stars Fully Comprehensive Guide for All Diabetics!
Reviewed in the United States on December 8, 2020
Verified Purchase

"The Secret to Controlling Diabetes in 90 days" is discovered, illustrated and explained in detail in this fully comprehensive guide, and I urge all diabetics to read through and benefit from this revolutionary diabetes control treatment. If you understand that "secret," as explained in this book, you will be victorious in controlling your diabetes in 90 days, and then live like a normal person for the rest of your life.

The author of this book, being a seriously diabetic person himself, is the living example. He published his official blood test results in this book for the past 10 plus years, taken once every 3 months. His hemoglobin A1c result has been consistently normal for more than 10 years, indicating the fact that he accomplished "Permanent Diabetes Control."

We the diabetics on the other hand should learn from his experience, and start implementing the awesome diabetes control method illustrated with many easy-to-understand examples in this wonderful book titled "Permanent Diabetes Control: The Complete Guide to Living Like A Normal Person Forever."

Steve_M
5.0 out of 5 stars How to Manage Diabetes and Live Like A Normal Person!
Reviewed in the United States on June 10, 2021
Verified Purchase

If you are struggling to keep your diabetes under control, and if you want your A1c level be under 7%, you must read and practice the procedures so nicely outlined with worked-out examples in this comprehensive guide.

This book is for all diabetic people (type2, type 1 & gestational) in the field of diabetes management. This book has the motivating information about diabetes basics, and diabetes control. Diabetics will be inspired by reading through this book, and commit themselves to control diabetes, and lower their haemoglobin A1c level to normal, which must be the ultimate goal of every diabetic person.

You will learn how to eat well, count calories of the foods you eat, how to take oral medication or how to inject insulin shots and how to exercise to lower after-meal glucose spikes, how to do record keeping, and more importantly how to control type 2 diabetes, type 1 diabetes or gestational diabetes, and achieve normal A1c in 90 days. Amazingly you will learn how to live like a normal person for the rest of your life.

Rakib
5.0 out of 5 stars Extraordinary Diabetes Control Book!
Reviewed in the United States on December 12, 2020
Verified Purchase

In my family circle, many of my relatives suffer from chronic diabetes, and they are all using this book "Permanent Diabetes control," and they all appreciated all contents of this book. This book teaches how to control the chronic diabetes in 90 days, and reveals the necessary secret that every diabetic patient should be aware of in order control diabetes effectively.

Doctors don't teach all those diabetes controlling skills presented in this. This book taught me very clearly with many worked out examples on how to calculate the daily average blood glucose level correctly. If I know how to do that correctly, I can easily control my diabetes, and achieve normal hemoglobin A1c under 7%. I enjoyed all 12 chapters. Every chapter has important information related to diabetes.

Permanent Diabetes Control book is the comprehensive guide, and I highly recommend it to all people living with diabetes, either type 2 or type 1. Diabetics should stop living with uncontrolled diabetes, and start learning "how control diabetes in 90 days". It is indeed possible to control diabetes in 90 days as this book convinces us with scientific reasoning.

Sea salt
5.0 out of 5 stars Must read.
Reviewed in the United States on February 26, 2020
Verified Purchase

This book "Permanent Diabetes Control" is extremely extraordinary guide to control diabetes in 90 days, and to live like a normal person thereafter. This book explains clearly 3 methods to accomplish permanent diabetes control:
a. How to Control Type 2 Diabetes With Diet & Exercise,
b. How to Control Type 2 Diabetes With Diet, Oral Medication & Exercise, and
c. How to Control Type 2 or Type 1 Diabetes with Diet, Insulin Shots & Exercise.

We know that "knowledge is power" so the diabetics should equip their minds with as much knowledge as possible on diabetes control by reading through this comprehensive guide. If we do so, our minds would guide us on how to control diabetes daily, and how to maintain hemoglobin A1c level always normal. This book will inspire you, provide you and guide you with all that powerful knowledge on how to achieve normal hemoglobin A1c. In the 2nd part of the book, the author gave all the tools and knowledge necessary on "Food & Nutritional Control, Diabetes Oral Medications & Insulin, and How to Exercise" to fight and control diabetes. There is a Chapter dedicated on Heart Disease. This is a well-organized and well-written book (packed with 12 chapters of extensive knowledge) to help diabetics. I am certain that this book will help many people with diabetes, highly recommended.

Anamaría Aguirre Chourio
5.0 out of 5 stars Genius Diabetes Control Book
Reviewed in the United States on February 27, 2020
Verified Purchase

Diabetes is a dangerous disease that cannot be controlled unless you master the topic and possess the extraordinary knowledge. This book "Permanent Diabetes Control" is packed with that "powerful knowledge" if you want to swallow and digest at least some of it.

Understanding Hemoglobin A1c Chart is the key to controlling diabetes. In this wonderfully designed book, the author explains "Hemoglobin A1c and Hemoglobin A1c Chart" so well like no one else with easy-to-understand experiments conducted at home along with the self-blood glucose monitoring data. Thanks to the author!

Give yourself 90 days to see outstanding results in controlling your diabetes (but you should control diabetes every day). I urge you to read this book, and learn all the contents without procrastinating. It can not only change your life with diabetes, but also can save your life from diabetic complications that you could develop over time. Diabetic complications are extremely dangerous and life-threatening.

If you have diabetes, take action before it is too late, read this book all 12 chapters, and master the diabetes controlling skills. I am the genuine admirer of this wonderful book!

Sammantha
5.0 out of 5 stars Permanent Diabetes Control
Reviewed in the United States on February 28, 2020
Verified Purchase

The title says it all: "Permanent Diabetes Control, The Complete Guide to Living Like A Normal person Forever". This is the comprehensive diabetes guide, and every diabetic person should read and benefit from it. No doctor could teach you the kind of tips and tricks, methods and procedures to control diabetes presented in this book, and there is no other book like this. This book is written to help you achieve permanent diabetes control in 90 days, and to live like a normal person thereafter.

By reading this book, anybody whether diabetic or not can learn how to count calories, how to eat well with appropriate proportions of protein, fat and carbohydrate, how to exercise, how to find your daily average blood glucose level, and how to achieve your haemoglobin A1c level equal to or lower than 7%. There are many examples with self-blood glucose monitoring data using a simple self-monitoring glucometer (the meter that monitors your blood glucose level every day at home).

Permanent Diabetes Control book overall is an amazing, comprehensive and extremely useful guide created to help you live like a normal person without facing long-term complications. There is a lot of useful information about diabetes and the treatment of diabetes that every diabetic person should be aware of by reading this book. If you want to control your diabetes in 90 days, either type 2 diabetes or type 1 diabetes, this is the best book to consult with. I strongly recommend this book to every newly diagnosed and veteran diabetic.

Jack mckeever
5.0 out of 5 stars   All a diabetic person needs is this book!
Reviewed in the United Kingdom on May 10, 2020
Verified Purchase

All a diabetic person needs is this book to self-control diabetes, and to live like a normal person for the rest of his/her life. This book teaches how to research on rising and falling blood glucose level by frequently self-monitoring with a fingerstick blood glucometer at home. This book teaches how to implement appropriately healthy diet, exercise, oral medication or insulin shots, and how to lower after-meal blood glucose spikes, and achieve daily average blood glucose level close to or under 7 mmol/L or 126 mg/dl depending on in which country a diabetic person resides. If you can do so every day for 90 consecutive days, you can easily achieve normal A1c level. There are many worked-out examples illustrated in Chapter 3 of this book. Chapter 3 contains everything a diabetic person ever needs to understand diabetes, and control it perfectly in order to achieve normal haemoglobin A1c. Achieving normal haemoglobin A1c is the key to controlling diabetes permanently.

Whether you are a newly diagnosed or veteran diabetic person, you must take advantage of this comprehensive diabetes control book. You can learn everything about the fundamentals of diabetes such as the function of pancreas, lack of insulin production, controlling diabetes with healthy diet, exercise along with pills or insulin injections. This book offers many strategies and secrets of controlling diabetes effectively, which you could not have learned by visiting family physicians and/or endocrinologists. All you need is this book if you are diabetic!

----

stacy anderson
5.0 out of 5 stars Achieve Normal A1c Level Using This Complete Guide!
Reviewed in the United Kingdom on June 9, 2021
Verified Purchase

Say "goodbye" to high blood sugar levels and high hemoglobin A1c level by reading and practicing the method illustrated in this book. This book is the primer for those diabetics who want to control their diabetes in 90 days, achieve normal A1c, and live like a normal person for the rest of their lives.

Lowering Hemoglobin A1c is the Key to Controlling Diabetes. Hemoglobin A1c Chart is made with Average Blood Glucose Level in 90 Days Versus Hemoglobin A1c. If we know the average blood glucose level in 90 days, we can determine the hemoglobin A1c, and vice versa. If hemoglobin A1c is not normal, a diabetic person needs to lower his/her average blood glucose level in 90 days.

This book teaches very clearly with examples how to calculate the daily average blood glucose level every day, and then how to calculate the global average in 90 days. By slashing the after-meal glucose spikes on a daily basis, it is possible to lower the average glucose level in 90 days, thereby lowering the hemoglobin A1c to normal. This book has provided the proof with a Real Life Case Study in Chapter 4. Achieving normal hemoglobin A1c must be the primary goal of a diabetic person. This is the book that must be consulted to educate yourself on this matter.

I have learned many important diabetes control strategies, tips and tricks in this powerfully inspiring book "Permanent Diabetes Control."

kaitlyn Jeffries
5.0 out of 5 stars Impressive Guide to Control Diabetes in 90 Days!
Reviewed in the United Kingdom on December 19, 2020
Verified Purchase

This book has taught me many diabetes controlling skills, and I am certainly benefited by its powerful contents. The "SECRET" developed by the author in this book to control either type 2 diabetes or type 1 diabetes, and to achieve normal A1c in 90 days is very effective.
By examining the hemoglobin A1c chart carefully, any person can realize that what this author says about that secret is scientifically valid.

After reviewing and examining all 12 chapters of this book, I can confirm that it is true that "Permanent Diabetes Control" book certainly guides you on how to control your diabetes perfectly in 90 days, and how to live like a normal person for the rest of your life.

Health & Well Being
5.0 out of 5 stars My Favorite Diabetes Control Guide
Reviewed in India on March 1, 2020
Verified Purchase

This book teaches us the most important aspect in diabetes control "how to determine the hemoglobin A1c level comfortably at home" without going to a laboratory blood test, but just by using the daily finger-stick blood glucose monitoring data from the glucometer that we use at home. I have never heard about it, no doctor told me about it, and no diabetes specialist would teach us about it.

If we learn how to determine the haemoglobin A1c level at home manually daily, we can master the diabetes control concept, and control diabetes easily in 90 days, and live like a normal person afterwards as long as we stick to the concepts outlined in this book.

If you are diabetic, suffering from either type 2 diabetes or type 1 diabetes, you should read this book cover to cover, master all the concepts outlined in this book, you will be amazed to see your hemoglobin A1c dropping like a rock to normal. In my opinion, this is the best book on this important topic "diabetes control".

Leslie C
5.0 out of 5 stars Did a great job.....
Reviewed in the United States on October 31, 2019
Format: Kindle Edition
Fantastic guide for all of us. I found it from Amazon. In a diabetic person, due to pancreatic deficiency, the body does not monitor glucose levels as adequately as needed nor does it supply sufficient insulin in the bloodstream to maintain normal glucose levels. Recommended!

Mahbub
5.0 out of 5 stars   Extremely well founded book.
October 12, 2019
Format: Kindle EditionVerified Purchase
The book is very good and I'm glad I bought it. I am not quite pre-diabetic but am getting close and must do what I can to prevent diabetes. I spent HOURS on the American Diabetic Assn website and did not learn very much. I did learn a lot from this book. So far in my quest for information on Diabetes, this book rates as the most informative, reliable, well organized, well written material on Diabetes. I recently found out I have the disease and use this book to educate myself. I have it on my Kindle which goes everywhere I go - in the car, to a doctor's appointment, etc. I learn a little bit at a time and the way the book is written makes it easy to remember. Anyone wanting information on how to control diabetes - to learn, to teach - in whatever capacity would benefit from having this book.

DAVIDSON
5.0 out of 5 stars   Diabetes control treatment with healthy diet!
Reviewed in the United States on November 3, 2019
Format: Kindle Edition
By this book you can learn about the hidden secret in the hemoglobin a1c chart. Author also include how to find out your daily average blood glucose level. You can also learn how to control type 2 diabetes with diet oral medication & exercise.

Max Banks
5.0 out of 5 stars Important for leading a normal healthy life.
Reviewed in the United States on October 9, 2019
Format: Kindle Edition

Diabetes is a common disease in today's world. All people are facing this problem. Someone's level is high someone is low. People who are suffering most can't control the level. The reason behind this is the proper guideline. This book will help them to follow all the rules and to lead a healthy life.

Lisa Anthony
5.0 out of 5 stars   Amazing !
Reviewed in the United States on October 31, 2019
Format: Kindle Edition

This is amazing guide book. This book shows lot's of tip & the tips are good for diabetes present. For read this book present learn perfectly how to recovery from diabetes. Thanks to writer who wrote this book.

AUTHOR'S OTHER PUBLICATIONS
REVIEWS: DRINKING WATER GUIDE by Rao Konduru, PhD

RE: Drinking Water Guide (book)   **www.DrinkingWaterGuide.com**

REVIEW: I was indeed thrilled to read through and learn the amazing descriptions about the formation of our Universe after the Big Bang, formation of stars, planets, galaxies, formation of our solar system, including our Sun and our planet Earth. Chapter 1, Chapter 13, Chapter 17, Chapter 18 & Chapter 19 contain the most valuable information. In a nutshell, this book teaches that we should avoid tap water, well water & bottled water, and drink only purified water that is either neutralized or slightly alkalized, and remineralized up to a TSD (Total Dissolved Solids) level of 200 ppm. The book teaches how to neutralize, slightly alkalize, fully alkalize and remineralize the purified water with sample experiments conducted at home. The book teaches healthy water-drinking habits, and gives recommendations at the end of each chapter. I greatly admire and recommend this highly researched, well-documented, and fully comprehensive guide on drinking water to every adult living on our planet Earth.   -- Prime Publishing Co., New Westminster, British Columbia, Canada.

Deanna Maio
5.0 out of 5 stars   Comprehensive Drinking Water Guide
Reviewed in the United States on February 17, 2020
Verified Purchase

NIKOLA TESLA said it all: "only a lunatic will drink unsterilized water". Very many people are still drinking unsterilized tap water and contaminated bottled water, jeopardizing their health, and developing strange diseases, and making many trips to hospitals and board-certified doctors. The tap water disaster incident that occurred in Flint, Michigan, USA in 2014 is a typical example of lead contamination that affected more than 100,000 residents.

This book describes about all kinds of drinking water available for human consumption, their defects, and appropriate "recommendations" in order to rectify those defects, and how to drink clean and healthy water in order to protect your health in the current day circumstances. This book Drinking Water Guide teaches many drinking water strategies:

(i) I must be wise and cautious all the time and should not take chances. I must not drink tap water, well water or bottled water of any kind, and make my own distilled water by purchasing and using a home distiller. Or, I must purchase RO water from a nearby supermarket, and I must always drink only purified water.
(ii) I would add very little Himalayan pink salt, Celtic sea salt or a few drops of ConcenTrace mineral drops to remineralize the purified water before drinking.
(iii) I would add a tiny bit of baking soda or a few drops of ConcenTrace mineral drops in order to improve the alkalinity and the presence of minerals in the purified water.
(iv) I would use pH strips or digital pH meter, monitor my drinking water pH, every now and then, and make sure that the purified water I drink is either neutralized (pH=7) or slightly alkalized (pH=7 to 7.5).

(v) I would use a TSD meter, and monitor the TDS level of my drinking water, and make sure that TDS level is always below 200 ppm. I will also research and find out the ideal TDS level that suits my body. I can do that by adjusting the tiny amount of Himalayan pink salt.
I am very grateful that I learned all the above-mentioned valuable information from this book "Drinking Water Guide". What an impressive book! I urge you to get this book without any hesitation.

PERMANENT DIABETES CONTROL
The Complete Guide to Living Like A Normal Person Forever

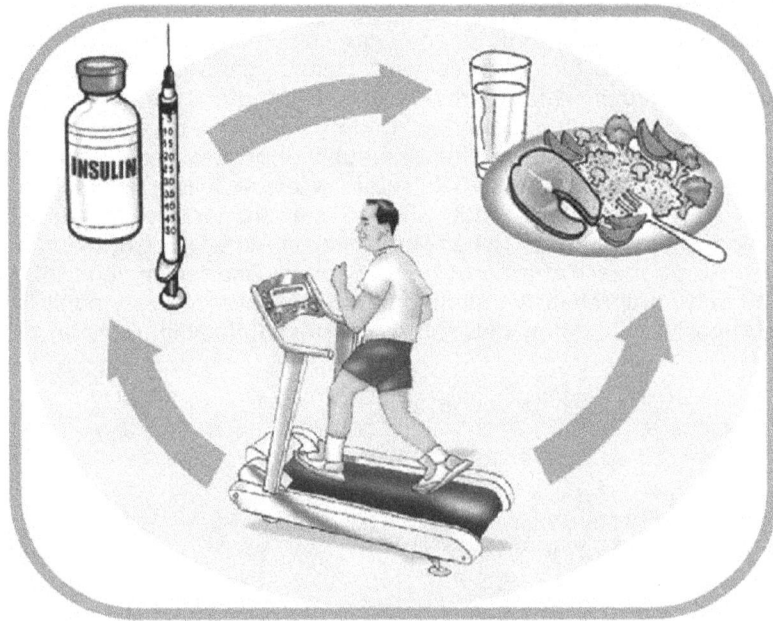

Permanent Diabetes Control Book Teaches
- **How to Eat Well and Control Diabetes (Do-It-Yourself)!**
- **The Hidden Secret in The Hemoglobin A1c Chart!**
- **How to Find Out Your Daily Average Blood Glucose Level!**
- **How to Control Type 2 Diabetes With Diet & Exercise!**
- **How to Control Type 2 Diabetes With Diet, Oral Medication & Exercise!**
- **How to Control Type 2 Diabetes With Diet, Insulin Shots & Exercise!**
- **How to Control Type 1 Diabetes With Diet, Insulin Shots & Exercise!**
- **How to Lower Your Hemoglobin A1c to Perfectly Normal!**
- **How to Slash After-Meal Glucose Spikes & Achieve Normal A1c!**
- **How to Prevent High Cholesterol and Heart Disease!**

REAL-LIFE CASE STUDY
- **Permanent Diabetes Control Accomplished!**
- **Rapid Acting Insulin (Humalog) Dose Cut By 60%!**
- **Hemoglobin A1c Dropped From A High-Risk 12%**
   To a Stunning 6.2%, 5.5%, 5.3%, 5.0%, Etc!
- **Reversed Critical Heart Disease Without Surgery!**

Rao Konduru, PhD

FOREWORD

Most people with diabetes focus their attention on fasting glucose levels in order to control diabetes rather than on lowering after-meal glucose spikes. If your blood glucose level from a fingerstick blood test early in the morning is normal, it doesn't mean your diabetes is controlled. Hemoglobin A1c is a parameter that directly reveals "the degree of diabetes control" during the preceding 90 days. Red blood cells live in the bloodstream for 90 days. Every 90 days, new red blood cells are born. Hemoglobin is a protein molecule that is present in red blood cells and carries and supplies oxygen from the lungs to the trillions of body's cells wherever it is needed. Hemoglobin also carries glucose along with it, because glucose can stick to all kinds of proteins in your body. While the blood circulates, depending on how high or how low the blood glucose level is, a certain amount of glucose is attached to the hemoglobin molecules to form glycated hemoglobin. Different doctors and scientists call it with different names: glycated A1c, hemoglobin A1c, HbA1c, or simply A1c. Therefore, by measuring the hemoglobin A1c level in a laboratory from the patient's blood sample, it is possible to know the average blood glucose level and the degree to which it has been controlled over the preceding 90 days. By lowering the hemoglobin A1c level to perfectly normal, and by keeping it normal for the rest of your life, you control your diabetes.

This book "Permanent Diabetes Control" guides you on how to control your diabetes perfectly in 90 days, and live like a normal person for the rest of your life.

"The Secret to Controlling Diabetes in 90 days" is discovered, illustrated and explained in detail in this fully comprehensive guide. All diabetics should read through and benefit from this revolutionary diabetes control treatment. If you understand that "SECRET," as explained in this book, you will be victorious in controlling your diabetes in 90 days, and then live like a normal person for the rest of your life.

Prediabetes or borderline diabetes can be controlled with healthy diet and daily exercise. Mild or moderate Type 2 diabetes can be controlled with healthy diet, oral medication(s) and daily exercise. For severe Type 2 diabetes or Type 1 diabetes, oral medications do not work, and so it should be controlled with healthy diet, insulin shots and daily exercise.

If you are on insulin, be aware that the insulin dose must be optimized. This book teaches everything about finding out the optimal insulin dose. Insulin is synthesized in such a way that it acts more quickly and much more effectively with exercise. After-meal exercise, either treadmill or walking, should be introduced into the diabetes control plan in order to burn fat, lose calories and optimize both the insulin dose and insulin action. After-meal exercise minimizes the insulin dose and maximizes insulin action and prevents after-meal glucose levels from rising too high, thus keeping the diabetes under tight control.

The research conducted by the author revealed the fact that by calculating the "Daily Average Blood Glucose Level" accurately for 90 days consecutive days, and by slashing the after-meal glucose spikes consistently every day for 90 consecutive days, it is possible to control diabetes perfectly and achieve normal hemoglobin A1c in 90 days. It is indeed possible to control diabetes in 90 days as this book convinces us with scientific reasoning (see hemoglobin A1c Chart).

The author of this book, by being a seriously diabetic person himself, is the living example. He published his official blood test results in this book for the past 10 plus years, taken once every 3 months. His hemoglobin A1c test result has been consistently normal for the past 10 plus years, revealing the fact that he accomplished "Permanent Diabetes Control."

-- Prime Publishing Co.

COPYRIGHT

Book Title: Permanent Diabetes Control
Subtitle: The Complete Guide to Living Like a Normal Person Forever
Author: Rao Konduru, PhD (Also Called Dr. RK)
Publisher: Prime Publishing Co.
Address: 720 – Sixth Street, Unit: 161
                 New Westminster, BC, Canada, V3L-3C5
Website: www.mydiabetescontrol.com
ISBN #:   ISBN 9780973112009

This book "Permanent Diabetes Control" has been properly registered under ISBN Number "ISBN 9780973112009" with the National Library of Canada Cataloguing in Publication, Ottawa, Ontario, Canada. The original manuscript has been submitted to the Legal Deposits, Library and Archives Canada, Ottawa, Ontario, Canada. All right reserved!

DISCLAIMER

The author of the books titled "Permanent Diabetes Control" and "The Secret to Controlling Type 2 diabetes" assumes no liability or responsibility including, without limitation, incidental and consequential damages, personal injury or wrongful death resulting from the use of any treatment method presented in this book. The reader should take a training course in a local diabetes clinic (diabetes education center) on the insulin-dependant diabetes, and should learn all the aspects on how to inject rapid-acting insulin (such as Humalog), and how to exercise by running on a treadmill, biking, or regular walk in order to lower after-meal blood glucose level to perfectly normal. Without acquiring pertinent training and knowledge to use the treatment procedures illustrated in these books, it is warned not to act alone without supervision. The examples in this book mimic reality but were created for illustrative purposes. All contents in this book are for the educational purposes only and do not in any way represent the professional medical advice.

Dr. Rao Konduru's Publications	
1. Permanent Diabetes Control	www.mydiabetescontrol.com
2. The Secret to Controlling Type 2 Diabetes	www.mydiabetescontrol.com
3. Reversing Obesity	www.reversingosleepapnea.com/ebook2.html
4. Reversing Sleep Apnea	www.reversingsleepapnea.com
5. Reversing Insomnia	www.reversinginsomnia.com
6. Drinking Water Guide	www.drinkingwaterguide.com

The paperbacks (softcover book) and Kindle eBook are available for purchase on Amazon.com for US residents, and on Amazon.ca for Canadian residents.

TABLE OF CONTENTS

CHAPTER 1 DIABETES FACTS & STATISTICS

TABLE OF CONTENTS

AROUND THE WORLD

In 2017, the International Diabetes Federation (IDF) reported the following facts and statistics about people living with diabetes, after studying the prevalence and incidence of prediabetes or borderline diabetes, type 1 diabetes and type 2 diabetes, risk factors for complications, acute and long-term complications, deaths, and costs: [1]

● About 425 million adults are now living with diabetes around the world. By the year 2045, this number could rise to 619 million people. [1]

● More than 1,106,500 children have been living with type 1 diabetes. [1]

● Diabetes is a major public health problem that is approaching epidemic proportions globally. In general, 1 in 2 people with diabetes live undiagnosed. Type 2 diabetes is more rapidly growing, spreading and becoming an epidemic than type 1 diabetes. [1]

● Diabetes caused 4 million deaths during 2017 alone. [1]

● Diabetes caused at least $727 billion US dollars in health expenditure in 2017, which is 12% of total spending on adults. [1]

● The International Diabetes Federation (IDF) reported in 2005 in an article that type 2 diabetes affects a staggering 25 million European adults, adding another 6 million cases by the year 2025. IDF also reported that about 65 million European adults (one in 7 people) have impaired glucose tolerance syndrome due to which blood glucose levels jump too high after meals and remain normal or near-normal a few hours after meals or while fasting. The total healthcare expenditures for diabetes in Europe is estimated between 28 billion and 53 billion Euros per year. [1, 2]

● About 5 to 10% of diabetic people have type 1 diabetes. The remaining 90 to 95% of diabetic people have type 2 diabetes. About 90% of type 2 diabetic people are overweight or obese, as obesity and type 2 diabetes go hand in hand. A lot of type 2 diabetics are on insulin. [2, 4]

● About 3 to 20% of pregnant women develop gestational diabetes, depending on their risk factors. A diagnosis of gestational diabetes may increase the risk of developing diabetes later in life for both mother and child. [5]

● By the year 2025, developing countries such as India, China, Pakistan, Indonesia, Russia, Mexico, Brazil, Egypt, and Japan respectively are those most likely to be affected by diabetes in increased numbers as their people tend to adopt western lifestyles. [2, 3]

● Type 1 diabetes occurs equally in males and females. The World Health Organization project stated that type 1 diabetes is rare in most Asian, African and American Indian populations. But in Scandinavia, particularly in Sweden and Finland, type 1 diabetes rates are higher. The reason for this discrepancy is unknown. [2]

IN THE USA

● In 2017, The Centers for Disease Control and Prevention (CDC) released its diabetes statistics report with the following information: There are 30.3 million people with diabetes (9.4% of the US population) including 23.1 million people who are diagnosed, and 7.2 million people (23.8%) undiagnosed. The numbers for prediabetes indicate that 84.1 million adults (33.9% of the adult U.S. population) have prediabetes, including 23.1 million adults aged 65 years or older (the age group with highest rate). The estimated percentage of individuals with type 1 diabetes remains at 5% among those with diabetes. The statistics are also provided by age, gender, ethnicity, and for each state/territory so you can search for these specifics. [6]

● In 2015, The American Diabetes Association in 2015, published its diabetes statistics report with the following information: There are 30.3 million Americans (9.4% of the population) are living with diabetes. Approximately 1.25 million American children and adults have type 1 diabetes. Of those 30.3 Americans with diabetes, 23.1 million were diagnosed, and 7.2 million were undiagnosed. [7]

● Every year, another 1.5 million Americans are diagnosed with diabetes. [7]

● Diabetes was the seventh leading cause of death in the United States in 2015 based on the 79,535 death certificates. In 2015, diabetes was mentioned as a cause of death in a total of 252,806 certificates. Diabetes may be underreported as a cause of death. Studies have found that only about 35% to 40% of people with diabetes who died had diabetes listed anywhere on the death certificate and about 10% to 15% had it listed as the underlying cause of death. [7]

● In 2107, the total cost of diagnosed diabetes in the United States is $327 billion (USD), $237 billion was for direct medical costs, and $90 billion was in reduced productivity. [7]

● Despite the fact that in most cases most of the risk factors are preventable, the following staggering numbers occur in the USA: [2]

Kidney Disease: About 38,000 diabetic people face kidney failure every year, and more than 100,000 people are treated with a form of kidney disease. Over 50% of these cases are preventable. People with diabetes are 17 times more prone to kidney disease after being diabetic for 20 years or more.
Blindness and Eye Disease: As many as 12,000 to 24,000 diabetic people become blind every year while 90% of these cases could have been prevented.
Amputations: About 82,000 diabetic people undergo leg amputations every year while 85% of these cases could have been prevented.
Heart Disease and Stroke: Among the deaths of people with diabetes, more than 80% are due to heart disease and stroke though proper diabetes-care could have reduced 35% of deaths.
Gestational Diabetes: About 135,000 expectant mothers are diagnosed with gestational diabetes every year, and the babies thus born experience an increased risk of serious complications in the future. Appropriate care during pregnancy could significantly reduce such risk.
Flu and Pneumonia: Between 10,000 and 30,000 diabetic people die every year due to complications related to flu and pneumonia. People with diabetes are three times more likely to die from flu and pneumonia than those without diabetes.

IN CANADA

● In Canada, over 3 million people live with and have diabetes, that's just over 9% of our total population. Unfortunately, that number is expected to rise. Diabetes Canada estimates that by the year 2025, a staggering 5 million people (12% of the population) will have diabetes. [8]

● Currently, there are 11 million Canadians living with prediabetes or borderline diabetes. That means that almost one in three people in Canada are affected by this condition. Prediabetes is a condition in which blood glucose levels are higher than normal, but haven't reached the level required for a diagnosis of type 2 diabetes. If prediabetes is undiagnosed or untreated, it can eventually lead to type 2 diabetes. [8]

● Statistics Canada in 2017 reported that 7.3% of Canadians aged 12 and older (roughly 2.3 million people) were diagnosed with diabetes. Between 2016 and 2017, the proportion of males who reported being diagnosed with diabetes increased from 7.6% in 2016 to 8.4% in 2017. The proportion of females remained consistent between the two years. [9]

● Canadians with type 1 diabetes have been living with their diagnosis for an average of 20.2 years, compared to 12.2 years for type 2 diabetes. Overall, males (8.4%) were more likely than females (6.3%) to report that they had diabetes. Diabetes increased with age for males, with the highest prevalence among those 75 years and older. The percentage of females reporting diabetes increased with age up to the age of 64, the prevalence did not increase significantly for those aged 75 and older. [9]

● Canadian adults, older than 18, who were either overweight or obese were more likely than those who were classified as having a normal weight to report that they had been diagnosed with diabetes. The prevalence of diabetes among obese Canadians was 13.7% in 2017, compared with 6.8% among overweight Canadians and 3.6% among those classified as having a normal weight. [9]

DIABETES STATISTICS RESULTED FROM HEART DISEASE [2]

Believe it or not, the following staggering information is true:

● Diabetes (living with high blood glucose levels) is the major reason of heart disease.

● More than 80 percent of people with diabetes die from some form of heart or blood vessel disease.

● The World Health Organization (WHO), the International Society and Federation of Cardiology (ISFC) and the United Nations Educational, Scientific and Cultural Organization (UNESCO) jointly reported in a press release in 1997 that cardiovascular diseases kill more than any other disease around the world. Every year, an estimated 15 million deaths are reported, which is about 30% of total deaths around the world, and many more millions of people are disabled due to heart and blood vessel diseases.

● Cardiovascular disease has been the number one killer in the USA since 1900 (heart disease being the first leading cause of death and stroke being the 3rd leading cause of death).

● About 61 million Americans (about one-fourth of the population) live with the complications of heart disease and stroke. In 2001, the cost for all cardiovascular diseases in the USA alone was $300 billion.

● Every 33 seconds, a person dies from cardiovascular disease in the USA alone.

● Every 34 seconds, a person dies from a form of heart disease in the USA alone.

● Every day, more than 2500 Americans die from heart disease.

● Every year, more than 250,000 people die of heart attack in the USA before they reach a nearby hospital.

● In 1991, 923,000 Americans died from heart and blood vessel diseases.

● Also, in countries like Russia, Romania, Bulgaria, Hungary, Bulgaria, Czechoslovakia and Poland, heart disease contributes to the highest number of deaths. The lowest death rates of heart disease were in Japan, France, Spain, Switzerland and Canada.

GOOD NEWS

● However, the good news is that many celebrities, famous athletes, Hollywood stars, wealthy people, politicians and highly qualified professionals of all types educational background, including doctors, engineers, lawyers, businessmen and businesswomen have experienced type 1 or type 2 diabetes, treated themselves successfully with proper knowledge and care and lived long and healthy. They demonstrated that they have willpower (knowledge is power) to fight and control diabetes.

● Controlling diabetes which is the only subject matter of this book as a matter of fact is a very interesting and enjoyable task. Please refer to Chapter 3 and Chapter 4, and learn how to control your diabetes permanently.

REFERENCES

1. Diabetes Facts & Figures (Statistics) by International Diabetes Federation (IDF)
https://www.idf.org/aboutdiabetes/what-is-diabetes/facts-figures.html

2. Permanent Diabetes Control (Book), Subtitle: The Complete Guide to Living Like A Normal Person Forever, Authored by Rao Konduru, MS, PhD, Reviewed and Endorsed by Dr. Marshal Dahl, MD, PhD., Endocrinologist, Faculty of Medicine, University of British Columbia, Vancouver, British Columbia, Canada, First Published in 2003.
www.mydiabetescontrol.com

3. Eve Gehling, M.Ed, The Family & Friends' Guide to Diabetes, John Wiley & Sons, New York, NY, USA, page 39, 2000.

4. Diabetes: Facts, Statistics, and You by Healthline.
https://www.healthline.com/health/diabetes/facts-statistics-infographic#1

5. What is diabetes? Types of Diabetes by Canadian Diabetes Association, 2019.
https://www.diabetes.ca/diabetes-basics/what-is-diabetes

6. The 2017 National Diabetes Statistics by American Association of Diabetes Educators by by Karen Kemmis, PT, DPT, MS, CDE, FAADE, Posted on July 26, 2017.
https://www.diabeteseducator.org/news/aade-blog/aade-blog-details/karen-kemmis-pt-dpt-ms-cde-faade/2017/07/26/the-2017-national-diabetes-statistics-report-is-here

7. Diabetes Statistics by American Diabetes Association, The Data Collected in 2015.
http://www.diabetes.org/diabetes-basics/statistics/
https://www.diabetes.org/resources/statistics/statistics-about-diabetes

8. Living Well With Diabetes by Diabetes Care Community.
https://www.diabetescarecommunity.ca/living-well-with-diabetes-articles/managing-diabetes-canada/

9. Diabetes-2017, Heath Fact Sheets by Statistics Canada.
https://www150.statcan.gc.ca/n1/pub/82-625-x/2018001/article/54982-eng.htm

CHAPTER 2 OVERVIEW OF DIABETES

TABLE OF CONTENTS

ARE YOU DIABETIC?
UNDERSTAND HOW GLUCOSE BUILDS UP IN THE BLOODSTREAM! [1]

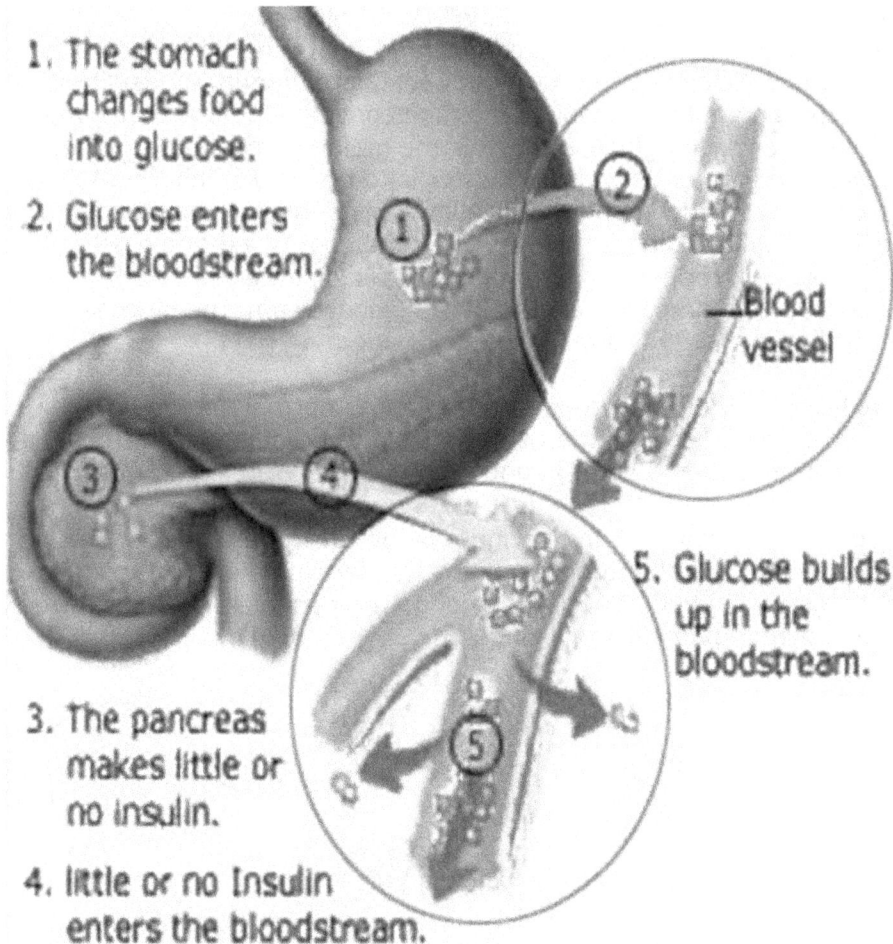

1. The stomach changes food into glucose.

2. Glucose enters the bloodstream.

Blood vessel

5. Glucose builds up in the bloodstream.

3. The pancreas makes little or no insulin.

4. little or no Insulin enters the bloodstream.

Figure 2.1 Glucose buildup in the blood stream.

1. The stomach changes food into glucose immediately after digestion.
2. Glucose enters the blood stream.
3. The pancreas makes little or no insulin if you are diabetic.
   Insulin is essential for aiding glucose transport into the trillions of body's cells.
   Insulin drives glucose molecules through the bloodstream.
4. Little or no insulin enters the bloodstream if you are diabetic.
5. Glucose builds up in the bloodstream because of the lack of insulin flow, and so a person with uncontrolled diabetes would be living with high blood glucose levels throughout the day, or his/her body's cells become unable to absorb glucose molecules due a kind of metabolic disorder, and therefore that person will be diagnosed with diabetes.
⦿ Diabetes over time damages essential components in your body, mostly your blood vessels in all parts of your body, arteries, nerves, and many other parts. The long-term side effects or complications of uncontrolled diabetes can be very serious, and some of them could eventually be fatal. So take action immediately if you have diabetes, and control it with healthy diet, oral medication or insulin and after-meal exercise.

DIABETES AND PANCREAS [1]

Diabetes Mellitus means "sweet urine" being siphoned through the urinary system out of the body. Diabetes is a Greek word meaning "to siphon", and Mellitus is a Latin word meaning "honey". Diabetes, when uncontrolled, is a chronic and fatal condition or disease developed due to the pancreatic deficiency in producing an adequate amount of insulin or due to the body's inability to properly utilize insulin. The food consumed is broken down by digestive juices into a simple sugar called glucose which is the main source of energy. The insulin drives glucose via the bloodstream into the body's cells to be used as energy. When the beta cells of the pancreas are destroyed and produce little or no insulin, the glucose builds up in the bloodstream, leading to diabetes. Also, when the body's cells become unable to respond to insulin secretion due to a a kind of metabolic disorder, diabetes develops. When the glucose level is markedly elevated in the bloodstream, the glucose overflows into the urine thus losing the body's main source of energy.

When the person's glucose levels in the bloodstream are no longer normal and unusually high, the person is diagnosed with diabetes or the person is said to be diabetic. The good news is that diabetes is not contagious and is fully controllable.

The pancreas of the human body as shown in the figure below is situated on the left side of the body underneath the stomach just beneath the liver. The pancreas is a soft, pinkish-gray colored banana-shaped gland of about 15 to 25 cm long. The pancreas is connected to the upper part of the small intestine by means of a duct.

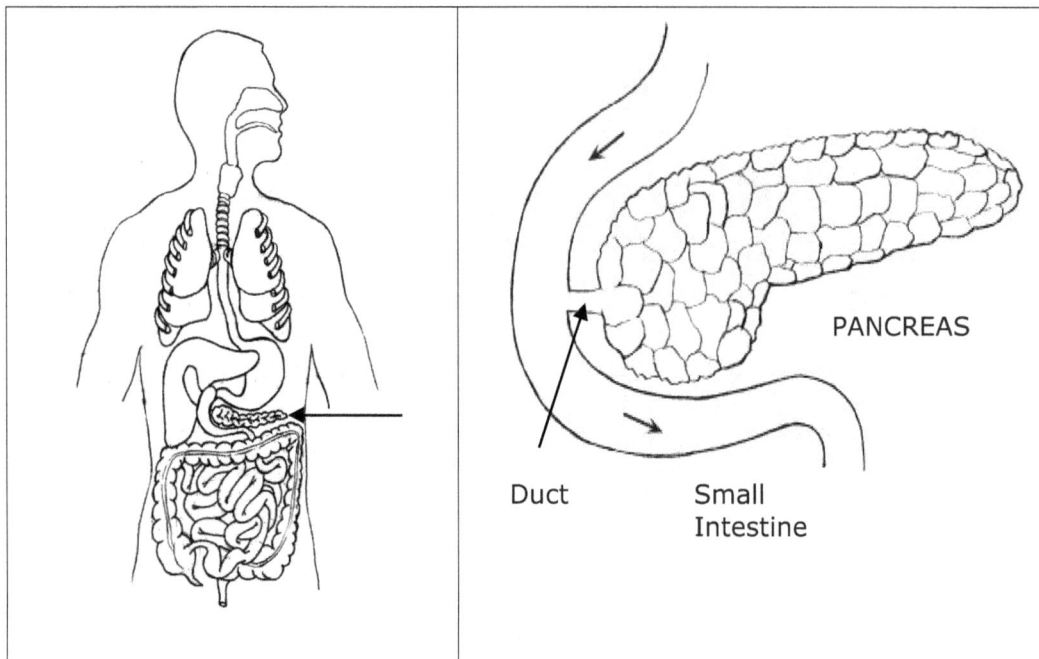

Figure 2.2 Picture of the human pancreas.

The Human Pancreas Serves Two Major Functions: [1]
(i) Exocrine Function (to produce digestive juices)
(ii) Endocrine Function (to produce insulin and glucagon)

In 1869, Dr. Paul Langerhans first identified that endocrine cells under low power magnification appear to be islands (islets) and since then they were named "Islets of Langerhans." Exocrine cells do not secrete any product into the bloodstream while endocrine cells do. A normal pancreas contains about 1 million cells, 1 to 2% of which are islets of Langerhans, very small bits of tissue at the tail end of the pancreas, embedded in exocrine pancreatic acinar tissue.

Each islet of Langerhans is made up of four different cells: alpha cells to secrete glucagon, beta cells to secrete insulin, gamma cells to secrete pancreatic polypeptide and delta cells to secrete somatostatin. The amazing beta cells are capable of sensing and measuring the blood glucose level within seconds and secrete an adequate amount of already stored insulin instantly.

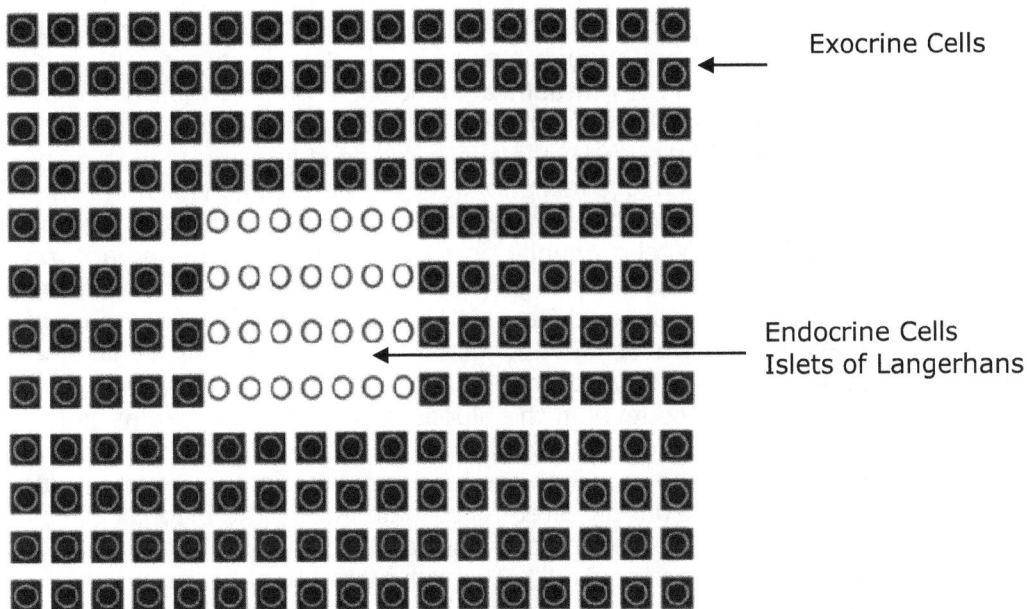

Exocrine Cells

Endocrine Cells
Islets of Langerhans

Figure 2.3 Cross Section of Pancreas (For Illustration Purpose Only).

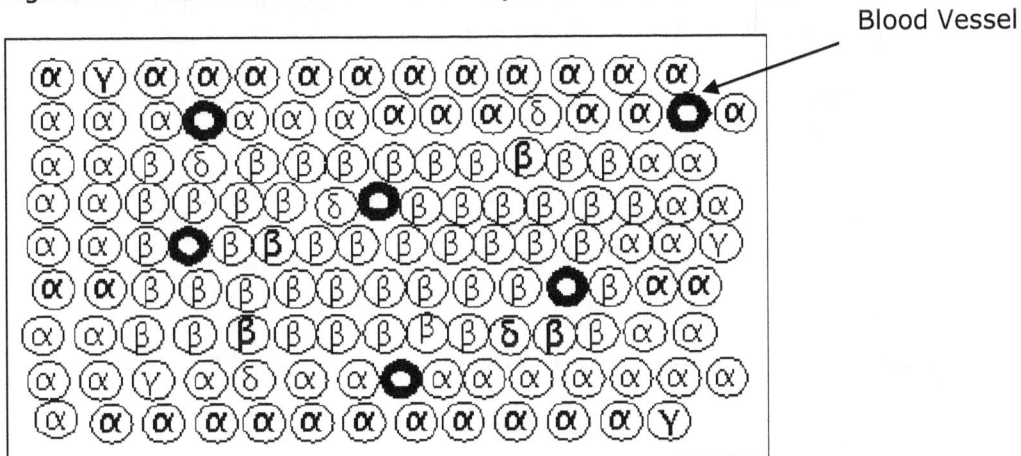

Blood Vessel

Figure 2.4   ISLET OF LANGERHANS (Beta cells, Alpha cells and blood vessels).

The Exocrine function of the pancreas is to produce a digestive alkaline juice that is enriched with about 15 different enzymes. This digestive juice passes through a duct as shown in Figure 1.1 and mixes with finely chewed and crushed food that is coming through the stomach and enters into the small intestine for further digestion. These enzymes break down different types of food into small particles in order to promote digestion. Some enzymes digest protein, some digest fat and others digest carbohydrate. The liver receives all sugars from the intestine walls and converts them into glucose—the body's main source of energy. The glucose is then distributed via the bloodstream to all cells of the body. When the exocrine function fails, enzymes lack and indigestion develops.

The Endocrine function of the pancreas is to control and regulate glucose level in the bloodstream by secreting the appropriate amount of insulin. The function of the islets of Langerhans is to produce two important hormones called insulin and glucagon. Beta cells produce insulin while alpha cells produce glucagon. Glucagon stimulates the cells of liver, muscle and kidney tissue to break down the already stored glycogen. Glycogen is the long chains of glucose stored in the liver, muscles and kidneys for future use. Whenever there is excess glucose in the bloodstream from digested food, the excess glucose is converted into glycogen. As shown in Figure 2.3, there are enough blood vessel inlets to receive either insulin or glucagon. Insulin and glucagon act mutually against each other to maintain normal glucose levels in the bloodstream. Whenever food is consumed, glucose from digested food is absorbed by the small intestine walls and is released into the bloodstream and blood glucose levels rise. Higher glucose levels stimulate the beta cells, which in turn secrete insulin into the bloodstream, and at the same time inhibit glucagon release from pancreatic alpha cells. Thus the insulin level gradually rises in the bloodstream and acts on the liver, fat and muscle cells to absorb the incoming molecules of glucose, amino acids and fatty acids. This action prevents the glucose level from rising too high. After a few hours of meal consumption or while fasting, the glucose level begins to drop. At this particular time, the pancreatic alpha cells secrete glucagon, which stimulates the liver to break down glycogen and release glucose. The glucose level in the bloodstream therefore begins to rise automatically. This counter-action of glucagon against insulin prevents the glucose levels from falling too low for a non-diabetic person. When the food is consumed next time during the day, the higher amounts of glucose from digested food again enters the bloodstream, beta cells get stimulated and the insulin secretion controls the glucose level, and so on. This is called the principle of "negative feedback control". This is how the healthy pancreas of a non-diabetic person maintains automatic counter-balance between the actions of insulin and glucagon and normal glucose levels all the time. Any defect caused by the poor functioning of the pancreas contributes to a lack of insulin supply or metabolic disorder due to which the body's cells become unable to utilize the insulin secretion properly, and the end result is a life-threatening build up of elevated glucose levels in the bloodstream causing a chronic and possibly fatal disease called ***diabetes mellitus.***

The amazing counter-action between β-Cells and α-Cells situated in the islets of Langerhans is responsible to maintain normal blood glucose levels for healthy non-diabetic people. β-Cells produce insulin while α-Cells produce glucagon.

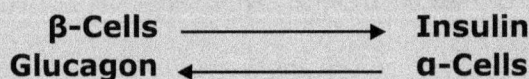

β-Cells ──────────→ Insulin
Glucagon ←────────── α-Cells

YouTube Videos About Pancreas

Watch the following YouTube videos to better understand the function of pancreas of the human body. [3, 4]

3. YouTube Video, Title: What is Pancreas?, Published by Rahul Azad, Aug 24, 2009
https://www.youtube.com/watch?v=1I2GTGEwZOY&feature=youtu.be
4. YouTube Video, Title: How the Body Works: The Pancreas, Published by Daniel Izzo, Aug 3, 2017
https://www.youtube.com/watch?v=j5WF8wUFNkI&feature=youtu.be

THE PRODUCTION OF INSULIN IN THE HUMAN BODY [1]

The production of insulin in the beta cells of a non-diabetic person is a two-step process. Beta cells first produce preproinsulin which is cleaved to produce pro-insulin, which is further cleaved to produce equal amounts of insulin and C-peptide. The insulin thus produced in beta cells has a half-life of about four minutes in the bloodstream (Half-life means the time required to decay one-half of the insulin produced). C-peptide lasts about 30 minutes.

The amazing beta cells of the pancreas sense and measure blood glucose within seconds and secrete the appropriate amount of insulin into the bloodstream in order to maintain normal glucose level all the time.

A VERY IMPORTANT NOTE: A healthy non-diabetic person's pancreas stores about 200 units of insulin, measures blood glucose level 500 times a day, and automatically secretes the appropriate amount of insulin into the bloodstream in order to maintain normal blood glucose level throughout the day. If you are diagnosed with diabetes, you should monitor and adjust insulin supply as frequently as possible and take action to adjust the insulin flow. But the problem is that the most diabetic people don't monitor even 5 times a day.

In a diabetic person, due to pancreatic deficiency, the body does not monitor glucose levels as adequately as needed nor does it adjust or supply sufficient insulin in the bloodstream to maintain normal glucose levels. So a diabetic person is required to monitor glucose levels as frequently as possible with an intention to control them. Only in this way, can diabetes be self-controlled.

CAUSES OF DIABETES [1]

• Heredity is the major reason. The defects associated with the function of the pancreas are duplicated from parents to children.
• Destruction of body's immune system leads to pancreatic dysfunction.
• Viruses could play a role in damaging the pancreas causing diabetes.
• Obesity can cause insulin resistance leading to diabetes.
• Some medications cause steroid-induced diabetes.
• Women who do not get enough to eat during first three months of their pregnancies give birth to babies who have short legs and who later develop Type 2 diabetes.
• Pregnant women could develop diabetes during the stress of pregnancy, and then both the mother and child could develop diabetes within 15 years after the pregnancy.

SYMPTOMS OF DIABETES [1, 5]

The following are the symptoms of diabetes a person experiences during and after the development of prediabetes or diabetes. A person should get tested for diabetes when experiences any of the following symptoms, and take appropriate action to treat diabetes.

- Frequent urination & Increased thirst,
- Fatigue or tiredness due to loss of glucose through urine,
- Disorientation or Irritability,
- Unexplained weight loss or weight gain,
- Extreme hunger,
- Presence of ketones in the urine (ketones are a byproduct of the breakdown of muscle and fat that happens when there is not enough insulin available in blood vessels),
- Blurred vision due to low blood sugars,
- Frequent infections on gums, skin, feet and vaginal infections, and slow healing from infections.

HYPERGLYCEMIA VERSUS HYPOGLYCEMIA [1]

Hyperglycemia and hypoglycemia are two extreme symptoms of diabetes. All people with type 1, type 2 and gestational diabetes may experience both symptoms of hyperglycemia and hypoglycemia. The following table shows the major differences between them.

Table 2.1 Hyperglycemia versus hypoglycemia.

HYPERGLYCEMIA	HYPOGLYCEMIA
Symptoms	**Symptoms**
Extreme thirst, urination, weakness, loss of appetite, nausea, vomiting.	Nervousness, sweating, hunger, blurred vision, imbalance.
Indications	**Indications**
High levels of glucose in blood and urine (over 13 mmol/L or 230 mg/dL).	Low levels of glucose in blood (below 4 mmol/L or 72 mg/dL).
Too little insulin in the blood.	Too much insulin in the blood.
Treatment	**Treatment**
Monitor glucose in the blood.	Monitor glucose in the blood.
Monitor glucose and ketones in urine.	Eat sugar, candy, orange juice,
Drink sugar-free fluids or water.	coke, etc. to raise glucose levels.
Exercise to bring glucose level down.	Inject glucagon if unconscious.
Inject insulin or take pill to treat hyper.	

REASONS WHY YOU HAVE UNCONTROLLED DIABETES [10]

● If your hemoglobin A1c result from a laboratory blood test is found to be over 7% or 0.07, your diabetes is said to be uncontrolled. Most diabetics don't know how to control diabetes, and live with elevated A1c level for decades despite trying hard a variety of oral medications, despite the daily insulin injections, and many trips to diabetes specialists.

● You are not monitoring enough and not researching enough to understand your elevated after-meal glucose spikes, and not supplementing your body with enough artificial insulin as you lack fine tuning skills.

● Did you know a healthy non-diabetic person's pancreas monitors blood glucose level 500 times a day, and automatically adjusts the insulin secretion to keep up the normal blood glucose levels throughout the day? This is called the "fine-tuning" skill of the pancreas. A diabetic person should monitor as many times as possible, and supplement insulin, to keep up the normal blood glucose levels. If you are a beginner in controlling your diabetes, you should monitor 10 times a day (5 fasting glucose levels and 5 after meal glucose levels), and analyse the data to better understand how your blood glucose levels are being fluctuated and how to control them. If you don't do that, your diabetes will remain uncontrolled.

● Even the doctors, endocrinologists and board-certified specialists are not equipped with the appropriate knowledge and training skills to transmit the real concept of controlling diabetes to their patients' minds, except leaving their patients in a dilemma of uncontrolled diabetes.

● The doctors don't teach their patients how to understand the hemoglobin A1c chart with clear concept. As a matter of fact, the secret to controlling diabetes lies in understanding the hemoglobin chart. And nobody ever told you about it, and nobody ever taught you that secret!

● You have been on oral medications for a long time, and did not think about switching to insulin shots because nobody convinced you that insulin is the best medicine to treat diabetes.

● Your hemoglobin A1c is not normal because you are not injecting enough insulin at appropriate times except some scheduled doses recommended by your doctor or nurse, and you are not exercising enough to lower after-meal spikes. And your doctors have been giving you full freedom to live like the way you want with unhealthy lifestyle.

● You are partying too much and eating too much with your family and friends every now and then. Your temptation to eat something delicious would lead to loss of control on dietary guidelines, causing you to overeat delicious foods that are made from processed and refined foods. Your unhealthy eating habits contribute to high blood glucose levels throughout the day, which further contribute to elevated A1c level.

● Most importantly, you lack self-efficacy, self-discipline, motivation, willpower, and a strong desire to fight and control your diabetes, and to achieve normal hemoglobin A1c level.

LONG-TERM COMPLICATIONS (SIDE-EFFECTS) OF DIABETES
[UNCONTROLLED DIABETES IS DANGEROUS!] [1, 5]

Do not simply rely on oral medications, waste year after year, and live with uncontrolled diabetes. Living with uncontrolled diabetes, and neglecting your health by inadequately managing your chronic diabetes means you are living with high glucose levels in the bloodstream, and high levels of hemoglobin A1c. At elevated blood glucose levels over a long time, the glucose sticks to the surface of the cells and it is then converted into a poison called "sorbitol", which damages the body's cells and blood vessels, leading to long-term side effects such as:

- High cholesterols (total cholesterol & LDL cholesterol) and high blood pressure,
- Heart attack, heart failure, coronary heart disease, stroke,
- Hardening of arteries or what is known as atherosclerosis,
- Peripheral artery disease (PAD), narrowing of arteries,
- Painful neuropathy (nerve damage and poor blood flow),
- Burning foot syndrome, numbness in feet and knees, intermittent claudication,
- Amputation (due to nerve damage in the feet),
- Kidney disease, kidney damage, loss of kidney,
- Erectile dysfunction (ED) and/or Impotence,
- Cataracts, blurred vision, retinopathy, blindness,
- Deafness (hearing impairment),
- Diseases of the small blood vessels in the eyes, kidneys, legs and nerves,
- Gum disease and bone loss (dental problems),
- Bladder and prostate problems,
- Skin diseases (bacterial and fungal infections),
- Dementia such as Alzheimer's disease,
- Depression develops over time if diabetes is left untreated,
- and many other strange problems and complications.

If your hemoglobin A1c from a blood test is more than 7%, your diabetes in uncontrolled, so take action immediately! When the after-meal blood glucose spike is too high after eating and remain elevated for more than two hours, this presents a significant mortality risk factor, and the person should switch to insulin shots, and should learn how to slash after meal spikes by incorporating exercise.

Learn how to control your diabetes permanently by reading through this book thoroughly.

TYPES OF DIABETES (Brief Description)

In Short, the Following are the Types of Diabetes: [2]

Prediabetes or Borderline Diabetes: Blood glucose levels are higher than what's considered normal, but not high enough to qualify as diabetes disease.
Type 1 diabetes: The pancreas produces no insulin, and so you need to inject insulin.
Type 2 diabetes: The pancreas doesn't make enough insulin or your body can't use it effectively, thereby developing type 2 diabetes.
Gestational Diabetes: Expectant or pregnant women are unable to make and use all of the insulin they need during pregnancy.

TYPES OF DIABETES (Elaborated Description) [1]

There are 3 types of diabetes:
(i) Type 1 Diabetes,
(ii) Type 2 Diabetes, and
(iii) Gestational Diabetes

Type 1 Diabetes Mellitus or insulin-dependent diabetes mellitus or adult diabetes, also called juvenile diabetes, is developed when the pancreas produces little or no insulin because the beta cells of the pancreas may have been totally damaged or destroyed. Type 1 diabetes is developed mostly in infants, children and young adults under the age 30 years. About 10% to 15% of the diabetics belong to the type 1 group. Insulin shots are required to treat type 1 diabetes.

Type 2 Diabetes or non-insulin dependent diabetes, also called adult-onset diabetes, is developed when the pancreas produces insufficient insulin because the beta cells of the pancreas may have been partly damaged. Even if the pancreas produces insulin well, the body tissues do not respond adequately to the insulin, becoming resistant to insulin. This is called insulin resistance. Insulin resistance is the underlying problem with type 2 diabetic people. About 85% to 90% of diabetics belong to type 2. Type 2 diabetics take oral medications. Some type 2 diabetics take insulin shots when the pills don't work. A lot of type 2 diabetics are now getting used to insulin shots to quickly offset the elevated glucose levels. Diabetes can be more precisely controlled with insulin as it acts much more effectively than pills.

Gestational Diabetes is developed temporarily in women during pregnancy mostly during the last three months. All pregnant women must be checked for diabetes several times during pregnancy. If diagnosed with gestational diabetes, nearly 40% of women usually develop type 2 diabetes later in life within 15 years. A non-diabetic woman, diagnosed with diabetes during pregnancy, should control diabetes to its fullest extent to protect herself and for the sake of a healthy child. A diabetic woman who is pregnant needs to take extra care. A pregnant woman is said to be diagnosed with gestational diabetes when she is tested positive for any two of the following:

   a. A fasting plasma glucose level of more than 5.8 mmol/L or 105 mg/dL.
   b. One-hour after-meal level of more than 10.6 mmol/L or190 mg/dL.
   c. Two-hour after-meal level of more than 9.2 mmol/L or 165 mg/dL.
   d. Three-hour after-meal level of more than 8.1 mmol/L or 145 mg/dL.

MEDICAL CHECK-UP AND DIAGNOSIS [1, 6]

If the pancreas of a person does not function properly, firstly the person experiences indigestion problem because of the lack of enzymes. Poor absorption of food causes weight loss and diarrhea. Secondly, there would be not enough insulin production, resulting in frequent urination, loss of glucose through urine, increased thirst and weight loss. In order to diagnose a person with diabetes, the following tests are performed:

● **The Chemcard Glucose Test:** It is a simple FDA approved screening test for diabetes, being used to quickly identify an abnormally high fasting plasma glucose level. It is a 3-minute test that requires a single drop of blood from a fingerstick. This unit is for both home use and in doctors' offices. This test kit does not require any laboratory analysis and is still 94 to 99.95% accurate. When a person approaches a physician with these symptoms of frequent urination and increased thirst, the physician readily suspects that the problem is related to diabetes. After a physical examination, and after obtaining information regarding symptoms and family history, the physician could instantly test the urine and blood from a fingerstick, and from these test results, the physician could tentatively determine if the person is diabetic or not.

● **The Oral Glucose Tolerance Test**: It is an important test in which the physician asks the patient to come back early in the morning after fasting for 10 hours but not greater than 16 hours. The patient is asked to consume 75 grams of glucose (dissolved in purified water), and the glucose levels are then monitored at intervals of 15 minutes or 30 minutes for a period of 2 to 3 hours. A non-diabetic person's glucose level gradually drops to normal in 2 hours (under 7.8 mmol/L or 140 mg/dL), whereas a diabetic person's glucose levels remain significantly higher (more than 11.1 mmol/L or 200 mg/dL) and the levels do not drop to normal until and after 6 hours, confirming that the person has diabetes.

● **Random Blood Glucose Test:** Regardless of when you last ate, a blood sample showing that your blood sugar level is 200 mg/dL (11.1 mmol/L) or higher suggests diabetes, especially if you also have signs and symptoms of diabetes, such as frequent urination and extreme thirst.
● **Fasting Blood Glucose Test.** A blood sample is taken after an overnight fast. A reading of less than 5.6 mmol/L or 100 mg/dL is normal. A level from 5.6 to 6.9 mmol/L or 100 to 125 mg/dL is considered prediabetes. If your fasting blood glucose level is more than 7 mmol/L or 126 mg/dL on two separate tests, you will be diagnosed with diabetes.
● **More Tests:** The physician could conduct more useful tests. The level of amylase in the blood could reveal inflammation of the pancreas. An excess quantity of fat present in the blood sample indicates that the pancreas is not producing enough enzymes. An ultrasound scan test gives pictures of the pancreas gland to see any physical damage. The physician, by carefully inserting a needle, collects a small piece of pancreas gland and sends it to a pathologist for further examination. There are also more tests available such as CT Scan, endoscopic retrograde cholangiopancreatography (ERCP) to see if the pancreas is damaged.

● **C-peptide Test:** It is also important to find out if the pancreas is producing any insulin or not. By measuring the amount of C-peptide present in the blood, it is possible to determine the amount of insulin produced by the pancreas. Type 1 diabetic people have decreased levels of insulin and C-peptide while type 2 diabetic people have normal or increased levels of C-peptide.

● **Hemoglobin A1c Test:** Ultimately, a hemoglobin A1c blood test would precisely reveal the average blood glucose level of a person over the preceding 90 days, based on which a physician can easily understand if the patient being tested is diabetic or non-diabetic, and take appropriate steps to control or treat diabetes if the patient is diagnosed with diabetes.

SELF-BLOOD GLUCOSE MONITORING DEVICES [1]

If you are diagnosed with diabetes, it is time to purchase a self-blood glucose monitoring device for home use, learn how to use it, and start monitoring and recording your daily blood glucose levels throughout the day (not just fasting glucose level in the morning). The best advice is that a diabetic patient must monitor at least 3 fasting blood glucose levels and 3 after meal blood glucose levels, meaning 6 times a day. The more frequently you monitor, the better you diabetes control could be. Whenever you monitor, if the blood glucose level is too high or not normal, you must take action by exercising or taking a medication (either oral medication or insulin). Only by doing so, you can better manage your daily blood glucose levels, and keep your diabetes under tight control.

GLUCOMETER FOR HOME USE: CONTOUR NEXT METER [7]

Traditional Blood Glucometer. [Also called patient's glucose meter] A simple and inexpensive glucometer for home use that suits everybody to do self-blood glucose monitoring every day. It comes with fingerstick test strips and lancets.	**Up-to-Date Glucometer** Meter can be hooked up to your smartphone.
Figure 2.5 Contour Next One Meter. Courtesy of Ascensia Diabetes Care Canada Inc.	Figure 2.6 Contour Next One Meter. Courtesy of Ascensia Diabetes Care Canada Inc.

You can better manage your diabetes by hooking up this up-to-date glucometer to your smartphone, and keep a record of all your blood glucose results and understand how your activities impact them, and take action in order to keep your diabetes under tight control. Contour next one meter would take the hassle out of your diabetes management, and help you understand your diabetes control. If you purchase this meter, the manufacturer (Bayer or Ascensia Diabetes Care Canada Inc.) trains you over the phone on how to use it, and even send you a meter for free. Or, a local pharmacist could teach you how to use the meter correctly.

IMPORTNANT NOTE: Whenever you go to do your diabetes panel blood tests in a laboratory (once every 3 months), take this meter with you to the laboratory, and get it tested, and make sure it is working perfectly. Compare your meter reading with the result obtained from the lab analysis.

CONTINUOUS GLUCOSE MONITORING DEVICES

1. Dexcom G6 Continuous Glucose Monitoring (CGM) System [8] (Noninvasive Glucose Monitoring System Without Finget Prick)

Continuous Glucose Monitoring (CGM) is a noninvasive method to track glucose levels throughout the day and night without finger-poking. A CGM system takes glucose measurements at regular intervals, up to 24 hours a day, and translate the readings into dynamic data, providing complete information on how your blood glucose levels are fluctuating throughout the day. A CGM can also contribute to improve diabetes management by helping to minimize the guesswork that comes with making treatment decisions based solely on a number from a blood glucose meter reading. Studies have shown that Dexcom CGM systems help lower hemoglobin A1c level to normal with minimal efforts, and reduce hypoglycemia, whether users are on oral medications, insulin injections or pump therapy.

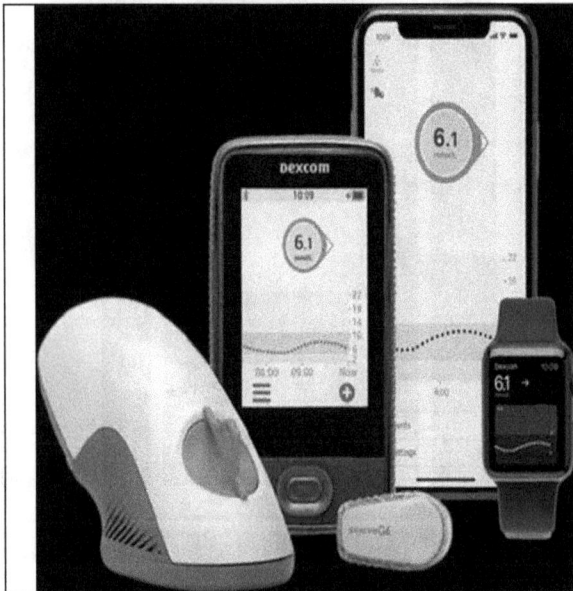

Figure 2.8 Dexcom G6 CGS System. Courtesy of Dexcom Inc.

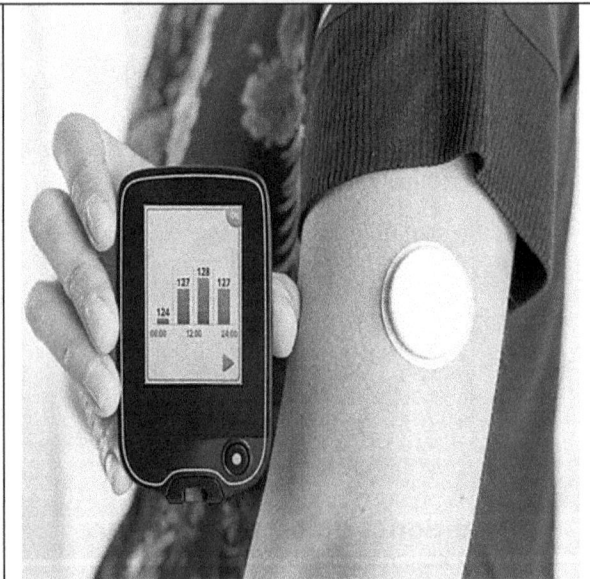

Figure 2.7 FreeStyle Livre 14-Day System. Courtesy of Abbott Laboratories

2. FreeStyle Livre Continuous Device With A 14-Day Sensor [9]

A small sensor automatically measures and continuously stores glucose readings day and night. The sensor lasts up to 14 days. Every 14 day, a new sensor has to be used. It records the glucose concentration every 15 minutes, storing that data in a rolling 8 hour log. With every scan you get your current glucose reading, the last 8 hours of glucose data and an arrow showing the direction your glucose is heading. The FreeStyle Libre system is designed to be water-resistant and can be worn while bathing, showering, swimming or exercising.

Advantages: With a continuous device, you can very easily control diabetes, and achieve normal hemoglobin A1c. By watching the glucose level throughout the day, and by injecting the appropriate amount of insulin whenever the glucose level is too high, you can slash glucose spikes, and achieve normal average blood glucose level on a daily basis.

Disadvantages: The sensors are very expensive, and the people with low income cannot afford to purchase them. The people with low income can still use the traditional glucometer, and can still control diabetes by monitoring frequently, recording and analysing the blood glucose data manually without purchasing those expensive devices.

ROUTINE TESTS FOR DIABETICS [1]

If a person is diagnosed with diabetes (type 1, type 2, or gestational diabetes), he/she must perform the following tests in a laboratory, with the physician's requisition in your area, once every 3 months or at least every 6 months, depending on the severity of the situation. Either a family physician or an endocrinologist (diabetes specialist) can order the following tests:

PART-I

1. Fasting Glucose and Hemoglobin A1c: Fasting glucose and Hemoglobin A1c tests must be performed once every 3 months in order to know if your diabetes is controlled or not. Get your home glucometer tested whenever you go to a laboratory blood test, and compre your glucometer reading with the result obtained from lab test.

2. Hematology Tests: A series of tests to understand the blood and diseases in the blood. WBC, RBC, Hemoglobin, Hematocrit, MCV, MCH, MCHC, RDW, Platelet Count.
Differential: Neutrophils, Lymphocytes, Monocytes, Eosinophils, Basophils, Granulocytes Immature.

3. Cholesterols Panel Tests (Lipids): Total cholesterol, LDL cholesterol, HDL Cholesterol, Chol-HDL Ratio, Non HDL-Cholesterol, Apolipoprotein B100, Triglycerides level. All these tests should be normal.

4. Liver Test: ALT (Alanine Aminotrabsferase), AST (Aspartate Aminotransferase), LD (Lactate dehydrogenase), Alkaline Phosphatase & Gamma GT. These tests pre-indicate the liver disease or liver damage. During the trial of a new cholesterol-lowering drug (such as statin drugs), these tests must be performed and results verified once every month until the drug suits the patient's body. After the statin drug suits the patient's body without serious side effects, liver test should be performed once every 3 months for diabetic people.

5. Thyroid Tests: The TSH test is essential once every 3 months if you have thyroid problems. If TSH is not normal then do the tests Free T3 & Free T4.

6a. Urine Test for Kidneys Function: MicroAlbumim in Unine, Creatinine in Urine, and ACR (Microalbumin/Creatinine Ratio).

6b. Blood Test for Kidneys Function: Estimated GFR (Glomerular Filtration Rate) test tells how quickly the kidneys are clearing waste from your body. Creatinine & Urea suggest a kidney problem. In addition, find out the levels of Sodium, Potassium, Chloride, Bicarbonate, Calcium, Magnesium, Phosphate, Iron (Ferritin), etc. in the blood.

7. PSA Test for Prostate: A Urologist examines the prostate gland and orders a urine test and PSA test to make sure that the prostate is normal. Bladder tests are to be performed if the patient have urinary problems.

8. Testosterone Test: Most people with diabetes develop erectile dysfunction (ED) problems. It is important to take testosterone test once every 3 months, and make sure it is normal. If the testosterone level is below 10, then do the bioavailable testosterone test.

9. Muscles Enzimes Creatine Kinase (CK) Test: Most people with diabetes develop muscle pain problems. Those who take cholesterol-lowering statin drugs develop muscle pain. In order to understand how serious the inflammation is, it in important to take CK test once every 3 months.

PART-II

10. Blood Pressure: Between 60 and 65% of diabetic people suffer from high blood pressure. Frequent self-blood pressure testing is necessary at least once every week. Many BP monitors indicate false or exaggerated BP reading. Also many people experience and live with "white coat syndrome." Try to understand what white coat syndrome is. Be careful and do the appropriate research in order to make sure that the BP device is reliable and trustworthy. Please do not take high blood pressure medication unless you are one 100% certain that you have high blood pressure.

11. Stress Test: A Cardiologist usually organizes a stress test: Running on a treadmill to evaluate the heart condition. One can self-organize this treadmill test by going to a gym.

12. Vision Test: An Optometrist or Eye Specialist performs eye examination to check the development of cataracts, and to make sure that the Retina is normal and that there is no diabetes-related vision impairment. Cataracts needs surgery upon maturity. Several months or years after cataracts surgery, it is very common that people experience floaters and flashes. A retina-tear needs immediate surgery.

Periorbital Dermatitis: Some older people with diabetes develop itching around the eyes (external itching). This itching is often mistakenly confused by eye doctors and treat that as a problem related to "dry eyes," and give eye drops to their patients. If the itching is outside the eyes (not inside the eyes), this problem should be recognized as "periorbital dermatitis," which is chronic disease in older patients (which has nothing to do with dry eyes). In order to treat this external itching on your eyes and/or nose, you need a prescription called Elocom Cream (Taro-Mometasone Cream), which is a corticosteroid. This cream should be applied very carefully outside the eyes without touching inside the eyes.

13. Foot Care: The Family Physician, Endocrinologist or Neurologist organizes a physical examination to check the numbness in feet and knees, and to make sure that the feet are not affected by neuropathy or peripheral neuropathy. Plantar fasciitis is a serious problem for some diabetics. A simultaneous heat and cold therapy on daily basis relieves the pain.

14. Doppler Test: A Vascular Specialist organizes a Doppler test to confirm the leg arteries are not narrowed (claudication) due to diabetes, which causes pain in lower legs while walking. This test confirms whether or not narrowing of leg arteries occurred.

15. SCAN Test: A Neurologist organizes a scan test, along with a physical examination, to make sure that neuropathy (nerve damage) is not caused by diabetes.

16. Skin Care: An Endocrinologist or Dermatologist could identify skin problems related to diabetes and recommend a treatment.

17. Dental Care: A General Dentist or a Specialist in periodontics could check for gum disease developed due to diabetes. Regular dental hygiene cleaning (deep gum cleaning) with a hygienist along with the appropriate dental fillings once every 3 months is recommended for diabetic people.

HOW IS THE BLOOD GLUCOSE LEVEL EXPRESSED FOR DIABETES? [1]

• In Canada, UK, Australia, New Zealand, South Africa & in some other countries around the world, the blood glucose level is expressed in mmol/L.

• In USA, India, China, and in many other countries around the world, the blood glucose level is expressed in mg/dL.

• If a diabetic person travels to other countries, and gets the blood test done, he/she should be educated enough to understand the test result in both units of measurement. The conversion factor is 18.

If you simply multiply the value in mmol/L by 18, you get the value in mg/dL.
If you simply divide the value in mg/dL by 18, you get the value in mmol/L.

For example, the blood glucose level in Canada = 7 mmol/L
The same blood glucose level in USA, India & China = (7 mmol/L)(18) = 126 mg/dL

For example, the blood glucose level in USA = 160 mg/dL
The same blood glucose level in Canada & UK = (160 mg/dL)/(18) = 8.9 mmol/L

• So a diabetic person must be familiar with both units, and should know how to convert the blood glucose level of any test result from one unit to the other.

WHY IS THE GLUCOSE CONVERSION FACTOR 18? [1]
Notation: dL = deciliter (1 liter = 10 deciliters); mg = milligram (1 gram = 1000 milligrams); mmol = millimole (1 mole = 1000 millimoles); L = liter

Here Is the Scientific Explanation:
Molecular Formula of Glucose is: $C_6 H_{12} O_6$

Molecular Weight = (6)(12) + (12)(1) + (6)(16) = 72 + 12 + 96 = 180 mg/mmol (approximately)

Molecular Weight of Glucose (precisely) = 180.16 mg/mmol

Suppose the blood glucose level is reported by a laboratory in Canada as 5.8 mmol/L. Convert the blood glucose level value to mg/dL as expressed in the USA.

To convert from mmol/L to mg/L, multiply by molecular weight.
To convert from mg/L to mg/dL, divide by 10 (1 liter is equal to 10 deciliters).
  5.8 mmol/L = (5.8 mmol/L) (180.16 mg/mmol) / (10 dL/L)
       = 104.49 mg/dL
Or, simply multiply by the conversion factor 18.
  5.8 mmol/L = (5.8 mmol/L) (18) (mg/dL) / (mmol/L) = 104.49 mg/dL

Conversion Factor = (180.16 mg/mmol) / (10 dL/L)
       = 18 (mg/dL) / (mmol/L)

• To convert mmol/L of glucose level to mg/dL, simply multiply it by 18.
• To convert mg/dL of glucose level to mmol/L, simply divide it by 18.

NORMAL BLOOD GLUCOSE LEVELS [1, 11, 12]

A diabetic person should be familiar with the normal blood glucose levels, and should make sure from a fingerstick blood test that the glucose levels are within the normal range. Frequent self-blood glucose tests are necessary to make sure that the diabetes is under tight control.

Table 2.2 Normal blood glucose levels of healthy (non-diabetic) people.

Normal Blood Glucose Levels of Healthy Non-Diabetic People [Courtesy of Joslin Diabetes Center, Adapted from One Touch Meter Manual]		
	Glucose (mmol/L)	Glucose (mg/dL)
Between 2 am and 4 am	> 3.9	> 70
Before breakfast (fasting)	3.9 to 5.8	70 to 105
Before lunch or before dinner	3.9 to 6.1	70 to 110
1 hour after meals	< 8.9	< 160
2 hours after meals	< 6.7	< 120

Table 2.3 Normal level of hemoglobin A1c.

Hemoglobin A1c	Normal Range
(i) Healthy Non-Diabetic People	4.5% - 6.2%
(ii) Diabetic People	< 7%

An Example of Diabetes Control

A diabetic person committed to control his/her diabetes and achieve normal hemoglobin A1c in 90 days. He/she started self-monitoring 7 times a day (4 fasting glucose levels and 3 after-meal glucose levels) as shown below:

Table 2.4

Time	7:15	9:00	12:00	14:00	18:45	19:45	22:00	Average
Glucose (mmol/L)	5.8	8.9	6.5	8.5	5.9	13.8	7.7	8.2
Glucose (mg/dL)	104.4	160.2	117	153	106.2	248.4	138.6	146.8

He/she calculated the daily average glucose level as 8.2 mmol/L or 146.8 mg/dL.

He/she calculated the daily average glucose level as 8.2 mmol/L or 146.8 mg/dL. He/she took action to lower after meal glucose levels with the aid of the healthy diet, oral medication or insulin shots, and daily exercise. After 90 days of consistent and serious efforts, the after-meal blood glucose levels and therefore the daily average glucose level dropped significantly as shown below:

Table 2.5

Time	7:15	9:00	12:00	14:00	18:45	19:45	22:00	Average
Glucose (mmol/L)	5.2	7.5	6.5	7.2	5.9	10.5	6.7	7.1
Glucose (mg/dL)	93.6	135	117	129.6	106.2	189	120.6	127.3

HERE IS THE SECRET: If the daily average blood glucose level of a diabetic person is maintained at or below 7 mmol/L or 126 mg/dL for 90 consecutive days, the hemoglobin A1c would automatically be normal. You can see this secret in the Hemoglobin A1c Chart (Chapter 3, Table 3.1).

REFERENCES

1. Permanent Diabetes Control (Book), Subtitle: The Complete Guide to Living Like A Normal Person Forever, Authored by Rao Konduru, MS, PhD, Reviewed and Endorsed by Dr. Marshal Dahl, MD, PhD., Endocrinologist, Faculty of Medicine, University of British Columbia, Vancouver, British Columbia, Canada, First Published in 2003. www.mydiabetescontrol.com

2. Diabetes: Facts, Statistics, and You by Healthline. https://www.healthline.com/health/diabetes/facts-statistics-infographic#1

3. YouTube Video, Title: What is Pancreas?, Published by Rahul Azad, Aug 24, 2009 https://www.youtube.com/watch?v=1l2GTGEwZOY&feature=youtu.be

4. YouTube Video, Title: How the Body Works: The Pancreas, Published by Daniel Izzo, Aug 3, 2017 https://www.youtube.com/watch?v=j5WF8wUFNkI&feature=youtu.be

5. Diabetes Overview by Mayo Clinic Staff, 2019. https://www.mayoclinic.org/diseases-conditions/diabetes/symptoms-causes/syc-20371444

6. Type 2 Diabetes by Mayo Clinic, 2019. https://www.mayoclinic.org/diseases-conditions/type-2-diabetes/diagnosis-treatment/drc-20351199

7. Contour Next One Meter Hooked Up to Smartphone by Ascensia Diabetes Care Canada Inc. https://www.contournextone.ca/

8. What is Continuous Glucose Monitoring (CGM)? by Dexcom.com. https://www.dexcom.com/en-CA/what-cgm

9. FreeStyle Libre Continuous Glucose Monitor Without A Finger Prick by abbott Laboratories. https://www.freestyle.abbott/ca/en/products/libre.html

10. The Secret to Controlling Type 2 Diabetes, Subtitle: Addendum to Permanent Diabetes Control, Authored by Rao Konduru, Published in 2019, ISBN # 9780973112054, Available on Amazon.com, www.mydiabetescontrol.com

11. Krall, L.P, MD, and Beaser, R.S, MD, Joslin Diabetes Manual, Philadelphia, Lea and Febiger, Pages 3-6, 135, 138, 1989.

12. Glucose Ranges in People Without Diabetes, Lifescan's One Touch Profile Blood Glucose Monitoring Manual, Table on Page 51, Lifescan, Printed in USA, 1996.

CHAPTER 3 DIABETES CONTROL

TABLE OF CONTENTS

ATTENTION DIABETICS!

● **"The Secret to Controlling Diabetes in 90 days"** is discovered, illustrated and explained in detail in this fully comprehensive guide. All diabetics should read through and benefit from this revolutionary diabetes control treatment. If you understand that "SECRET," as explained in this book, you will be victorious in controlling your diabetes in 90 days, and then live like a normal person for the rest of your life.

● The author of this book, by being a seriously diabetic person himself, is the living example. He published his official blood test results in this book for the past 10 plus years, taken once every 3 months. His hemoglobin A1c test result has been consistently normal for the past 10 plus years, revealing the fact that he accomplished "Permanent Diabetes Control."

DIABETES CONTROL BASICS

INTRODUCTION TO DIABETES CONTROL [1]

When the pancreas of the human body produces little or no insulin, diabetes develops. Due to this insulin deficiency, the human body becomes unable to supply and control insulin flow into the bloodstream, thereby allowing elevated blood glucose levels. Either an effective oral medication or an artificial insulin is therefore essential to combat insulin deficiency. In order to properly optimize the effectiveness of the medication, diabetes should be controlled by mutually adjusting the food intake, daily exercise, and the dosages of the medication. For a given major meal, the dosage of either oral medication or insulin dose and exercise should be mutually adjusted, which is a complex task to be practiced by any diabetic patient. It is not possible to adjust the dosage of a oral medication on a daily basis, but the dosages of artificial insulin can be easily adjusted daily or whenever needed. Diabetes control can be simplified by keeping exercise as a constant factor (one hour a day), and by adjusting the dosage of artificial insulin in an attempt to lower the after-meal glucose spikes. The dosage of artificial insulin for a given major meal can be approximately determined, cut in half, or cut in even less than half by introducing after-meal exercise, and by frequently monitoring, recording and researching after-meal blood glucose levels. Attaining such an extensive monitoring and researching experience is not impossible, but it takes diligence, self-discipline, commitment, determination, and a strong desire to achieve normal hemoglobin A1c level.

Diabetes control is considered to be a matter of controlling the following three parameters:

a. Fasting Glucose Level Before All Meals
b. After-meal Glucose Level (Within and After 2 Hours of the Meal)
c. Hemoglobin A1c (Monitored Once Every 3 Months)

An extensive study of after-meal meal glucose levels is essential in the beginning, for a period of 3 to 6 months, in order to research and understand the body's response with a variety of heavy meals against insulin dose and exercise. This research is unavoidably required to control diabetes that has long been forgotten and was left uncontrolled. After the hemoglobin A1c has been successfully brought close to normal value for the first time, the earned research experience helps guide the individual to further control diabetes without finger-poking as frequently. The individual who earns extensive research experience in the beginning for 3 to 6 months will be rewarded for the rest of his/her life.

A diabetic person should have a thorough knowledge about the normal blood glucose levels, and should be able to recognize how high or how low the glucose level is at any particular time. The blood glucose level of a non-diabetic person after 2 hours of a heavy meal consumption drops to normal range. For a diabetic person, it is indeed possible to lower the blood glucose level close to normal value within 2 hours of meal consumption through injecting appropriate insulin dose and introducing an after-meal exercise for one hour.

Normal Blood Glucose Level In General
Between 4 mmol/L and 7 mmol/L
    (In Canada, UK, Australia, New Zealand, South Africa & in some other countries).
Between 72 mg/dL and 126 mg/dL
    (In USA, India, China, and in many other countries around the world).

CONTROL YOUR DIABETES IN 90 DAYS: Why 90 Days? [1]

Most people with diabetes focus their attention on fasting glucose levels in order to control diabetes rather than on lowering after-meal glucose spikes. If your blood glucose level from a fingerstick blood test early in the morning is normal, it doesn't mean your diabetes is controlled. Hemoglobin A1c is a parameter that directly reveals the degree of "diabetes control" during the preceding 90 days. Red blood cells live in the bloodstream for 90 days. Every 90 days, new red blood cells are born. Hemoglobin is a protein molecule that is present in red blood cells and carries and supplies oxygen from the lungs to the trillions of body's cells wherever it is needed. Hemoglobin also carries glucose along with it, because glucose can stick to all kinds of proteins in your body. While the blood circulates, depending on how high or how low the blood glucose level is, a certain amount of glucose is attached to the hemoglobin molecules to form glycated hemoglobin. Different doctors and scientists call it with different names: glycated A1c, hemoglobin A1c, HbA1c, or simply A1c. Therefore, by measuring the hemoglobin A1c level in a laboratory from the patient's blood sample, it is possible to know the average blood glucose level and the degree to which it has been controlled over the preceding 90 days. Which obviously means that it takes at least 90 days to see any significant improvement in the hemoglobin A1c level from a laboratory blood test. By lowering the hemoglobin A1c level to perfectly normal, and by keeping it normal for the rest of your life, you control your diabetes. This book "Permanent Diabetes Control" guides you on how to control your diabetes perfectly in 90 days, and live like a normal person for the rest of your life.

HEMOGLOBIN A1c EXPLAINED [1]

Human blood, referred to as the river of life, is pumped from the heart through a network of large and small blood vessels. If all blood vessels and capillaries were joined together in one line, they would stretch to 300 million feet. Blood runs at different speeds depending on how fast the heart beats. A normal adult possesses about 5 to 6 liters of blood that is approximately 7 to 8 % of body weight. Blood is a liquid stored in the heart, blood vessels and in the sinusoids of the bone marrow, liver and spleen. About 55% of blood is plasma, a clear yellowish liquid. The other 45% of blood is made of red blood cells, white blood cells and platelets. Platelets coagulate when the skin is cut and form a clot to stop bleeding. Plasma is watery, consisting of 93% water and 7% solid proteins the majority of which is albumin. Bone marrow is a soft tissue located in bones that produces red blood cells, platelets and white blood cells. Plasma transports red blood cells, white blood cells and platelets through the blood vessels. Plasma delivers nutrients to trillions of cells and also picks up waste including carbon dioxide from the cells.

The blood carries oxygen from the lungs to all the body's cells where it is burned. But the oxygen could react quickly in blood and burn prematurely before it reaches the body's cells. This premature burning is prevented by a protein molecule. The blood in the human body contains about 30 trillion red blood cells, and each red blood cell has about 270 million protein molecules. Each protein molecule represents a ring composed of carbon, nitrogen and hydrogen atoms. The ring floats in the bloodstream and a cluster of 4 iron atoms that sit in the center of each ring protects a pair of oxygen atoms from premature burning. **This incredibly designed protein molecule is called "hemoglobin".**

Hemoglobin carries oxygen with it and drops it off whenever and wherever oxygen is needed in order to promote all sorts of chemical reactions that occur every instant in the body. Red blood cells live in the bloodstream for 60 to 90 days. Every 90 days, new red blood cells are generated in the bloodstream. While the blood circulates, glucose is attached to hemoglobin depending on how much glucose is present in the bloodstream. This attachment takes place in different ways and all the hemoglobin that is attached to glucose in the red blood cells is called "glycohemoglobin," roughly 6% of the hemoglobin in the blood. [2] The hemoglobin that is attached or bound to glucose is also called glycosylated hemoglobin. The more glucose is in the blood, the more glycohemoglobins or glycosylated hemoglobins form. Glycohemoglobin remains in the blood for 60 to 90 days. Glycohemoglobin is divided into 3 types such as A1a, A1b and A1c. Two-thirds of this glycohemogobin is called hemoglobin A1c, and one-third is made up of A1a and A1b. Hemoglobin A1c that is present in the red blood cells has special characteristics and is easily identifiable by laboratory techniques. This suggests that hemoglobin A1c reflects the total amount of glucose attached to it in red blood cells over the preceding 90 days. The measurement of hemoglobin A1c therefore indicates how high the average blood glucose level has been and how good/poor the blood glucose control has been over the preceding 90 days.

Analytical methods have been developed to readily test the diabetic person's blood and report the results of hemoglobin A1c test in "gm of A1c per gm of total hemoglobin" or in percentage (%). Medical scientists developed a correlation between hemoglobin A1c levels and the corresponding average blood glucose levels as shown in the table below. They found that lowering blood glucose level by 30 mg/dL (1.67 mmol/L) would lower hemoglobin A1c by approximately 1%, and decrease the diabetes risk probability by up to 25%.

For non-diabetic people, the normal level of hemoglobin A1c is between 4% and 6%. For diabetic people, a value less than 7% is considered "normal." Between 7% and 8% is considered fair, but not normal (you should try to lower it to 7). The following table or conversion chart shows the relationship between hemoglobin A1c and the average blood glucose level over the preceding 90 days.

HEMOGLOBIN A1c CHART [1]
[A Very Important Table to Keep in Mind if You Are Diabetic]

Table 3.1 **Hemoglobin A1c Chart** (Hemoglobin A1c Versus Average Blood Glucose).

HbA1c	Average Blood Glucose Level in 90 Days		
[%]	(mg/dL)	(mmol/L)	Assessment
4.0	60	3.3	It is Too Low, Try to Keep It Higher Immediately!
5.0	90	5.0	The Perfect Control! Extremely Difficult to Achieve!
6.0	120	6.7	Normal & Excellent Control (Congrats!)
6.2	126	7.0	Normal & Excellent Control (Reference Level!)
7.0	150	8.3	Fair or Moderately Good Control, Keep It Steady!
8.0	180	10.0	Too High, Take Action to Lower Immediately!
9.0	210	11.7	Poor Control, Take Action to Lower Immediately!
10.0	240	13.3	Poor Control, Take Action to Lower Immediately!
11.0	270	15.0	Very Poor Control, Take Action Immediately!
12.0	300	16.7	Very Poor Control, Take Action Immediately!
13.0	330	18.3	Very Poor Control, It Is Dangerous To Live Like That!
14.0	360	20.0	Very Poor Control, It Is Dangerous To Live Like That!
Courtesy of www.Bayer.com			

From this hemoglobin A1c chart, if you know the value of hemoglobin A1c from a laboratory blood test, you can determine the average blood glucose level in 90 days. Or, if you know the average blood glucose level in 90 days, you can determine the hemoglobin A1c level.

NORMAL BLOOD GLUCOSE LEVELS AND NORMAL A1c LEVELS [1, 3, 4]

Table 3.2 Normal blood glucose levels of healthy (non-diabetic) people.

Normal Blood Glucose Levels of Healthy Non-Diabetic People [Courtesy of Joslin Diabetes Center, Adapted from One Touch Meter Manual]		
	Glucose (mmol/L)	Glucose (mg/dL)
Between 2 am and 4 am	> 3.9	> 70
Before breakfast (fasting)	3.9 to 5.8	70 to 105
Before lunch or before dinner	3.9 to 6.1	70 to 110
1 hour after meals	< 8.9	< 160
2 hours after meals	< 6.7	< 120

Table 3.3 Normal level of hemoglobin A1c.

Hemoglobin A1c	Normal Range
(i) Healthy Non-Diabetic People	4.5% - 6.2%
(ii) Diabetic People	< 7%

The Secret to Controlling Diabetes Successfully [1]

Most diabetics don't know how to control diabetes, and live with uncontrolled diabetes, with elevated A1c level, for decades. Even the doctors and specialists are not equipped with the appropriate knowledge and training tools to transmit the real concept on controlling diabetes to the minds of their patients, except leaving their patients in a dilemma of uncontrolled diabetes. Read this section carefully and grasp the concept. If you understand this "secret", your diabetes control would be more rewarding than ever before, and this "secret" could save your life if you are seriously diabetic!

The secret lies in understanding the "Hemoglobin A1c Chart (Table 3.1)" conceptually! Think like a mathematician by looking at the hemoglobin A1c chart "Average Blood Glucose Level Versus A1c", and try to understand the relationship between "Average Blood Glucose Level" and "Hemoglobin A1c." You should be able to find out "Hemoglobin A1c" from the chart (Table 3. 1) by interpolation if you know the "Average Blood Glucose Level". Practice it and understand it.

HERE IS THE SECRET: If you can maintain your daily average blood glucose level at or below 7 mmol/L or 126 mg/dL every day for 90 consecutive days, your hemoglobin A1c would automatically be normal. You can see this secret in the Hemoglobin A1c Chart (Table 3.1).

Think about this concept over and over again, and program your mind to manage your daily average blood glucose level at or below 7 mmol/L or 126 mg/dL every day for 90 consecutive days, and then take the laboratory blood test. You will be surprised to learn that your hemoglobin A1c result is normal (close to 7% or 0.07).

Most people live with uncontrolled diabetes just because they were never taught this secret. Whenever your glucose level jumps above and beyond 7 mmol/L or 126 mg/dL, you need to compensate that excess by lowering it to below 7 mmol/L or 126 mg/dL, and by staying close to the lowest possible level so that the daily average glucose level would always be 7 mmol/L or 126 mg/dL. If you can do, your hemoglobin A1c would automatically be normal.

IF YOU UNDERSTAND THESE 2 EXAMPLES, THEN YOU MASTER DIABETES CONTROL

EXAMPLE-I: For example, your after-meal glucose level rose to 10 mmol/L or 180 mg/dL and stayed there for 2 hours. Immediately after 2 hours, if you can lower that spike to 5 mmol/L or 90 mg/dL, and keep it lowered for another 3 hours, your average glucose level during the preceding 5 hours would be precisely 7 mmol/L or 126 mg/dL. If your daily average blood glucose level is 7 mmol/L or 126 mg/dL for 90 consecutive days, your hemoglobin A1c would automatically be normal. You can understand this from basic arithmetics by simply calculating the average of 5 numbers (the total of 5 numbers divided by 5). This is a very simple example. If you can understand this simple example and solve this simple problem, you will be able solve much complex problem, by calculating average glucose level for all 24 hours. You don't need to calculate the average for all 24 hours, but just grasp the concept through your imagination, and think like a mathematician.

EXAMPLE-II: For example, your after-meal glucose level rose to 10 mmol/L or 180 mg/dL and stayed there for 4 hours. Immediately after 4 hours, if you can lower that spike to 5 mmol/L or 90 mg/dL, and keep it lowered for another 6 hours, your average glucose level during the preceding 10 hours would be precisely 7 mmol/L or 126 mg/dL. If your daily average blood glucose level is 7 mmol/L or 126 mg/dL for 90 consecutive days, your hemoglobin A1c would automatically be normal. This is a very simple example. If you can understand this simple example and solve this simple problem, you will be able solve much complex problem, by calculating average glucose level for all 24 hours. You don't need to calculate the average for all 24 hours, but just grasp the concept through your imagination.

Bottom Line

Whenever the glucose level spikes above and beyond 7 mmol/L or 126 mg/dL, you should immediately lower that spike to 5 mmol/L or 90 mg/dL, and keep it lowered by staying close to lowest possible level so that the daily average glucose level would always be 7 mmol/L or 126 mg/dL. In other words, you need to compensate any excess glucose level in intervals of time throughout the day by lowering your glucose level to lowest possible value. It doesn't matter whether you are type 1 diabetic or type 2 diabetic, if you could master this concept, and could maintain you daily average at 7 mmol/L or 126 mg/dL for 90 consecutive days, your A1c would automatically be normal (< 7% or < 0.07). Your hemoglobin A1c is normal means your diabetes is tightly controlled. If you live with tightly controlled diabetes, all complications would be minimized.

Can The Hemoglobin A1c be Determined At Home? [1]
If You Understand This Example, Then You Understand A1c Chart!

It may sound unbelievable, but yes, hemoglobin A1c can be manually determined at home, without going to a laboratory for a blood test, up to a certain degree of accuracy using your fingerstick blood glucose meter. This kind of self-monitoring would help you control your diabetes on your own at home without anybody's help. You don't need to go to your doctor, get a requisition for blood test, and go to a laboratory to have the blood test done. You can approximately determine your hemoglobin A1c at home if you are knowledgeable, and eager to do it.

The following experiment will show you how to do it at home using your glucometer.
A diabetic person recorded his/her blood glucose levels (4 fasting glucose levels and 4 after-meal glucose levels) in a typical day as shown below using the glucometer at home:

Table 3.4

Time	7:15	9:00	12:00	14:00	18:45	19:45	22:00	23:00	Average
Glucose (mmol/L)	5.8	8.9	6.5	8.5	5.9	15.8	12.7	7.7	9.0
Glucose (mg/dL)	104.4	160.2	117	153	106.2	248.4	174.6	138.6	150.3

He/she then calculated the average glucose level as 9.0 mmol/L or 150.3 mg/dL. **IMPORTANT NOTE:** By exercising high self-discipline and high willpower, he/she thus monitored blood glucose levels every day continuously, at least 6 to 8 times a day, without any interruption for 90 consecutive days, and calculated the average blood glucose value in 90 days as 9.2 mmol/L or 165.6 mg/dL.

From the aforementioned A1c Chart (Table 3.1), he/she noted down the hemoglobin A1c value.

Average glucose level in 90 days = 9.2 mmol/L or 165.6 mg/dL
From the Hemoglobin A1c Chart (Table 3.1), Hemoglobin A1c = 7.5% = 0.075

The more fingerstick blood glucose data a person collects, the more accurate the value of hemoglobin A1c would be. If you monitor 10 times a day (5 fasting glucose levels and 5 after-meal glucose levels for 90 consecutive days), your self-monitored hemoglobin A1c value would be more accurate (but it is still an approximate value, and not an exact value which is obtained from a laboratory blood test). If you can monitor every hour (24 times a day) for 90 consecutive days, and calculate the average blood glucose level, then your A1c would be reasonably accurate.

IMPORTANT NOTES (CAUTION)
🌑 However, please be noted that the hemoglobin A1c test should be done in a laboratory once every 3 months to make certain that your diabetes is precisely controlled. The above-mentioned calculations would help you manage your diabetes tentatively and to lower your A1c to normal but do not provide you with accurate A1c value. You cannot always trust your glucometer at home and suppose that it is working perfectly. Your glucometer might be broken, you probably didn't even notice, and your glucometer could be producing erroneous results. If that happens, you will end up determining a wrong result of A1c. You cannot simply rely on the A1c value determined at home all the time. So it is very important that you need to find out your hemoglobin A1c value from a laboratory test once every 3 months, and compare it with your self-monitored A1c value.

🌑 Also get your glucometer tested and make sure it is working perfectly whenever you go to a laboratory for your diabetes panel blood test. You should make sure that your glucometer at home is not giving erroneous glucose level due to malfunctioning. By comparing your blood glucose level generated by your glucometer with the lab test result, you can find out if your meter is working perfectly or broke down.

How to Calculate the Daily Average Blood Glucose Level From The Self-Blood Glucose Monitoring Data?
[THESE BASIC ARITHMETICS COULD SAVE YOUR LIFE!]

⊕ In Canada, UK, Australia, New Zealand, South Africa & in some other countries around the world, the blood glucose level is expressed in mmol/L as shown in the following tables.

⊕ In USA, India, China, and in many other countries around the world, the blood glucose level is expressed in mg/dL as shown in the following tables. The conversion factor is 18.

Table 3.5

Glucose	Breakfast		Lunch		Dinner		During Night	
Units	Before Meal	After Meal	Before Meal	After Meal	Before Meal	After Meal	10 pm	2 am
mmol/L	5.6	12.9	7.5	14.5	6.9	18.5	7.7	7.2
mg/dL	100.8	232.2	135.0	261.0	124.2	333.0	138.6	129.6

$$\text{Daily Average} = \frac{5.6 + 12.9 + 7.5 + 14.5 + 6.9 + 18.5 + 7.7 + 7.2}{8} = 10.1 \text{ mmol/L}$$

$$\text{Daily Average} = \frac{100.8 + 232.2 + 135.0 + 261.0 + 124.2 + 333.0 + 138.6 + 129.6}{8} = 181.8 \text{ mg/dL}$$

IF THE DAILY AVERAGE GLUCOSE LEVEL IS TOO HIGH, WHENEVER THE DAILY AVERAGE GLUCOSE LEVEL IS MORE THAN 7 mmol/L or 126 mg/dL, a diabetic person must take action, and slash the after-meal glucose spikes until the daily average glucose level drops to 7 mmol/hr or 126 mg/dL. A diabetic person must lower his/her after-meal glucose levels every day with the aid of the healthy diet, oral medication or insulin shots, and after-meal exercise. After 90 days of consistent and serious efforts, the after-meal glucose levels would drop significantly, and therefore the daily average glucose level would reach a value close to 7 mmol/L or 126 mg/dL as shown below:

Table 3.6

Glucose	Breakfast		Lunch		Dinner		During Night	
Units	Before Meal	After Meal	Before Meal	After Meal	Before Meal	After Meal	10 pm	2 am
mmol/L	4.7	8.4	5.5	9.0	5.8	9.1	7.1	6.5
mg/dL	84.6	151.2	99.0	162.0	104.4	163.8	127.8	117.0

$$\text{Daily Average} = \frac{4.7 + 8.4 + 5.5 + 9.0 + 5.8 + 9.1 + 7.1 + 6.5}{8} = 7.0 \text{ mmol/L}$$

$$\text{Daily Average} = \frac{84.6 + 151.2 + 99.0 + 162.0 + 104.4 + 163.8 + 127.8 + 117.0}{8} = 126.2 \text{ mg/dL}$$

⊕ From the Hemoglobin A1c Chart (Table 3.1), you can see that when the daily average glucose level is 7 mmol/L or 126 mg/dl, hemoglobin A1c = 7%.

HERE IS THE SECRET: If you can maintain your daily average blood glucose level at or below 7 mmol/L or 126 mg/dL every day for 90 consecutive days, your hemoglobin A1c would automatically be normal. You can see this secret in the Hemoglobin A1c Chart (Table 3.1).

HOW TO CALCULATE DALILY AVARAGE BLOOD GLUCOSE LEVEL? [2]
GIVEN BELOW ARE MORE EXAMPLES:
[THESE BASIC ARITHMETICS COULD SAVE YOUR LIFE!]

EXAMPLE-I: Calculate the average of 2 glucose levels
(1 fasting glucose level and 1 after-meal glucose level).

For example, fasting glucose level = 4 mmol/L
For example, after-meal glucose level = 10 mmol/L

$$\text{Daily Average} = \frac{4 + 10}{2} = 7 \text{ mmol/L}$$

For example, fasting glucose level = 72 mg/dL
For example, after-meal glucose level = 180 mg/dL

$$\text{Daily Average} = \frac{72 + 180}{2} = 126 \text{ mg/dL}$$

From the Hemoglobin A1c Chart (Table 3.1), A1c = < 7% (which is normal).

If you know the average blood glucose level for 90 consecutive days, you can find out A1c from the A1c chart. The more times you monitor throughout the day, the more accurate your A1c would be. If your daily average is close to 7 mmol/L or 126 mg/dL for 90 days, your A1c will be normal.

EXAMPLE-II: Calculate the average of 4 glucose levels
(2 fasting glucose levels and 2 after-meal glucose levels).

For example, 2 fasting glucose levels are = 4 & 5 mmol/L
For example, 2 after-meal glucose levels are = 10 & 12 mmol/L

$$\text{Daily Average} = \frac{4 + 10 + 5 + 12}{4} = 7.75 \text{ mmol/L}$$

For example, fasting glucose levels = 72 & 90 mg/dL
For example, after-meal glucose levels = 180 & 216 mg/dL

$$\text{Daily Average} = \frac{72 + 180 + 90 + 216}{4} = 139.5 \text{ mg/L}$$

From the Hemoglobin A1c Chart (Table 3.1), A1c = < 7% (which is normal).

If you know the average blood glucose level for 90 consecutive days, you can find out A1c from the A1c chart. The more times you monitor throughout the day, the more accurate your A1c would be. If your daily average is close to 7 mmol/L or 126 mg/dL for 90 days, your A1c will be normal.

EXAMPLE-III: Calculate the average of 6 glucose levels
(3 fasting glucose levels and 3 after-meal glucose levels).

For example, 3 fasting glucose levels are = 4, 5 & 6 mmol/L
For example, 3 after-meal glucose levels are = 10, 12 & 15 mmol/L

$$\text{Daily Average} = \frac{4 + 10 + 5 + 12 + 6 + 15}{6} = 8.7 \text{ mmol/L}$$

For example, 3 fasting glucose levels = 72, 90 & 108 mg/dL.
For example, 3 after-meal glucose levels = 180, 216 & 270 mg/dL

$$\text{Daily Average} = \frac{72 + 180 + 90 + 216 + 108 + 270}{6} = 156 \text{ mg/dL}$$

From the Hemoglobin A1c Chart (Table 3.1), A1c = > 7%   which is not normal!

If you know the average blood glucose level for 90 consecutive days, you can find out A1c from the A1c chart (Table 3.1). The more times you monitor throughout the day, the more accurate your A1c would be. If your daily average is close to 7 mmol/L or 126 mg/dL for 90 days, your A1c will be normal.

Similarly you can calculate the average glucose level by monitoring 10 times a day, and determine haemoglobin A1c value from the A1c chart. The more times you monitor, the more accurate your A1c would be. If you monitor every hour (24 times a day) for 90 consecutive days, you haemoglobin A1c value would be reasonably accurate.

IMPORTANT INFORMATION: You can determine the daily average blood glucose level more accurately, and find out your hemoglobin A1c level at home without going to a laboratory blood test by using a continuous glucose monitoring device such as:
(i) Dexcom System, or
(ii) FreeStyle Livre 14-Day System.

For example Dexcom system is capable to monitor and record your blood glucose level every 5 minutes. Which means you can collect 12 glucose readings per hour, or 288 glucose readings per day. If you can calculate the daily average from 288 readings, it would be a lot more accurate. An accurate daily average blood glucose level would result in the accurate hemoglobin A1c by using Hemoglobin A1c Chart (Table 3.1) without going to a laboratory blood test.

HERE IS WHAT YOU SHOULD DO TO CONTROL YOUR DIABETES
Find out the after-meal glucose spikes from the glucose data, and slash them immediately or as soon as possible by taking the appropriate action so that your daily average glucose level would be close to 7 mmol/L or 126 mg/dL. You can do that:
(i) by changing the current diet, and by introducing a new healthy diet,
(ii) by changing and adjusting the dosage of the oral medication, and
(iii) by means of an effective after-meal exercise that quickly lowers after-meal glucose spike.

If your daily average glucose level is close to 7 mmol/L or 126 mg/dL for 90 consecutive days, your hemoglobin A1c would automatically be normal (Please refer to Table 3.1).
ATTENTION DIABETICS: If you understand the calculation of the average blood glucose level, and how to determine hemoglobin A1c from the Hemoglobin A1c Chart with clear concept, you can very easily become a master of diabetes control, and achieve normal A1c!

MOST COMMONLY ASKED QUESTION

DO I REALLY NEED TO MONITOR 8 TIMES A DAY TO CONTROL DIABETES?
[That is a lot of work and tedious to monitor so many times every day]

Every diabetic person, while reading this book, might be wondering and worried about monitoring so many times every day in order to determine the daily average blood glucose level, and the hemoglobin A1c (from Table 3.1) at home.

HERE IS THE ANSWER: The answer is "Not Really." You don't need to poke your finger and monitor your blood glucose level so many times for the rest of your life. You monitor 6 to 8 times a day "only during the research phase" until you understand your after-meal blood glucose spikes for the first 3 to 6 months. If you are capable to do the research precisely, you can complete the research phase in 90 days, and achieve normal A1c by the end of 90 days. During the research phase, the more times you monitor, the more accurate your "Daily Average Glucose Level" would be, and the better you understand about your diabetes and your after-meal blood glucose spikes throughout the day. After you completed the research phase, you will be rewarded by your own monitoring and researching experience, and you will start monitoring skilfully only a few times a day. From your extensive monitoring experience, you can easily guess your glucose level, if it is too high or too low, and take appropriate action.

For example, Dr. RK used to monitor 10 times a day during the research phase until he understood his body's response with insulin shots and until he understood his after-meal blood glucose spikes. He was then rewarded by his own monitoring and researching experience. After 3 to 6 months of his research phase, he started monitoring only a few time a day. Dr. RK now monitor only 2 times a day, his diabetes is perfectly controlled, and his most recent hemoglobin A1c is 5.5%. He just guesses his blood glucose spike, and inject the exact amount of insulin to offset the spike and exercise. Exercise is required only after consuming every large or heavy meal, and for small meals no exercise is required.

WHO CAN USE ORAL MEDICATIONS & WHO CAN USE INSULIN SHOTS?
[1, 2, 3]

The International Diabetes Federation (IDF) reported in 2017 that there are approximately 425 million adults worldwide (ranging 20-79 years of age) living with diabetes. About 5 to 10% of these people suffer from type 1 diabetes, and the remaining 90 to 95% suffer from to type 2 diabetes. [3]

Type 1 Diabetes: Type 1 diabetes mellitus or insulin-dependent diabetes mellitus or adult diabetes, also called juvenile diabetes, is developed when the pancreas produces little or no insulin because the beta cells of the pancreas may have been totally damaged or destroyed. Type 1 diabetes is developed mostly in infants, children and young adults under the age 30 years. Insulin shots are certainly required to treat type 1 diabetes. As explained above, in order to optimize the insulin dose and insulin action, type 1 diabetics also need to exercise after every major meal consumption in order to slash the after-meal spikes and to tightly control diabetes.

Type 2 Diabetes: Nearly 40% of the adults in USA alone suffer from prediabetes or borderline diabetes, and at least some of them would soon be diagnosed with type 2 diabetes. The people with type 2 diabetes around the world can be categorized into 3 groups based on the severity of the disease: (i) mild, (ii) moderate and (iii) severe.

⊕ For those people with prediabetes or borderline diabetes, or mild type 2 diabetes, diabetes can be controlled without any oral medication or insulin, but with healthy lifestyle (dietary changes) and regular exercise or physical activity. However high self-discipline is required to maintain healthy lifestyle.

⊕ For some people with moderate type 2 diabetes, diabetes can be controlled with healthy lifestyle (dietary changes), and oral medication (s) along with regular exercise or physical activity. However high self-discipline is required to maintain healthy lifestyle.

⊕ For those people with severe type 2 diabetes, and for some people with moderate type 2 diabetes, oral medications do not work effectively, and it would be difficult to achieve normal hemoglobin A1c. And so this group of diabetic people are advised to switch to insulin shots (both long-acting insulin and rapid-acting) along with after-meal exercise. Those diabetics who use insulin shots need after-meal exercise because insulin dose needs to be optimized. Injecting too much insulin without exercise has adverse side effects, and therefore insulin dose should be cut in half by incorporating an appropriate after-meal exercise plan.

⊕ Some diabetic people with expert knowledge go easy on the dietary guidelines and still manage to control diabetes with insulin shots, keep their A1c perfectly normal, and live like a normal person. These people with expert knowledge know how to inject the right amount of rapid-acting insulin, by trial and error and exercise, and lower after-meal blood glucose spike quickly to normal, and know how to achieve normal A1c.

▶ Insulin is the best medicine to treat diabetes, and insulin shots always work for any kind of diabetes (either type 1 diabetes or type 2 diabetes). That is why, many doctors recommend their patients to switch to insulin shots.

HOW TO CONTROL DIABETES

The next question pops up on your mind is how to lower that high after-meal blood glucose spike immediately to normal, and how to control diabetes?

There are three methods being discussed in this course with easy-to-understand examples: Method 1, Method 2 & Method 3.

THE SECRET TO CONTROLLING DIABETES IN 90 DAYS: If you can lower your after-meal blood glucose spikes to normal every day for 90 consecutive days in an attempt to lower your "Daily Average Blood Glucose Level" close to 7 mmol/L or 126 mg/dL, your hemoglobin A1c comes down to normal in 90 days. THIS IS THE SECRET YOU NEED TO LEARN AND PRACTICE. Dr. RK has been doing this successfully for the past 20 years.

Method 1: Type 2 Diabetes Control
HEALTHY DIET & EXERCISE WITHOUT ANY MEDICATION

Method 2: Type 2 Diabetes Control
HEALTHY DIET ALONG WITH ORAL MEDICATION & EXERCISE

Method 3: Type 2 Diabetes Control | Type 1 Diabetes Control
HEALTHY DIET ALONG WITH INSULIN SHOTS & EXERCISE

WHY ARE AFTER-MEAL BLOOD GLUCOSE LEVELS NOT TOO HIGH? AN IMPORTANT CLARIFICATION
By examining the self-blood glucose monitoring data in Method 1, Method 2, Method 3, a reader might wonder and raise a question such as "why are the after-meal blood glucose levels not significantly high enough in the collected glucose data?". Most of the data showed in this book have after meal-glucose levels under 13 mmol/L or 234 mg/dL.

HERE IS THE EXPLANATION
(i) All the fingerstick blood glucose data were collected after consuming the healthy diet (low carbohydrate diet) so the collected glucose levels were not too high, but however they are high enough to significantly raise or elevate hemoglobin A1c level.

(ii) In order to prevent the ketones formation, a diabetic person should not exercise when the blood glucose level is over 13 mmol/L or 234 mg/dL unless the exercise suits a person without forming ketones. Each person is different so each person should find out if exercise is causing ketones formation or not by doing the ketones test. To understand this, please refer to Method 3 where "Ketones Formation" and "Ketoacidosis" are explained. A diabetic person should be cautious beforehand and should not exercise when the after-meal glucose levels are higher than 13 mmol/L or 234 mg/dL, unless the exercise suits his/her body without forming ketones. A diabetic person should inject the correct amount of insulin just before consuming a major meal so that the after-meal glucose spike would be close to or below 13 mmol/L or 234 mg/dL, and then exercise in order to lower his/her after-meal blood glucose level to perfectly normal (5 mmol/L or 90 mg/dL). That is why in all the self-blood glucose monitoring data, you will find the after-meal blood glucose levels below 13 mmol/L or 234 mg/dL.

Method 1: Type 2 Diabetes Control
WITH HEALTHY DIET & EXERCISE (NO MEDICATION)

DIETARY GUIDELINES

After-meal spike of the blood glucose level can be avoided by consuming a low-carbohydrate meal without medication:

● A balanced low-carbohydrate diet with lean meat (oven-baked skinless chicken, skinless turkey or fish), all kinds of vegetables, leafy greens, legumes, fruits (limited quantity only), either low-fat milk, or skim milk, or low-fat soy milk, and nuts and seeds (limited quantity) are safe and healthy for a diabetic person

● Every person, whether diabetic or non-diabetic, should eagerly try to find and eat a variety of vegetables, leafy greens and fruits available in the market, by changing them every day, and by covering all of them every week so that the body would get all kinds of vitamins, minerals and fiber.

● A whole-foods meal, without any processed or refined items in it, along with egg whites best suits a person with severe type 2 or type 1 diabetes. Egg white is one 100% protein and one 100% safe, and so it can be used to adjust the daily protein requirement while preparing a balanced meal.

● White rice spikes blood glucose level immediately after consumption, and therefore a diabetic person (who is not on insulin) should never eat white rice. Brown rice or wild rice is okay, but it still needs control.

● Salt consumption and oil consumption should be minimized in order to lose weight and to keep the blood pressure under control.

● A diabetic person should lose excess weight in order to control his/her diabetes. Weight loss could result in the reversal of type 2 diabetes for some people, and keeps the blood pressure and cholesterols under control.

● A low-carbohydrate diet or no-carbohydrate diet with excessive amount of red meat, processed meat, or breaded and deep-fried meats for a diabetic person is unsafe, unhealthy, and even dangerous, and therefore should be avoided.

● Hamburgers, cheeseburgers, deep-fried potatoes (so called fries), all kinds of processed and refined products of any kind, all kinds of bakery items, all kinds of ready-to-eat meals, all kinds of breads, anything made by adding starchy white flour or all-purpose white flour, all kinds of soups and soup mixes, all kinds of chips and snacks being sold in supermarkets, grocery stores and gas stations could unwillingly and unnoticeably make a diabetic person overweight or obese and could clog and damage arteries, and therefore should be avoided.

● Always read the label whenever you purchase any food item, focus your attention on whole foods (natural foods). Make sure the food is not altered, processed or refined, and make sure that it does not contain any additives, preservatives, artificial colors and flavors except the food itself, preserved in its natural form.

● Alcohol abuse increases the lipids in the blood, which is a type of fat that can harden arteries, increasing bad cholesterol (LDL cholesterol) and arterial plaque in the heart's blood vessels and arteries. Eventually the arteries could be clogged, resulting in heart attack or heart failure. Therefore a diabetic person should avoid regular alcohol drinking.

● Smoking poses greater risk for people with diabetes. Just like high blood glucose levels, the poisonous chemicals in cigarette smoke attack blood vessels, contributes to hardening of the arteries (or what is known as atherosclerosis) which impairs the blood's ability to carry oxygen to the trillions of the body's cells. Eventually the arteries could be clogged, causing heart disease, heart attack or heart failure. Therefore, a diabetic person should quit smoking immediately or as soon as possible.

▶ No medication is necessary if your diabetes is under control with healthy diet and exercise.

PHYSICAL ACTIVITY STIMULATES THE INSULIN PRODUCTION FROM PANCREAS

Physical Activity (Any Kind of Exercise) Boosts Insulin Production from Pancreas

● The function of the islets of Langerhans is to produce two important hormones called insulin and glucagon (long chains of glucose). Beta cells of pancreas produce insulin and alpha cells of pancreas produce glucagon. The amazing counter-action between beta cells and alpha cells situated in the islets of Langerhans is responsible to maintain normal blood glucose levels. Physical activity has a significant positive effect on insulin sensitivity. Any type of physical activity stimulates beta cells in order to release more insulin, and has the potential to make your body's insulin work better by flowing smoothly throughout the blood vessels.

● Diabetes Care (a monthly peer-reviewed medical journal of American Diabetes Association) published the following information: In a randomized study on type 2 diabetes, researchers asked 1,152 Mexican Americans about their physical activity, and took blood samples to analyze their beta cell function of pancreases, and levels of glucose and insulin. They found that people who said they exercised had better beta cell function, independent of weight, diet, and body fat. The researchers concluded that the physical activity (daily exercise) may boost beta cells function of pancreas, releases more insulin into the bloodstream, thereby lowering blood glucose levels.

EXAMPLE: 1 How to Control Type 2 Diabetes
With Healthy Diet and Exercise (Without Medication)

Mike was diagnosed with type 2 diabetes 5 years ago. But he has been living without diabetes care. He never tried to understand what diabetes is and never read a book about it. Even though his doctor warned him numerous times and insisted him to control diabetes, he has neglected all about his diabetes, and kept himself busy with his work, and has been eating greasy foods in all kinds of restaurants. Recently he had a minor heart attack and hospitalized for a few days. His doctors performed an angioplasty and told him that a bypass surgery is unnecessary at that time, and released him from the hospital.

After he came home from the hospital, he went to library and read as many diabetes books as possible. He also purchased several diabetes books online and read them all with curiosity. He most recently purchased "Permanent Diabetes Control", read it cover to cover, understood all the contents, and was indeed inspired to control his diabetes for the rest of his life. Now he has a clear concept on "how to control diabetes". He has also seen several diabetes nurses and endocrinologists, got answers to his questions, and also attended a diabetes course in his community diabetes center. He collected all the information, and equipped himself with all the tools necessary to control his diabetes. In other words, Mike awakened the giant within him, and committed to control his diabetes, starting today.

By consuming the same kind of meals (breakfast, lunch & dinner) he has been consuming during the past 5 years in a typical day, he monitored his blood glucose levels (4 fasting glucose levels and 4 after-meal glucose levels) using his self-monitoring glucose meter, and recorded as follows (just to do some research and to see what was going wrong):

Table 3.7

Time	7:15	9:00	12:00	14:00	18:45	19:45	22:00	23:00	**Average**	**A1c**
Glucose (mmol/L)	5.8	15.9	7.5	22.8	6.9	20.5	18.5	8.1	13.3	10%
Glucose (mg/dL)	104.4	286.2	135	410.4	124.2	369	333	145.8	238.5	10%

He then calculated the daily average blood glucose level as 13.3 mmol/L or 238.6 mg/dL.

By using the A1c Chart (show above), he determined the hemoglobin A1c level as approximately 10%.

MIKE'S DIETARY CHANGES & EXERCISE PROGRAM

Mike committed to make dietary changes, and to exercise high self-discipline and high willpower. He immediately stopped eating out in the restaurants, and started cooking and eating at home. His new diet is shown below:

Breakfast: Puffed wheat cereals, low-fat milk (or soy milk) and a banana.
Lunch: Oven-baked chicken breast, legumes, salad made from leafy greens & tomatoes. He walked 30 minutes after lunch.
Dinner: Oven-baked fish, brown rice (limited quantity), steamed vegetables & an apple. He walked another 30 minutes after dinner.
Snacks: Limited quantities of cottage cheese (dry curd), salad, Kamut puffs, cashews, nuts & seeds (limited quantity), etc.
Water: He started drinking 8 to 16 cups of purified water. He also learned how to remineralize purified water.

As a result of the dietary changes and exercise, he lost weight, and his body mass index dropped to normal in a few months, and he did not have major after-meal blood glucose spikes anymore. Within a few days, his blood glucose levels in general dropped significantly. He continued to live like that for 90 days. His daily blood glucose monitoring data in a typical day are shown below:

Table 3.8

Time	7:15	9:00	12:00	14:00	18:45	19:45	22:00	23:00	Average	**A1c**
Glucose (mmol/L)	5.2	10.8	6.4	10.9	6.9	13.5	7.3	7.2	8.5	7.2%
Glucose (mg/dL)	93.6	194.4	115.2	196.2	124.2	243	131.4	129.6	153.5	7.2%

After 90 days, from the hemoglobin A1c chart, he determined the value of hemoglobin A1c as approximately 7.2%.
After 6 months, from the hemoglobin A1c chart, he determined the value of hemoglobin A1c as approximately 7.0%.
After 1 year, from this hemoglobin A1c chart, he determined the value of hemoglobin A1c as approximately 6.7%.

Once every 3 months, he took diabetes panel blood test in a laboratory, and his hemoglobin A1c was found to be normal (< 7%).

Mike is happier than ever. His diabetes is reasonably controlled, and will remain controlled for the rest of his life as long as:

- He self-monitors and records his blood glucose levels every day, calculates daily average, and tries to keep his daily average close to 7 mmol/L or 126 mg/dL every single day,
- He eats healthy meals at home by following the dietary guidelines, and avoids eating junk foods (processed foods & refined foods) in restaurants,
- He walks or exercises in a gym every day after a major meal consumption,
- He exercises high self-discipline and high willpower to maintain the normal A1c level (<7%).

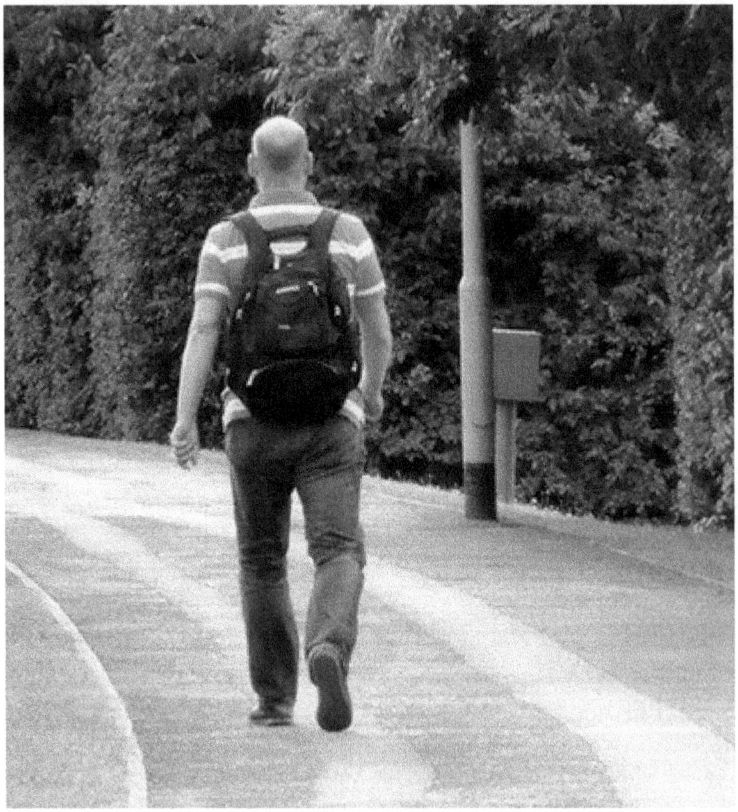

Figure 3.1 A type 2 diabetic is lowering his after-meal blood glucose level with the aid of healthy diet and exercise (walking on the road).

DISADVANTAGES OF METHOD 1 (WITHOUT MEDICATION)

- It works for some people only (mostly for pre-diabetics). It doesn't work for most people with diabetes. You need to try it out looking for successful results.
- Even if it works, after some time it may not work, and the person may eventually need an oral medication or insulin.
- It is extremely difficult to maintain high self-discipline and high will power, and so most people cannot maintain normal A1c level all the time. People eat out every now and then, tempt to eat snacks and other unsafe foods, and diabetes could easily go out of control.

Method 2: Type 2 Diabetes Control
WITH HEALTHY DIET, ORAL MEDICATION & EXERCISE

DIETARY GUIDELINES

After-meal spike of the blood glucose level can be avoided by consuming a low-carbohydrate meal along with medication:

● A balanced low-carbohydrate diet with lean meat (oven-baked skinless chicken, skinless turkey or fish), all kinds of vegetables, leafy greens, legumes, fruits (limited quantity only), either low-fat milk, or skim milk, or low-fat soy milk, and nuts and seeds (limited quantity) are safe and healthy for a diabetic person.

● Every person, whether diabetic or non-diabetic, should eagerly try to find and eat a variety of vegetables, leafy greens and fruits available in the market, by changing them every day, and by covering all of them every week so that the body would get all kinds of vitamins, minerals and fiber.

● A whole-foods meal, without any processed or refined items in it, along with egg whites best suits a person with severe type 2 or type 1 diabetes. Egg white is one 100% protein and one 100% safe, and so it can be used to adjust the daily protein requirement while preparing a balanced meal.

● White rice spikes blood glucose level immediately after consumption, and therefore a diabetic person (who is not on insulin) should never eat white rice. Brown rice or wild rice is okay, but it still needs control.

● Salt consumption and oil consumption should be minimized in order to lose weight and to keep the blood pressure under control.

● A diabetic person should lose excess weight in order to control his/her diabetes. Weight loss could result in the reversal of type 2 diabetes for some people, and keeps the blood pressure and cholesterols under control.

● A low-carbohydrate diet or no-carbohydrate diet with excessive amount of red meat, processed meat, or breaded and deep-fried meats for a diabetic person is unsafe, unhealthy, and even dangerous, and therefore should be avoided.

● Hamburgers, cheeseburgers, deep-fried potatoes (so called fries), all kinds of processed and refined products of any kind, all kinds of bakery items, all kinds of ready-to-eat meals, all kinds of breads, anything made by adding starchy white flour or all-purpose white flour, all kinds of soups and soup mixes, all kinds of chips and snacks being sold in supermarkets, grocery stores and gas stations could unwillingly and unnoticeably make a diabetic person overweight or obese and could clog and damage arteries, and therefore should be avoided.

● Always read the label whenever you purchase any food item, focus your attention on whole foods (natural foods). Make sure the food is not altered, processed or refined, and make sure that it does not contain any additives, preservatives, artificial colors and flavors except the food itself, preserved in its natural form.

● Alcohol abuse increases the lipids in the blood, which is a type of fat that can harden arteries, increasing bad cholesterol (LDL cholesterol) and arterial plaque in the heart's blood vessels and arteries. Eventually the arteries could be clogged, resulting in heart attack or heart failure. Therefore a diabetic person should avoid regular alcohol drinking.

● Smoking poses greater risk for people with diabetes. Just like high blood glucose levels, the poisonous chemicals in cigarette smoke attack blood vessels, contributes to hardening of the arteries (or what is known as atherosclerosis) which impairs the blood's ability to carry oxygen to the trillions of the body's cells. Eventually the arteries could be clogged, causing heart disease, heart attack or heart failure. Therefore, a diabetic person should quit smoking immediately or as soon as possible.

▶ **An oral medication** similar to "Metformin (Glucophage® XR)" has to be taken with the evening meal or according to the dosage instructions provided by the manufacturer. Sometimes, your doctor may also prescribe you a second oral medication such as Invokamet. Some doctors also prescribe insulin sensitizers such as Actos, which helps your body to use the insulin from the pancreas effectively and at the same time decreases the glucose released by the liver. However there are many oral medications for type 2 diabetes.

PHYSICAL ACTIVITY STIMULATES THE INSULIN PRODUCTION FROM PANCREAS
Physical Activity (Any Kind of Exercise) Boosts Insulin Production from Pancreas

● The function of the islets of Langerhans is to produce two important hormones called insulin and glucagon (long chains of glucose). Beta cells of pancreas produce insulin and alpha cells of pancreas produce glucagon. The amazing counter-action between beta cells and alpha cells situated in the islets of Langerhans is responsible to maintain normal blood glucose levels. Physical activity has a significant positive effect on insulin sensitivity. Any type of physical activity stimulates beta cells in order to release more insulin, and has the potential to make your body's insulin work better by flowing smoothly throughout the blood vessels.

● Diabetes Care (a monthly peer-reviewed medical journal of American Diabetes Association) published the following information: In a randomized study on type 2 diabetes, researchers asked 1,152 Mexican Americans about their physical activity, and took blood samples to analyze their beta cell function of pancreases, and levels of glucose and insulin. They found that people who said they exercised had better beta cell function, independent of weight, diet, and body fat. The researchers concluded that the physical activity (daily exercise) may boost beta cells function of pancreas, releases more insulin into the bloodstream, thereby lowering blood glucose levels.

EXAMPLE: 2 How to Control Type 2 Diabetes
With Healthy Diet, Oral Medication and Exercise

Both parents of Maria were diagnosed with type 2 diabetes when they were in their sixties. According to the Centers for Disease Control and Prevention (CDC), type 2 diabetes accounts for about 90 to 95 percent of all diagnosed cases of diabetes in adults, and type 1 diabetes accounts for the remaining 5 to 10 percent. Diabetes is known to be hereditary. The influence of family history on whether a person develops diabetes is better established with type 2 than it is with type 1. When Maria was 55 years old, she suffered from frequent urination problem, and was hospitalized for a couple of days. An endocrinologist (diabetes specialist), in the hospital, ordered a diabetes panel blood test, and diagnosed her with type 2 diabetes. The hospital staff asked Maria many questions concerning her family history and diabetes sufferers in her family, and concluded that the heredity was the reason why Maria's was diagnosed with type 2 diabetes. The laboratory blood test showed the following results:

Her fasting glucose level (from the laboratory blood test) was 9.5 mmol/L or 171 mg/dL
Her hemoglobin A1c (from the laboratory blood test) was 11.3%

On the same day, the nurses researched about her eating habits and the rise and fall of her daily blood glucose levels during 24 hours period. They gave Maria exactly the same kind of meals she has been consuming at her home in a typical day, and monitored her blood glucose levels (4 fasting glucose levels and 4 after-meal glucose levels). Maria's blood glucose levels in a typical day, when she was diagnosed with type 2 diabetes, are shown below:

Table 3.9

Time	6:00	9:00	12:00	14:00	18:45	19:45	22:00	23:00	Average	A1c
Glucose (mmol/L)	9.2	19.5	8.9	22.5	10.8	19.7	18.5	9.8	14.9	11.0%
Glucose (mg/dL)	165.6	351	160.2	405	194.4	354.6	333	176.4	267.5	11.0%

They calculated the average glucose level in a typical day as 14.9 mmol/L or 267.5 mg/dL.
From the same laboratory blood test, her hemoglobin A1c was 11%. It is dangerous to live with such a high A1c (11%). Maria was warned to take action immediately and lower A1c.

The endocrinologist in the hospital prescribed her Metformin alone (Glucophage® XR), 500 mg once a day with evening meal.

(i) Type 2 Diabetes Training Course
Maria was asked by her doctor to attend a type 2 diabetes training course in the same hospital. A nurse taught her in a 2-day session all about the dietary guidelines, how to eat healthy, how to count calories, how to take oral medication, and how to exercise every day after a major meal consumption. Maria is determined to control her diabetes seriously. She purchased the fingerstick blood glucose monitor (glucometer), strips and lancets. She purchased the medication Metformin alone (Glucophage® XR), 500 mg, enough for 3 months (to be re-filled once every 3 months).

(ii) Dietary Guidelines
Maria started following all the dietary guidelines as described in the above-mentioned section.

(iii) Self-Monitoring Daily Blood Glucose Levels
Maria started monitoring her blood glucose levels 8 times a day (4 farting glucose levels & 4 after-meal glucose levels). She learned how to calculate the daily average glucose level. She also learned how to estimate her hemoglobin A1c level roughly using A1c Chart (Table 3.1). She started taking diabetes panel tests once every 3 months in a laboratory. She is also scheduled to see her endocrinologist (diabetes specialist) once every 3 months. After 6 months of dieting along with oral medication and exercise, her blood glucose level data on a typical were recorded as follows:

Table 3.10

Time	6:00	9:00	12:00	14:00	18:45	19:45	22:00	23:00	Average	A1c
Glucose (mmol/L)	6.9	13.5	7.5	15.8	7.5	13.0	10.8	7.5	10.3	8.3%
Glucose (mg/dL)	124.2	243	135	284.4	135	234	194.4	135	185.6	8.3%

Maria calculated the average glucose level in a typical day as 10.3 mmol/L or 185.6 mg/dL.
Maria also determined her hemoglobin A1c (from A1c Chart) as roughly 8.3%.
Her fasting glucose level (from the laboratory blood test) was 6.5 mmol/L or 117 mg/dL
Her hemoglobin A1c (from the laboratory blood test) was 8.6% (It is still too high).
Her hemoglobin A1c dropped from 11.3% to 8.6% in 6 months.
That was a great improvement, but her A1c is still not normal. She needs further improvement.

So her endocrinologist (diabetes specialist) increased the dosage of her medication to 1000 mg. She took some extra care in implementing the dietary guidelines and exercise, and started consuming less calories, and lost some weight. After 6 more months of consistent and serious efforts, her blood glucose levels on a typical day were recorded as follows:

Table 3.11

Time	6:00	9:00	12:00	14:00	18:45	19:45	22:00	23:00	Average	A1c
Glucose (mmol/L)	5.3	10.2	7.5	10	5.8	9.7	7.5	6.0	7.8	6.8%
Glucose (mg/dL)	95.4	183.6	135	180	104.4	174.6	135	108	139.5	6.8%

Maria calculated the average glucose level in a typical day as 7.8 mmol/L or 139.5 mg/dL. Maria also determined her hemoglobin A1c (from A1c Chart) as roughly 6.8%.

Her fasting glucose level (from the laboratory blood test) was 4.9 mmol/L or 88 mg/dL. Her hemoglobin A1c from a laboratory blood test was 6.9%, close to the one she calculated. Her hemoglobin A1c dropped from 11.3% to 6.9% in 12 months, which is considered normal for a diabetic person.

Once every 3 months, she took diabetes panel blood test in a laboratory, and her hemoglobin A1c was found to be normal (< 7%) consistently for the following year.

IMPORTANT NOTE: It took 12 months for Maria to achieve normal A1c because she never understood and never used the "SECRET" as explained in this book (nobody told her about it). Had she used the SECRET with clear concept, she could have achieved normal A1c in 90 days.

HERE IS THE SECRET: If you can maintain your daily average blood glucose level at or below 7 mmol/L or 126 mg/dL every day for 90 consecutive days, your hemoglobin A1c would automatically be normal. You can see this "SECRET" in the Hemoglobin A1c Chart (Table 3.1).

Maria is happier than ever. Her diabetes is reasonably controlled, and will remain controlled for the rest of her life as long as:
꙳ She self-monitors and records her blood glucose levels every day, calculates daily average, and tries to keep her daily average close to 7 mmol/L or 126 mg/dL every single day.
꙳ She eats healthy meals at home by following the dietary guidelines described in the above-mentioned section, and avoids eating junk foods (processed foods & refined foods) in restaurants,
꙳ She takes her oral medication every day with her evening meal, and never forgets,
꙳ She walks or exercises in a gym every day after a major meal consumption,
꙳ She exercises high self-discipline and high willpower to maintain normal A1c level (<7%).

DISADVANTAGES OF METHOD 2 (WITH ORAL MEDICATION)
꙳ It is extremely difficult to maintain high self-discipline and high will power. Most people cannot maintain normal A1c level all the time. They eat out every now and then, tempt to eat snacks and other unsafe foods, and so diabetes could easily go out of control.
꙳ It works for some people and it doesn't work for other people with diabetes. You need to try it out looking for successful results.
꙳ It takes long time to see successful results (where as with insulin shots, you can see immediate results with perfection).
꙳ Even if it works, after some time it may not work, and the person may eventually need insulin.
꙳ For most diabetics, it is not possible to accomplish perfect diabetes control with consistent hemoglobin A1c level.
꙳ Pills don't work as effectively as insulin. Artificial insulin is the best medication for diabetes, as explained in Method 3. So if pills don't work, please switch to insulin shots.

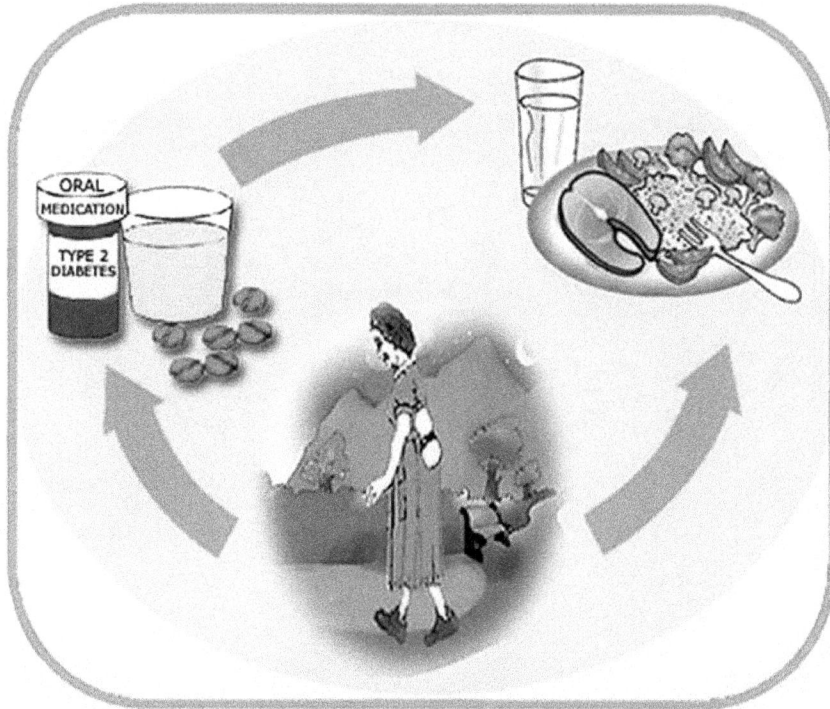

Figure 3.2 A type 2 diabetic is lowering her after-meal blood glucose level with the aid of healthy diet, oral medication and exercise (walking on the road).

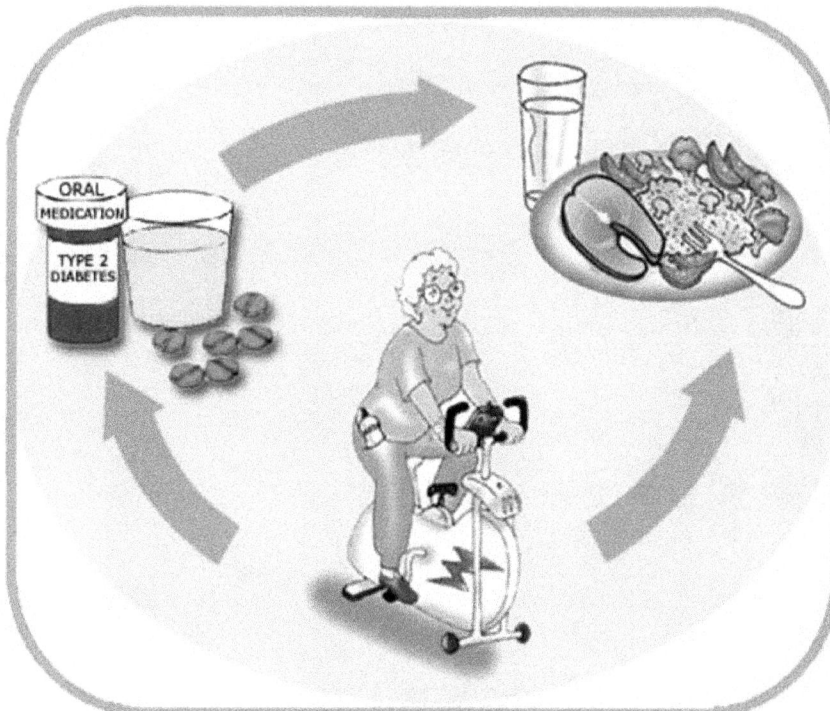

Figure 3.3 A type 2 diabetic is lowering her after-meal blood glucose level with the aid of healthy diet, oral medication and exercise (biking in a gym).

Method 3: Type 2 Diabetes Control
WITH HEALTHY DIET, INSULIN SHOTS & EXERCISE

INTRODUCTION: If the oral medication along with diet and exercise does not stabilize your blood glucose levels and if you are unable to maintain a consistently normal A1c (<7%), then you should switch to insulin injections, and your diabetes control would be more rewarding than ever. Pills don't work for many people. It is a slow process to see successful results of maintaining normal A1c. But insulin is guaranteed to work instantly. You can see results immediately within an hour in terms of lowering blood glucose levels. Even if you are type 2 diabetic, you can always switch to insulin shots any time without any fear or hesitation. Many type 2 diabetics around the world use insulin shots to control diabetes.

LONG-TERM SIDE EFFECTS OF DIABETES
[UNCONTROLLED DIABETES IS DANGEROUS]

Don't simply rely on oral medications, waste year after year, and live with uncontrolled diabetes. Living with uncontrolled diabetes, and neglecting your health by inadequately managing your chronic diabetes means you are living with high glucose levels in the bloodstream, and high levels of hemoglobin A1c. At elevated blood glucose levels over a long time, the glucose sticks to the surface of the cells and it is then converted into a poison called "sorbitol", which damages the body's cells and blood vessels, leading to long-term side effects such as:

- High cholesterols (total cholesterol & LDL cholesterol) and high blood pressure,
- Heart attack, heart failure, coronary heart disease, stroke,
- Hardening of arteries or what is known as atherosclerosis,
- Peripheral artery disease (PAD), narrowing of arteries,
- Painful neuropathy (nerve damage and poor blood flow),
- Burning foot syndrome, numbness in feet and knees, intermittent claudication,
- Amputation (due to nerve damage in the feet),
- Kidney disease, kidney damage, loss of kidney,
- Erectile dysfunction (ED) and/or Impotence,
- Cataracts, blurred vision, retinopathy, blindness,
- Deafness (hearing impairment),
- Diseases of the small blood vessels in the eyes, kidneys, legs and nerves,
- Gum disease and bone loss (dental problems),
- Bladder and prostate problems,
- Skin diseases (bacterial and fungal infections),
- Dementia such as Alzheimer's disease,
- Depression develops over time if diabetes is left untreated,
- and many other strange problems and complications.

If your hemoglobin A1c is more than 7%, your diabetes in uncontrolled, so take action immediately! When after-meal blood glucose spike is too high after eating and remain elevated for more than two hours, this presents a significant mortality risk factor, and the person should switch to insulin shots.

INSULIN IS THE BEST MEDICATION FOR DIABETES

A rapid-acting insulin such as Humalog or Novolog/NovoRapid, if combined with exercise, would help lower the blood glucose spike immediately and is guaranteed to work instantly if you know exactly how many units you needed to inject.

▶ A highly knowledgeable diabetic person can very easily lower his/her huge blood glucose spike to perfectly normal within 30 minutes by injecting the right amount of insulin and by running on a treadmill, or even by the regular walking.

You will not be able to lower a huge blood glucose spike with oral medications being prescribed. A rapid-acting inhaled insulin Afrezza is a new oral medication, but it is not yet widely known in all places (not available in Canada). Even if it is available, it cannot be divided into tiny portions. Whereas insulin dose can be divided into several portions, and inject several times (before and after a heavy meal consumption).

Even the biking or walking on the street, with insulin injected, would help lower the steep blood glucose spike. If you inject the right amount of insulin for a given meal you consumed, and run on a treadmill for 30 minutes, for example, your blood glucose spike drops immediately from a high-risk 20 mmol/L or 360 mg/dL to a stunning 5 mmol/L or 90 mg/dL. And then if you could keep this average glucose level at 7 mmol/L or 126 mg/dL for the rest of the day, your daily average would be perfectly normal. <u>If you can keep up the daily average blood glucose level close to 7 mmol/L or 126 mg/dL for 90 consecutive days, your A1c will automatically be normal</u>. You will become a master of diabetes control, your life will change, and you will be happier than ever.

IMPORTANT NOTE ON INSULIN

Rapid-acting insulin such as Humalog or Novolog alone doesn't work effectively. Rapid-acting insulin works only on the top of the long-acting insulin such as Humulin-N. Whenever you inject rapid-acting insulin such as Humalog, you should have long-acting insulin such as Humulin-N already injected into your body. Whenever you switch to insulin shots, you should always use both long-acting insulin (Humalog) and rapid-acting insulin (Humulin-N) together. You should master the concept of how insulin works, and how to inject. You should go to your community diabetes center, and take a "full course" on how to use insulin shots for diabetes. They will train you and teach you on how to calculate insulin doses and how to inject (it doesn't matter if you are type 1 diabetic or type 2 diabetic).

However, you need to research and find out which method (of the 3 methods discussed above) suits you the best, and stick to that treatment. Switching to insulin shots would be the best choice, it doesn't matter at all weather you are type 2 diabetic or type 1 diabetic. You can always switch from one method to the other.

DIETARY GUIDELINES & RAPID-ACTING INSULIN

After-meal spike of the blood glucose level can be avoided by consuming a low-carbohydrate meal along with insulin shots.

● A balanced low-carbohydrate diet with lean meat (oven-baked skinless chicken, skinless turkey or fish), all kinds of vegetables, leafy greens, legumes, fruits (limited quantity only), either low-fat milk, or skim milk, or low-fat soy milk, and nuts and seeds (limited quantity) are safe and healthy for a diabetic person.

● Every person, whether diabetic or non-diabetic, should eagerly try to find and eat a variety of vegetables, leafy greens and fruits available in the market, by changing them every day, and by covering all of them every week so that the body would get all kinds of vitamins, minerals and fiber.

● A whole-foods meal, without any processed or refined items in it, along with egg whites best suits a person with severe type 2 or type 1 diabetes. Egg white is one 100% protein and one 100% safe, and so it can be used to adjust the daily protein requirement while preparing a balanced meal.

● White rice spikes blood glucose level immediately after consumption, and therefore a diabetic person (who is not on insulin) should never eat white rice. Brown rice or wild rice is okay, but it still needs control.

● Salt consumption and oil consumption should be minimized in order to lose weight and to keep the blood pressure under control.

● A diabetic person should lose excess weight in order to control his/her diabetes. Weight loss could result in the reversal of type 2 diabetes for some people, and keeps the blood pressure and cholesterols under control.

● A low-carbohydrate diet or no-carbohydrate diet with excessive amount of red meat, processed meat, or breaded and deep-fried meats for a diabetic person is unsafe, unhealthy, and even dangerous, and therefore should be avoided.

● Hamburgers, cheeseburgers, deep-fried potatoes (so called fries), all kinds of processed and refined products of any kind, all kinds of bakery items, all kinds of ready-to-eat meals, all kinds of breads, anything made by adding starchy white flour or all-purpose white flour, all kinds of soups and soup mixes, all kinds of chips and snacks being sold in supermarkets, grocery stores and gas stations could unwillingly and unnoticeably make a diabetic person overweight or obese and could clog and damage arteries, and therefore should be avoided.

● Always read the label whenever you purchase any food item, focus your attention on whole foods (natural foods). Make sure the food is not altered, processed or refined, and make sure that it does not contain any additives, preservatives, artificial colors and flavors except the food itself, preserved in its natural form.

● Alcohol abuse increases the lipids in the blood, which is a type of fat that can harden arteries, increasing bad cholesterol (LDL cholesterol) and arterial plaque in the heart's blood vessels and arteries. Eventually the arteries could be clogged, resulting in heart attack or heart failure. Therefore a diabetic person should avoid regular alcohol drinking.

● Smoking poses greater risk for people with diabetes. Just like high blood glucose levels, the poisonous chemicals in cigarette smoke attack blood vessels, contributes to hardening of the arteries (or what is known as atherosclerosis) which impairs the blood's ability to carry oxygen to the trillions of the body's cells. Eventually the arteries could be clogged, causing heart disease, heart attack or heart failure. Therefore, a diabetic person should quit smoking immediately or as soon as possible.

▶ Rapid-acting insulin such as Humalog is to be injected just before or immediately after every meal consumption (breakfast, lunch, dinner, and all snacks). Long-acting insulin has to be injected once or twice a day. Rapid-acting insulin does not work effectively if there no long-acting insulin in your body.

If you master the concept of injecting rapid-acting insulin, you can go easy on the aforementioned dietary guidelines, and enjoy high carbohydrate meal once or twice a week. Some diabetic people with expert knowledge go easy on the aforementioned dietary guidelines and still manage to control diabetes with insulin shots, keep their A1c perfectly normal, and live like a normal person. You cannot do that with oral medications. So it is strongly advised to switch to insulin shots if you are type 2 diabetic.

PHYSICAL ACTIVITY STIMULATES THE INSULIN PRODUCTION FROM PANCREAS
Physical Activity (Any Kind of Exercise) Boosts Insulin Production from Pancreas

● The function of the islets of Langerhans is to produce two important hormones called insulin and glucagon (long chains of glucose). Beta cells of pancreas produce insulin and alpha cells of pancreas produce glucagon. The amazing counter-action between beta cells and alpha cells situated in the islets of Langerhans is responsible to maintain normal blood glucose levels. Physical activity has a significant positive effect on insulin sensitivity. Any type of physical activity stimulates beta cells in order to release more insulin, and has the potential to make your body's insulin work better by flowing smoothly throughout the blood vessels.

⦿ Diabetes Care (a monthly peer-reviewed medical journal of American Diabetes Association) published the following information: In a randomized study on type 2 diabetes, researchers asked 1,152 Mexican Americans about their physical activity, and took blood samples to analyze their beta cell function of pancreases, and levels of glucose and insulin. They found that people who said they exercised had better beta cell function, independent of weight, diet, and body fat. The researchers concluded that the physical activity (daily exercise) may boost beta cells function of pancreas, releases more insulin into the bloodstream, thereby lowering blood glucose levels.

PHYSICAL ACTIVITY ALSO STIMULATES THE FLOW OF ARTIFICIAL INSULIN INJECTED

⦿ Artificial insulin is synthesized in such a way that it works much more effectively and flows a lot more quickly throughout the blood vessels with physical activity (exercise). The amount of artificial insulin dosage must be minimized (optimized) because:

⦿ Too much insulin lowers blood glucose level too fast, causing hypoglycemia (a disorder of low blood glucose levels).

⦿ Too much insulin also constricts arteries, leading to heart attack and coronary heart disease.

⦿ Too much insulin also stimulates the brain so that a person feels hungry and eats more and causes the liver to manufacture fat in the belly.

⦿ Too little insulin on the other hand would not be enough to cover the entire meal and to maintain normal glucose levels.

⦿ **An optimum insulin dose is therefore crucial**. After-meal exercise, either treadmill, biking or walking, should be introduced into the diabetes control plan in order to burn fat, lose calories and optimize both the insulin dose and insulin action. After-meal exercise minimizes the insulin dose and maximizes insulin action and prevents after-meal glucose levels from rising too high, thus keeping diabetes under tight control.

HOW MUCH ARTIFICIAL INSULIN IS TO BE INJECTED TO CONTROL DIABETES? GENERAL RULE

▶ The insulin manufacturing company Eli Lily recommended that in general 1 unit of rapid-acting Humalog is necessary for 8 grams of carbohydrate in your meal in order to lower after-meal glucose level to normal. This rule is being used in all the diabetes clinics around the world.

⦿ If you consume 80 g of carbohydrate through your meals, you need to inject 10 units of Humalog insulin.

⦿ If you consume 100 g of carbohydrate through your meals, you need to inject 12.5 units of Humalog insulin.

⦿ If you consume 200 g of carbohydrate through your meals, you need to inject 25 units of Humalog insulin.

⦿ And so on.

PHYSICAL ACTIVITY (EXERCISE) CUTS INSULIN DOSAGE REQUIREMENT IN HALF

If you consume 80 g of carbohydrate through your meals, and if you are not exercising and staying home, you need to inject 10 units of Humalog insulin to lower your after-meal glucose level to normal or close to normal.

If you consume 80 g of carbohydrate through your meals, and are planning to exercise (running on a treadmill or biking in a gym, or walking on the road or in the shopping mall),

you need to inject only 5 units of Humalog insulin (insulin dose has to be cut in half). After 30 minutes of exercise, your blood glucose level drops to normal. Some people need to inject the remaining 5 units of Humalog (2nd shot) after completing the exercise in order to keep the after-meal glucose levels normal for a prolonged period of time. Some people don't need the second shot. You need to research on yourself, and find out the right rapid-acting insulin dose for any given meal.

HANDS ON TRAINING COURSE IN A DIABETES CLINIC IN YOUR AREA

If you are planning to switch to insulin shots, you should take a training course in a local diabetes clinic in your community or nearby hospital. The hands on training course is a diabetes clinic is usually organized by an endocrinologist (diabetes specialist), a nurses and a dietician, for a few days. They teach you:

a. How to inject insulin (both long-acting insulin and rapid-acting insulin) into the fatty tissue of your body,
b. How to find out the amount of carbohydrate in any meal,
c. How to count calories using measuring cups or by weighing foods with an electronic balance,
d. How to calculate the dosage of rapid-acting insulin for any meal, and
e. How to exercise to lower after-meal glucose levels to normal by running on a treadmill or by walking with rapid-acting insulin injected.

Once you have learned everything about diabetes control with insulin and exercise, you can go home and start controlling your diabetes with insulin shots. Your diabetes control would be more rewarding than ever (a lot better than the treatment with oral medications). You can achieve perfect diabetes control if you work hard.

FIVE IMPORTANT PRECAUTIONS
Every insulin-dependant diabetic should be aware of the following 5 precautions:

1. **HYPOGLYCEMIA (Low Blood Glucose Levels):** If you are going to try rapid-acting insulin shots with exercise (treadmill or other) in order to control your diabetes, in the beginning stages until you become accustomed to this treatment, you should monitor after every 15 minutes or as frequently as possible, and make sure your blood glucose level did not drastically drop to below normal 5 mmol/L or 90 mg/dL, and did not reach a condition called hypoglycemia (low blood glucose levels). If you inject too much insulin and run on a treadmill or walk, your blood glucose level may drop below normal, and you may be collapsed or knocked out due to hypoglycemia. Be aware and beware of this dangerous situation, and protect yourself by monitoring every 15 minutes or at least every 30 minutes. Always carry concentrated sugar solution or sugar jelly with you so that you swallow sugar and recover quickly from any such predicament. Chewing a candy sometimes helps raise blood glucose level.

2. **KETONES FORMATION:** If you exercise when your blood glucose level is above 14 mmol/L or 250 mg/dL, and if there is not enough insulin in your body because you are diabetic (either type 1 or type 2), your body becomes unable to use glucose as fuel and starts burning fat, releasing ketones into your body. Ketones (chemically known as ketone bodies) are byproducts of the breakdown of fatty acids. Glucose is the body's main source of energy. In order to transport glucose to trillions of body's cells, you need insulin. But when the body cannot use glucose for energy because of lack insulin, it burns fat instead, and uses as energy. When fats are broken down for energy, chemicals

called ketones appear in the blood and urine. When some obese people, who are seriously diabetic and whose blood glucose levels are too high after eating (above 14 mmol/L or 250 mg/dL), go on strenuous exercise, their bodies burn fat because of the lack of insulin in the body, and burning fat may lead to a serious condition called diabetic ketoacidosis (DKA), which requires immediate medical treatment.

The Symptoms of ketoacidosis (DKA) Are: nausea, feeling of illness, vomiting, abdominal pain, common cold or flu, tiredness all the time, thirsty or very dry mouth, flushed skin, difficulty breathing, confusion, and fruity breath. If you notice any of these symptoms when your blood glucose level is above 14 mmol/L or 250 mg/dL, and when exercising, you should immediately do a blood ketone test (you can also do urine ketone test, but it is not accurate), and find out if you have developed ketones formation in your body, and take action immediately. If ketones are present, you should stop exercising, and immediately inject a rapid-acting insulin such as Humalog to lower the blood glucose level to below 14 mmol/L or 250 mg/dL.

Some people do exercise with rapid-acting insulin injected when blood glucose level is above 14 mmol/L (or 250 mg/dL), and do not experience any formation of ketones or pertinent symptoms. Every person is different, and therefore you should research and be prepared to face such situation (how to avoid or handle the ketones formation).

● To avoid any such unsafe situation of ketones formation, you should inject rapid-acting insulin just before and during the high-carbohydrate meal consumption so that your after-meal glucose level will not be elevated above and beyond 14 mmol/L or 250 mg/dL. Then you can exercise without panicking about ketones formation.
● Or you should consume a well-planned healthy diet that will not raise your blood glucose level above 14 mmol/L or 250 mg/dL, and exercise thereafter without panicking about ketones formation.

3. **ARTIFICIAL INSULIN SENSITIVITY:** Artificial insulin sensitivity varies from person to person. Some people may need more units of insulin (both long-acting insulin and rapid-acting insulin), and some others may need less units insulin for the same amount of high-carbohydrate meal and for the same length of exercise to lower the after-meal glucose level to normal. Each person is different so he/she should research, and find out the appropriate insulin dose for a particular meal. By trial and error, and by monitoring every 15 minutes, you should be able to determine the right insulin dose for a particular high-carbohydrate meal, and stick to that insulin dose when repeating the same meal next day. As the experience builds up, you will be able to guess the insulin dose quickly for any given meal, and inject it to lower after-meal glucose level like an expert.

PLEASE NOTE: As the insulin manufacturing company Eli Lily suggested "1 unit of rapid-acting insulin Humalog is required for every 8 grams of carbohydrate being consumed", it may not be true for all people. One unit of Humalog per 8 grams of carbohydrate is a rough estimate to begin with. It could be a little more a little less depending on the body's ability to handle the artificial insulin. Some obese people may need more insulin to control after-meal glucose levels than the others. Every person has to research and find out, by trial and error, exactly how many units of rapid-acting insulin are to be injected for a particular meal. Rapid-acting insulin works on the top of long-acting insulin so you should not try using rapid acting insulin alone.

4. **ARTIFICIAL INSULIN RESISTANCE:** Artificial insulin resistance is very commonly encountered by the people with diabetes who inject rapid-acting insulin (Humalog) every day and exercise to lower after-meal glucose levels. Suddenly insulin stops working even if you double or triple the dosage (number of units of rapid-acting insulin) because the body developed insulin resistance. If that happens, the best natural remedy is to go on fasting for a couple of days to a week, and consume low-calorie and non-fat soups, organic apple cider vinegar with mother unfiltered and unpasteurized and lemon juice with cayenne pepper throughout the day, and you should lose weight at least a few pounds. After a few days to a week, you will notice yourself that the insulin resistance disappeared, and insulin starts working as usual.

5. **LIPOHYPERTROPHY (INSULIN SHOTS OVER TIME DEVELOP ABDOMINAL LUMPS):**
If you start using insulin shots, you better understand what "Lipohypertrophy" is. Lipohypertrophy is a medical term, meaning a lump under the skin, caused by the accumulation of extra fat at the site of many subcutaneous injections of insulin. It may be unsightly and mildly painful, and may interfere with insulin action. Insulin may not work as effectively as expected if you developed lipohypertrophy. It is a common complication caused due to carelessly managed injections on the abdominal. To avoid lipohypertrophy, never re-use the syringes (discard the syringe after every sigle use), and do not inject insulin repeatedly at the same site of your belly or any other body part. Keep rotating injection sites every day. Divide your abdominal into 4 quadrants. Inject on 1st quadrant during the first week, by leaving a half an inch between every two injection sites, and proceed to next quadrant during the next week, and so on. Many insulin-dependant diabetic people suffer from abdominal lumps because they were not properly trained when they started injecting insulin shots. So if you are new to insulin shots, you better be aware of this problem called "lipohypertrophy" beforehand.

If you have already developed lipohypertrophy, the following are the treatment methods:

(i) Massage the lumps with your hand regularly by applying baby oil (you will see improvement day by day). The lumps may not disappear completely, but you will see some improvement.
(ii) Seek laser treatment with a specialist (most likely a plastic surgeon could do it) if lumps are bothering you. If the lumps are not bothering, you can live with them.
(iii) Liposuction is also heard to be a quick and ideal treatment to remove a large abdominal lumps,
(iv) Ultrasound body fat reduction treatment is also being used by some doctors.
(v) Electricity therapy is also available to treat lipohypertrophy.

Longer Needles, Or Shorter Needles? [5]
In the past, diabetics have been using 12.7 mm needles to inject insulin. Most recently, research proved that a needle depth of 5 mm works fine for all people, including children. With shorter needles (4 to 5 mm), inject at a 90-degree angle with no pinching of the skin. If longer needles are used, pinch up the skin to avoid injecting into intramuscular tissue. Also, hold the needle in the skin for 5 to 10 seconds after you give the insulin (even longer with higher doses) so the medication doesn't leak from the site. For very lean people, pinching the skin and injecting at an angle are recommended even with shorter needles.

HOW TO ACHIEVE NORMAL A1c WITH INSULIN SHOTS & EXERCISE?
FIVE EXAMPLES DISCUSSED WITH DAILY DABETES CONTROL ROUTINE

EXAMPLE: 3 How to Control Type 2 Diabetes With Insulin & Exercise
This Is The Most Important Example If You Want To Enjoy
High-Carbohydrate Meals and Still Live With Normal A1c

INTRODUCTION: Adam was diagnosed with type 2 diabetes when he was 46 years old. Adam tried Method 1 (Dietary Guidelines Without Oral Medication) for a year. It did not work. Then he started using Method 2 (Dietary Guidelines Along With Oral Medication) for two more years. It did not work for him because he could not maintain high self-discipline and high will power, and has been cheating on his diet, and eating in restaurants every now and then. His hemoglobin A1c has been very high, and was unable to lower it significantly. He changed doctors and visited several endocrinologists, and also tried several kinds of oral medications in all possible dosages. Those oral medications did not work. He wasted altogether 4 to 5 years, trying oral medications, without any success. He could not lower his hemoglobin A1c to close to 7%. His hemoglobin A1c has always been above and beyond 9.5% all the time no matter how hard he tried.

Adam started experiencing shortness of breath and angina pain whenever he takes a walk on the street. His blood test showed that his cholesterols (both total cholesterol and LDL cholesterol) were elevated. He was hospitalized for a week and was placed in an intensive care unit. The angiogram test showed the plaque formation in his arteries (what is known as atherosclerosis). His doctor prescribed him a statin drug to lower cholesterols, but that high dosage of statin has been causing him severe muscle pain. When he was in the hospital, some of the nurses recommended him to switch to insulin shots to control his diabetes quickly and effectively. They also recommended him that he could take a diabetes course in his community's diabetes clinic where he lives.

LIFE-CHANGING EVENT TOOK PLACE
When he was 51 years old, Adam attended an insulin-dependant diabetes course in a diabetes clinic, located in his own community. Diabetes clinics are there in every community or hospital to offer hands on training courses on how to inject insulin shots and how to exercise to control diabetes. This diabetes course has changed Adam's life forever. In this diabetes course, an endocrinologist, several nurses and dieticians taught him the following aspects:
- How to inject insulin (both long-acting insulin and rapid-acting insulin) using a syringe and/or a pen,
- How to read labels on any food item to recognize and identify the amount of fat, protein & carbohydrate,
- How to count calories using measuring cups and electronic balance, and by making simple calculations,
- How to determine the amount of carbohydrate present in any meal,
- How to calculate the amount of rapid-acting insulin to be injected for any given meal (1 unit of Humalog insulin is required for 8 grams of carbohydrate),
- How to exercise (either running on a treadmill, biking, or regular walk) in order to lower the after-meal glucose level quickly to normal.

Adam took this course with a great interest, and fully focussed and committed on controlling his type 2 diabetes as quickly as possible. He also read books on diabetes and updated his knowledge in every possible way. He started Method 3 with insulin shots along with exercise, and he successfully controlled his diabetes, and achieved normal hemoglobin A1c level (below 7%) in 6 months.

Believe it or not, it is very easy to control diabetes with insulin shots along with exercise. With Method 3, you can go easy on dietary guidelines and can consume and enjoy high-carbohydrate meals whenever you feel like, and you can still control your diabetes successfully if you can equip your mind with proper knowledge.

The detailed schedule of Adam's diabetes control plan in a typical day, during the past 6 months, is shown below:

7:00 am   Adam wakes up and monitors his fasting blood glucose level early in the morning.
7:05 am   Blood glucose level: 4.8 mmol/L or 86.4 mg/dL.
            He takes coffee with 1% milk, and checks his emails, and listens to music on YouTube video.

7:30 am   He prepares his breakfast, and injects mixed dose of insulin when he is ready to eat.
            (25 units of long-acting insulin Humulin-N, and 8 units of rapid-acting insulin Humalog)

Breakfast (Daily Routine)
7:45 am   BREAKFAST
Adam eats an egg-white omelet (egg-white is one 100% protein) every day in the breakfast. Egg-white omelet is made with veggies (broccoli or cauliflower or spinach, mushrooms, onions, bell peppers with a few drops of extra virgin olive oil), whole wheat bread toasted (no butter added), mustard sauce, a small cup of low-fat yogurt, a small cup of fresh blueberries, and purified water. After the breakfast he goes outside and walks for 10 to 15 minutes and self-monitors his blood glucose level.

8:10 am   Blood glucose level usually at this time of the day : 5.5 mmol/L or 99 mg/dL.

Lunch (Eats Mostly At Home, and Eats Once or Twice a Week in a Restaurant)
11:30 am Adam went to a restaurant to eat lunch today.
Adam eats high-carbohydrate lunch once or twice a week in a restaurant to his fullest satisfaction.

11:45 am Adam injected 20 units of rapid-acting insulin Humalog from his pen,
            and started eating lunch in the restaurant.
LUNCH: Thai cashews chicken cooked with bell peppers, onions, peas & soy sauce, a bowl of white rice, one spring roll, and a glass of wine. After the lunch, he went into a 7-Eleven store, purchased Drumstick ice cream, and ate it.

12:30 pm Adam went to a gym to exercise. He monitored his glucose level again.
            It was 13.8 mmol/L or 248.4 mg/dL.
            Adam ran on a treadmill for 30 minutes, and monitored again.
1:05 pm   Blood glucose level dropped to: 8.5 mmol.L or 153 mg/dL.
1:10 pm   Adam injected 4 more units of rapid-acting insulin Humalog,
            and ran on treadmill for another 30 min, and monitored.
1:45 pm   Blood glucose level further dropped to: 5.2 mmol.L or 93.6 mg/dL. Adam went home.

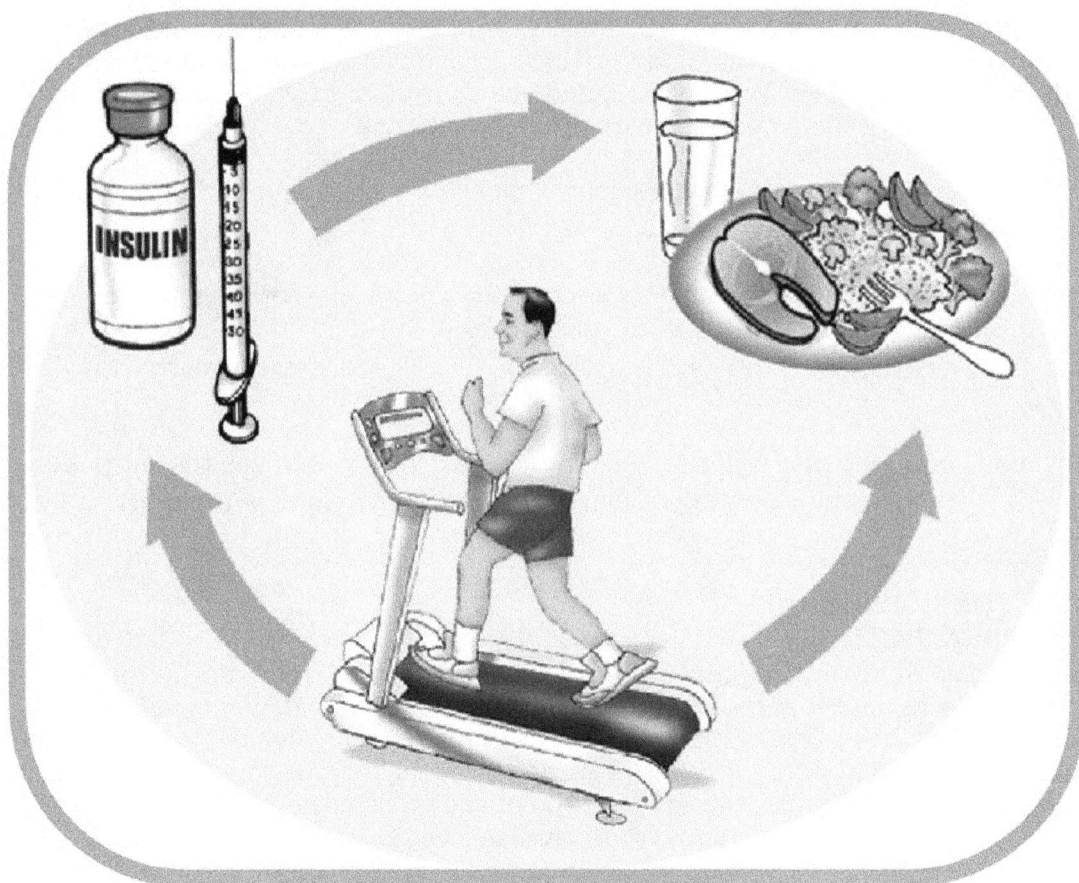

Figure 3.4 A type 2 diabetic is lowering his after-meal blood glucose level with the aid of healthy diet, rapid-acting insulin and exercise (running on a treadmill).

IMPORTANT POINTS TO REMEMBER

(i) It is important to note here that Adam managed to lower his after-meal spike to perfectly normal within 2 hours after eating a high-carbohydrate meal. Had he not done this, he could have been living with highly elevated blood glucose levels (levels above 20 mmol/L or 360 mg/dL) throughout the afternoon, contributing to elevated average blood glucose level, and in turn elevated hemoglobin A1c. Living like that for months and years could lead to all kinds of long term side effects of chronic and fatal disease called diabetes mellitus.

(ii) Adam injected 20 units of rapid-acting insulin Humalog just before the meal so that his after-meal glucose level would be under 14 mmol/L or 250 mg/dL because he learned that ketones formation occurs if he exercises with blood glucose level over 14 mmol/L or 250 mg/dL. It is important to inject the sufficient amount of rapid-acting insulin Humalog before eating so that your after-meal glucose level would be below 14 mmol/L or 250 mg/dL, and you can exercise without panicking about ketones formation. Ketones formation does not occur to everybody so you should find out if your body is sensitive to Ketones formation and its symptoms. If your body doesn't form ketones, you don't need to worry about this aspect, and can exercise immediately after a major meal consumption even if your after-meal glucose level is more than 14 mmol/L or 250 mg/dL.

2:30 pm   Adam monitored again. Blood glucose level rose to: 9.1 mmol/L or 163.8 mg/dL. Remember! Adam ate white rice in his lunch. White rice digests and raises blood glucose level for a long time.Therefore he injected another 10 units of rapid-acting insulin Humalog again after he came home, and this treatment kept his blood glucose level normal till 6 pm.

Had he eaten brown rice with his lunch, instead of white rice, his diabetes control could have been a lot easier. However, sometimes, you can enjoy white rice if you know how to control your diabetes by injecting more insulin. You can even eat a large bowl of desert as long as you know how to lower your after-meal glucose level to normal.

6:00 pm   Adam monitored just before dinner. Blood glucose level: 6.5 mmol/L or 117 mg/dL.

Dinner (Daily Routine)
6:05 pm   Adam prepares his dinner, and injects mixed dose of insulin when he is ready to eat dinner. He injected 25 units of Humulin-N and 5 units of rapid-acting insulin Humalog.
6:05 pm   Adam eats a low-carbohydrate meal in his dinner that would not raise his blood glucose level too high.
DINNER: Oven-baked fish, steamed vegetables, one slice of bread and one organic apple or organic banana. After eating, he goes out and walks for 10 to 15 minutes to lower his after-meal glucose level.
9:30 pm   Adam monitors just before going to bed.
        Blood glucose level typically: 6.9 mmol.L or 124.2 mg/dL.

In-Between Meal Snacks (Daily Routine)
Adam eats 3 times a day a few items of the following in-between meal snacks:
- Organic green cabbage cooked with onions, carrots, sweet potatoes, yams, fresh garlic & fresh ginger,
- Cottage cheese dry curd (It contains high protein, zero fat, very low carbohydrate, low sodium),
- Low-fat and low-sugar yogurt,
- Boiled chickpeas & boiled kidney beans,
- Kamut Puffs (crunchy and tasty),
- Fruits (organic banana or apple, avocados, pomelo, grape fruit, oranges, grapes, pears, papaya, lemons & limes, etc.),
- Nuts in limited quantities (cashews, blanched almonds, walnuts, peanuts, etc.).

Adam minimizes and consumes only a little sea salt and extra virgin oil in all his meals. Minimization of the salt consumption and oil consumption helps lose weight, and keeps the blood pressure under control.
Whenever he eats a snack, he injects a few units of Humalog insulin so that his blood glucose level remains normal. From his extensive experience on monitoring and controlling, he easily guesses the number of units of Humalog to be injected.

Adam's self-blood glucose monitoring data in a typical day are shown below:
Table 3.12

Time	7:00 AM	8:10 AM	12:30 PM	1:05 PM	1:45 PM	2:30 PM	6:00 PM	9:30 PM	Average	A1c
Glucose (mmol/L)	4.8	5.5	13.8	8.5	5.2	9.1	6.5	6.9	7.5	6.6%
Glucose (mg/dL)	86.4	99	248.4	153	93.6	163.8	117	124.2	135.7	6.6%

Adam calculated his daily average blood glucose level as 7.5 mmol/L or 135.7 mg/dL.
He also determined the hemoglobin A1c (from A1c Chart) as 6.6%.

Adam lost weight by following the dietary guidelines. His arteries are cleared and unclogged. He doesn't suffer from shortness of breath or angina pain anymore.

He does not need high doses of statin drug anymore so he doesn't suffer from muscle pain. He takes very low dosage of statin Zocor (5 mg or 10 g), and takes cholesterol-lowering supplement guggul.

His cholesterols are now perfectly normal. Adam is happier than ever.
Adam brought his health back to normal with diligence, knowledge and determination.
Adam has become a self-taught doctor of diabetes control.

EXAMPLE 4: A TYPE 2 DIABETIC HAS BEEN CONTROLLING HIS DIABETES LIKE AN EXPERT

Sam is a 51-year-old Type 2 diabetic. After every major high-carbohydrate meal consumption, his blood glucose level rises above 18 mmol/L o 324 mg/dL. His hemoglobin A1c is over 9.8%. During the past 2 years, he has been experiencing heart disease, angina and kidney disease.
He has been injecting too much insulin (25 units of Humalog) to lower his high blood sugar levels without incorporating exercise along with insulin shots. He has read a lot about diabetes and insulin. He learned that too much insulin stimulates the brain so that a person feels hungry and eats more and also causes the liver to add fat in the belly. He decided to optimize the insulin dose for the evening meal by implementing 1 hour of exercise. His diabetes control strategy is described below with his physical activity in the evening after dinner:

5:30 pm   Prepared a major meal of 900 kilocalories (150 gm of carbohydrate).Skinless chicken cooked with veggies and fat free soy milk, brown rice, sea salt & cayenne pepper.
6:00 pm   Monitored fasting glucose (see table below); consumed major meal.
6:30 pm   Monitored blood glucose level (see table below).
               He learned that he should not exercise if his level is over 13 mmol/L or 234 mg/dL.
               (Ketones formation could occur in the body if he exercises at high glucose levels)
               Injected 6 units of Humalog to bring his level down to 13 mmol/L.
7:00 pm   Blood glucose level dropped to 12.9 mmol/L or 232 mg/dL.
7:00 pm   Injected 4 more units of Humalog, and started walking.
               Walked precisely 7 ½ minutes, carefully looking at his wristwatch.
               Came home by walking another 7 ½ minutes (total 15 minutes).
               Monitored his glucose and spent 5 minutes for record keeping.
               Repeated the same 3 more times to complete 1 hour of exercise.

Speed: 4.0 mph; Calories burned: 300 Kcal

Table 3.13   ◄-------------- Walked --------------►

Time	6:00 PM	6:30 PM	7:00 PM	7:15 PM	7:35 PM	7:55 PM	8:15 PM
Glucose (mmol/L)	6	19.4	12.5	8.5	7.6	6.1	4.7
Glucose (mg/dL)	108	349	225	153	136.8	109.8	84.6

For 150 gm of carbohydrate in a meal, it would require 19 units of Humalog (1 unit for every 8 gm). But Ervin lowered his level to normal with 11 units only, cutting Humalog dose by 47%. He has controlled his after-meal glucose levels and minimized his Humalog insulin dose every day diligently for 6 months. His hemoglobin A1c has dropped from 9.8% to 6.7% in 6 months. Sam is now a happy man. He no longer suffers from angina pain from clogged arteries, and his kidney disease disappeared. He now monitors only a few times a day, and still his diabetes is tightly controlled (his hemoglobin A1c level is less than 7%). His own experience on injecting rapid-acting insulin with every meal on a daily basis has helped him master the concept of controlling diabetes. Sam has become a self-taught master of diabetes control.

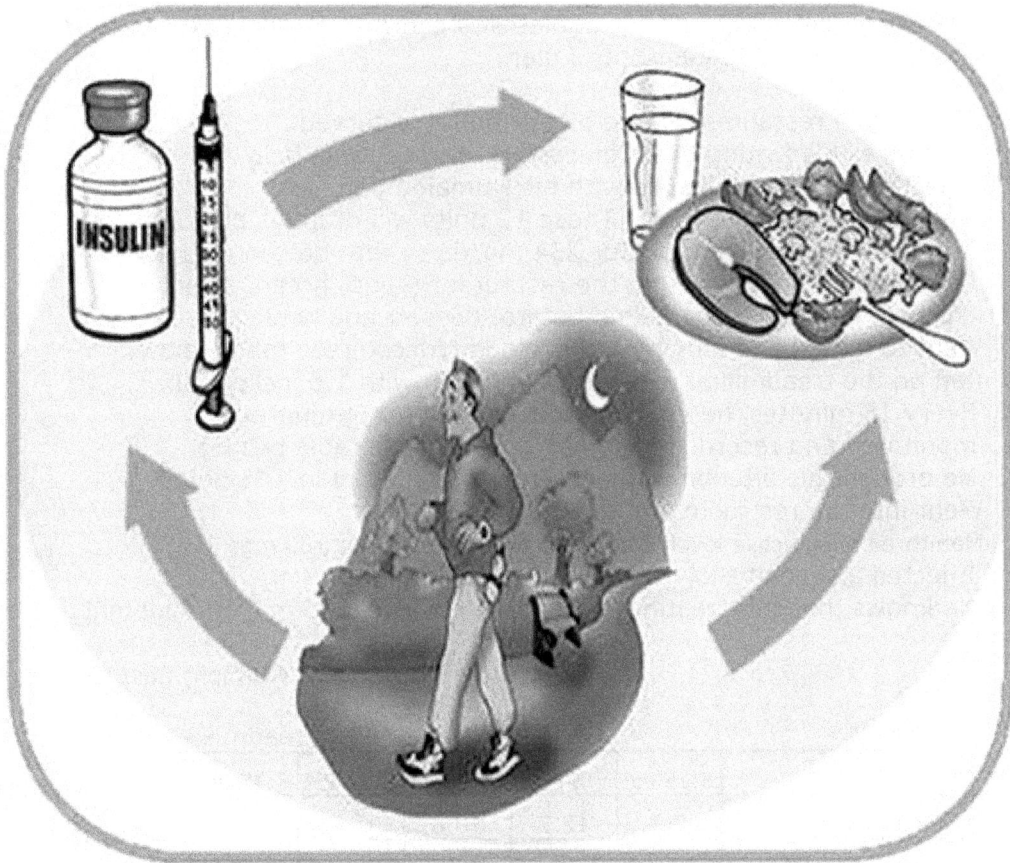

Figure 3.5 A type 2 diabetic is lowering his after-meal blood glucose level with the aid of healthy diet, rapid-acting insulin and exercise (walking on the road).

EXAMPLE 5: A TYPE 2 DIABETIC ATHLETE HAS BEEN CONTROLLING HIS DIABETES LIKE AN EXPERT

Ken is a 37-year-old Type 2 diabetic. He is an all-around athlete who exemplifies high achievement in sports, specializing in soccer. He eats in restaurants very often. His blood glucose level reaches over 20 mmol/L or 360 mg/dL after every heavy meal. He does not calculate the insulin dose but guesses how much insulin dose he should inject before and after exercise, with 1 hour of exercise, to keep his glucose level within the normal range. He plays soccer and other games every week¾no problem.

He diligently researched his elevated after-meal blood glucose levels against rapid-acting Humalog doses and exercise through consuming a variety of heavy meals. After a few months, he became a self-taught doctor of diabetes control. Here is a typical example of his one-day activity during his diabetes control plan:

5:15 pm   Went into a restaurant where dinner buffet is served.
             Monitored his fasting blood glucose level (see table below).
             Injected 12 units of insulin with his Humalog pen.
             He has already researched. These 12 units will drop his blood glucose
             level just below 13 mmol/L or 234 mg/dL so that he can exercise.
             Consumed a heavy meal in the restaurant (soup, bread, salad,
             chicken, rice, legumes, baked potato, dessert and beer).
5:50 pm   Went to a gym and monitored his blood glucose (see table below).
6:00 pm   Ran on the treadmill at a speed of 4.0 mph with 1.0 inclination.
             Every 15 minutes, he interrupted treadmill for 5 minutes,
             monitored and recorded his blood glucose (see table below).
             He brought his after-meal glucose level to normal in 1 ½ hours.
7:05 pm   Went into the restroom and took a shower.
7:25 pm   Monitored his glucose level; Increased to 10 mmol/L or 180 mg/dL.
             Injected a second shot, some 5 units of Humalog.
             He knows that this treatment will keep his levels normal till midnight.

Speed: 4.0 mph; Calories burned: 355

Kcal

Table 3.14	◀---------------- Treadmill ----------▶					
Time	5:15 PM	5:50 PM	6:15 PM	6:25 PM	6:45 PM	7:05 PM
Glucose (mmol/L)	5.3	12.7	10.8	7.5	6.8	5
Glucose (mg/dL)	95.4	228.6	194.4	135	122.4	104.4

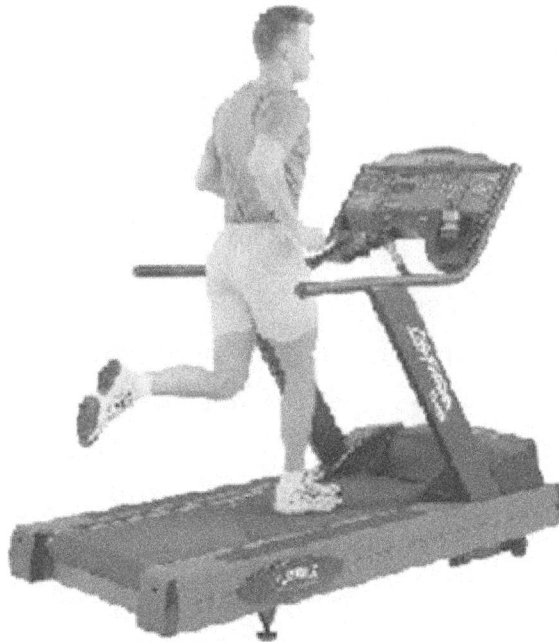

Courtesy of Life Fitness
Figure 3.6 A type 2 diabetic athlete is lowering his after-meal blood glucose level with the aid of healthy diet, rapid-acting insulin and exercise (running on a treadmill).

EXAMPLE 6: A TYPE 2 DIABETIC ATHLETE HAS BEEN CONTROLLING HIS DIABETES LIKE AN EXPERT

Anderson, a 52-year-old athletic person, used to be a very active football player and wrestler. Three years ago, he was diagnosed with Type-2 diabetes. Anderson chose to take insulin shots to control his diabetes effectively. Anderson was on his way home driving from Seattle, WA, United States to Vancouver, BC, Canada. It was 5:30 pm. It would take another hour to get home. He was hungry and decided to eat. He drove into a highway restaurant in Bellingham and ate a lot of food from the buffet (salad bar, pasta, chicken, sushi, tempura, fruit salad, dessert and beer). He injected 10 units of Humalog with his insulin pen just before the meal. He finished his meal by 6 pm. He got home at 7 pm, and monitored his blood glucose level. It was very high: 15.5 mmol/L or 279 mg/dL. He wanted to go to the gym and do treadmill. But he had already read the book Permanent Diabetes Control in which he learned that he should not do exercise if his blood glucose level is above 14 mmol/L or 250 mg/dL because ketones would form and accumulate in his body. He therefore injected another shot of Humalog, about 4 units, and drove to the gym in half an hour (7:30 pm), where he monitored his level again as 12.5 mmol/L or 225 mg/dL. He then exercised (ran on treadmill at high speed) for 1 hour, and found his glucose level dropped to 4.9 mmol/L or 88.2 mg/dL by 8:30 pm. He got home by 9 pm and monitored his level again. The level had risen to 8.1 mmol/L or 151.2 mg/dL. He injected another shot, 4 more units of Humalog, and watched TV. By 9:30 am his level had dropped to 5.3 mmol/L or 95 mg/dL and remained normal till 11:45 pm. He then injected 15 units of intermediate-acting insulin Humalog-N, ate fresh carrots and a few dried apricots (bedtime snack), and went to sleep. By 7 am the next morning, his level was 5.5 mmol/L or 98 mg/dL.

Anderson made clear notes on items he consumed in the restaurant and all insulin shots injected so that next time he can consume the same meal and manage his insulin shots comfortably. He eats in the restaurant to his fullest satisfaction twice a week, and his diabetes is still tightly controlled.

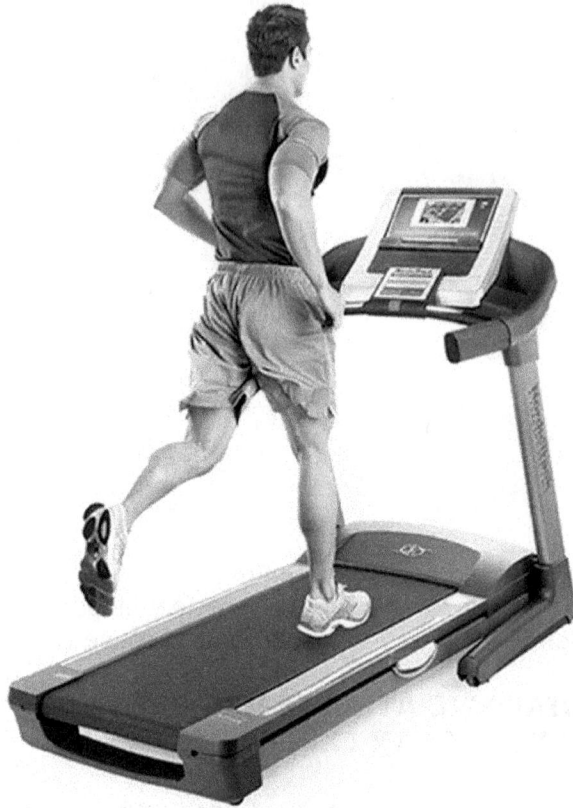

Courtesy of Life Fitness
Figure 3.7 A type 2 diabetic athlete is lowering his after-meal blood glucose level with the aid of healthy diet, rapid-acting insulin and exercise (running on a treadmill).

Example 7: A LADY WITH TYPE 2 DIABETES HAS BEEN CONTROLLING HER DIABETES LIKE AN EXPERT

Elza is a 64-year-old female. She has been Type 2 diabetic for 15 years and switched to insulin shots 2 to 3 years ago. She lives in New Westminster, BC, Canada, where she knew a restaurant called "Old Spaghetti Factory." She is cautious with her health and has been practicing diabetes control for the past 2 to 3 years. She ordered a Spaghetti meal in the restaurant brought it home at 5:15 pm. She separated all the meal items: baked chicken, spaghetti, soup, garlic bread, lettuce, tomatoes, and measured the weight of each item. From the calorie-counter tables, she noted the breakdown of fat, protein and carbohydrate for spaghetti, soup, garlic bread, lettuce and tomatoes (chicken has no carbohydrate). From the weight of each item, she calculated the carbohydrate content of each item, and added them up to obtain total carbohydrate content of her meal as approximately 150 g. She knew that 1 unit of Humalog is needed for 8 g of carbohydrate. So for 150 g of carbohydrate, she needed 19 units of Humalog. Because she planned to exercise, her insulin dose required was 9.5 units (half of 19 units). She injected 10 units of Humalog just before she ate at 5:30 pm. Her level rose to 12.6 mmol/L or 226.8 mg/dL 30 minutes after the meal. She walked for 1 hour in her neighborhood. She monitored her levels every half an hour. After 1 hour of walking, her blood glucose level dropped to 5.5 mmol/L or 102.6 mg/dL. She then injected a second shot, about 5.8 units of Humalog. Her levels remained normal until midnight. She then took 15 units of Humulin-N, ate one Savory Garlic Matzo (fat free and cholesterol free) and baby carrots as her bedtime snack, and went to sleep. By next morning, her level was 4.6 mmol/L or 82.8 mg/dL (perfectly normal).

Next time when she goes to the same restaurant (Old Spaghetti Factory), she can sit and eat in the restaurant without panicking, inject 19 units of Humalog, and eat the Spaghetti meal and still keep her after-meal blood glucose level normal. Or if she is planning to walk after the meal, she could cut the Humalog dose in half, inject it and eat the meal, and walk afterwards. She can order the same meal and inject 5.8 units of Humalog twice (before meal and after exercise). Elza mastered the concept of diabetes control with insulin and exercise. Her hemoglobin A1c has been normal (under 7%) for the past 2 to 3 years. Her diabetes has been permanently controlled, as she mastered the topic. She doesn't need any doctors to take care of her health, except for blood test requisitions and prescriptions. Elza has become an expert of diabetes control.

HOW TO CONTROL TYPE 1 DIABETES WITH INSULIN SHOTS & EXERCISE

The diabetes control for type 1 diabetes or type 2 diabetes remains exactly the same. A type 1 diabetic person needs more insulin dosages than a type 2 diabetic person. For type 2 diabetic or type 1 diabetic, insulin dosages vary from person to person and from meal to meal. Each person is different. Each person (either type 1 or type 2 diabetic) should use his/her own insulin dosages. But in terms of controlling diabetes, the method remains the same.

Refer to preceding examples. And suppose that the person in those examples is type 1 diabetic, and controlling his/her type 1 diabetes. Lifestyle changes (dietary guidelines), insulin shots, exercise program, and managing type 1 diabetes remain the same.

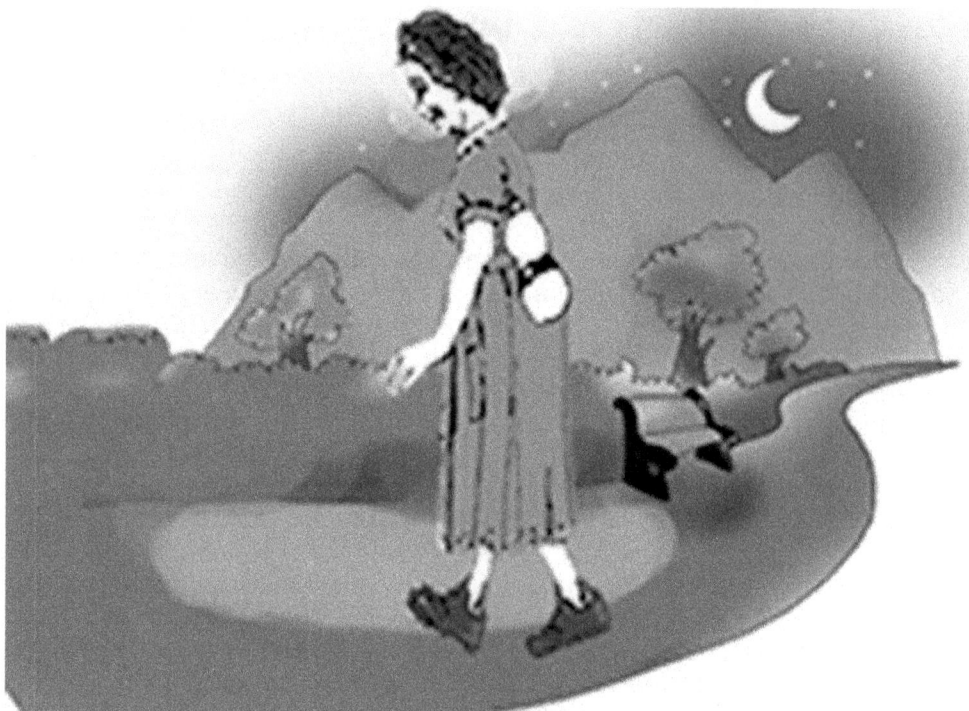

Figure 3.8 A type 2 diabetic is lowering her after-meal blood glucose level with the aid of healthy diet, rapid-acting insulin and exercise (walking on the road).

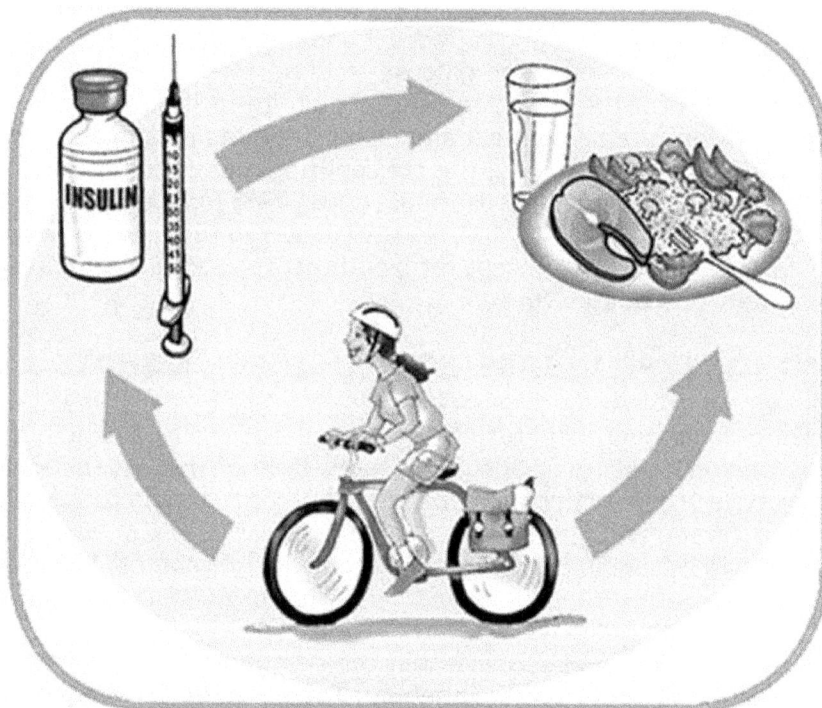

Figure 3.9 A type 1 diabetic is lowering her after-meal blood glucose level with the aid of healthy diet, rapid-acting insulin and exercise (cycling on the road).

ADVANTAGES OF METHOD 3 (WITH INSULIN SHOTS)

There is no such disadvantage in terms of controlling diabetes using Method 3.

⊃ You don't really need to worry about high self-discipline and high willpower. You can go easy on dietary changes as long as you know how to take insulin shots before or after every meal consumption (breakfast, lunch, dinner and all snacks). However, a healthy lifestyle is extremely important for a diabetic person. Eating out a high-carbohydrate meal in a restaurant once or twice a week is okay as long you master the concept of controlling the after-meal spike immediately after the consumption.

⊃ You can enjoy a large high-carbohydrate meal by eating in a buffet-serving restaurant, including a large bowl of desert, and can lower your after-meal glucose spike to normal, within 1 or 2 hours, if you know how to do it correctly by injecting the right amount of insulin, accompanied by an after-meal exercise.

⊃ A highly knowledgeable diabetic person can very easily lower his/her steep blood glucose spike to perfectly normal in 30 to 60 minutes by injecting the right amount of insulin and by running on a treadmill. Even a simple walking exercise on the road with insulin injected would lower the steep glucose spike.

⊃ It is the best method to achieve perfect diabetes control when your body produces a little or no insulin.

⊃ You can see immediate results, and achieve perfect control for the rest of your life if you master the subject matter.

⊃ Perfect diabetes control is not possible with pills (oral medications). When you are on pills and consume a large amount of high-carbohydrate meal and are faced by a steep glucose spike, there is nothing you can do about it, but wait until the next morning to see normal fasting glucose level. Whereas with rapid-acting insulin & exercise, you can immediately lower your after-meal blood glucose spike, and can keep your A1c level normal.

DISADVANTAGES OF METHOD 3 (WITH INSULIN SHOTS)

⊃ Some people are scared and don't feel comfortable to deal with needles every day because they are not accustomed to needles. They don't realize the fact that they can very easily learn how to inject insulin shots in order to lower the after-meal spike by taking a hands-on course in any diabetic clinic in their community.

⊃ Other than that, rapid-acting insulin (such as Humalog) along with exercise is the best treatment to control diabetes, it doesn't matter whether you are either type 2 diabetic or types 1 diabetic. Try it out!

WHY SHOULD THE INSULIN DOSE BE OPTIMIZED?

Evening meal or any major meal causes the highest blood glucose levels in people with diabetes. Elevated blood glucose levels are accumulated in the bloodstream soon after the major meal consumption, dominate in and largely contribute to establishing the average blood glucose level in 90 days.

Hemoglobin A1c is a parameter that directly reveals the degree of "diabetes control" during the preceding 90 days. Red blood cells live in the bloodstream 60 to 90 days. Every 90 days, new red blood cells are born. Hemoglobin is a protein molecule that carries and supplies oxygen from the lungs to the trillions of body's cells wherever it is needed. While the blood circulates, depending on how high or how low the blood glucose level is, a certain amount of glucose is attached to the hemoglobin molecules to form glycated hemoglobin. Different people call it with different names: glycated A1c, hemoglobin A1c (HbA1c), or simply A1c. Therefore, by measuring the hemoglobin A1c level in a laboratory from the patient's blood sample, it is possible to know the average blood glucose level and the degree to which it has been controlled over the preceding 90 days. The hemoglobin A1c chart was developed to show the influence of average blood glucose level in 90 days versus hemoglobin A1c.

From this A1c chart, one can firmly confirm that elevated average blood glucose level indicates the elevated hemoglobin A1c. Elevated hemoglobin A1c means the diabetes has been poorly controlled. Therefore elevated after-meal glucose levels must be slashed as quickly as possible and brought to normal within 1 or 2 hour of the major meal consumption in order to bring hemoglobin A1c close to its normal value. Normal hemoglobin A1c means the diabetes has been tightly controlled.

WHY SHOULD THE INSULIN DOSE BE OPTIMIZED (Continued)?

The artificial insulin dose must be optimized (and minimized), because too much insulin causes hypoglycemia and constricts arteries leading to heart attack and coronary heart disease. Too much insulin also stimulates the brain so that a person feels hungry and eats more and causes the liver to manufacture fat in the belly. Too little insulin on the other hand is not enough to cover the entire meal and to maintain normal glucose levels. An optimum insulin dose is therefore crucial. Insulin is synthesized in such a way that it starts flowing and working a lot more quickly and much more effectively with exercise.
A continuous exercise (30 to 60 minutes), either treadmill, biking or regular walk, should be introduced into the diabetes control plan in order to lower after-meal glucose level, burn fat, lose calories, and optimize both insulin dose and insulin action. If the exercise is introduced immediately after every heavy meal, it not only minimizes the insulin dose but in addition maximizes insulin action and prevents after-meal glucose levels from rising too high, thereby keeping the diabetes under tight control. The following procedures are being recommended by Dr. RK to optimize the insulin dose.

HOW TO OPTIMIZE THE INSULIN DOSE BY TRIAL AND ERROR PROCEDURE?

A diabetic person, before using the method described here, should have undergone an insulin-dependant diabetes course in a local diabetes clinic in his/her area. In this hands on course, they teach the following aspects:

- How to inject insulin (both long-acting insulin and rapid-acting insulin) using a syringe and/or a pen,
- How to read labels on any food item to recognize and identify the amount of fat, protein & carbohydrate,

- How to count calories using measuring cups and electronic balance, and by making simple calculations,
- How to determine the amount of carbohydrate present in any meal,
- How to calculate the amount of rapid-acting insulin to be injected for any given meal (1 unit of Humalog insulin is required for 8 grams of carbohydrate),
- How to exercise (either running on a treadmill, biking, or regular walk) in order to lower the after-meal glucose level quickly to normal.

A diabetic person should have a clear knowledge on the amount of carbohydrate content of a food item and/or a meal being consumed, and should be able to guess the insulin dose. With experience, over time, this guessing of insulin dose becomes an easy and enjoyable task.

TRIAL AND ERROR PROCEDURE: SIMPLIFIED APPROACH DIABETES COBTROL

a. Small Meal

Example: It could be a brown toast with 2 hash brown patties and a small cup of apple juice, and a coffee with 1% milk.

- Inject 5 units of rapid-acting insulin Humalog just before eating.
- Consume the meal, and start exercising (Just go out and walk) for 15 to 20 minutes. Or, if you have a bike at home, ride the bike.
- Monitor blood glucose level. It should be close to normal.
  Normal: 5 mmol/L or 90 mg/dL
- If the glucose level reached normal, you have done your job.
- If the glucose level did not reach normal, then inject a few more units of rapid-acting insulin Humalog so that the level would reach normal.
- Your goal is to lower your after-meal glucose level to normal as quickly as possible within 30 minutes, by guessing the insulin dose by trial and error.
- This experience will help you inject insulin more precisely from next day.

b. Mid-Sized Meal

Example: It could be a whole wheat bagel served with cream cheese, a soup and baked potatoes, and a herbal tea.
- Inject 10 units of rapid-acting insulin Humalog just before eating.
- Consume the meal, and start exercising (Just go out and walk) for 30 minutes. Or, if you have a bike at home, ride the bike.
- Monitor blood glucose level. It should be close to normal.
  Normal: 5 mmol/L or 90 mg/dL
- If the glucose level reached normal, you have done your job.
- If the glucose level did not reach normal, then inject 5 more units of rapid-acting insulin Humalog so that the level would reach normal.
- Monitor after 30 minutes. If the glucose level did not reach normal, then inject a few more units of rapid-acting insulin Humalog so that the level would reach normal.
- Your goal is to lower your after-meal glucose level to normal as quickly as possible within an hour, by guessing the insulin dose by trial and error.
- This experience will help you inject insulin more precisely from next day.

c. Large Meal (Low Carbohydrate)

It could be a large, carefully prepared low-carbohydrate meal consumed at home by following dietary guidelines.

Example: Baked skinless chicken, brown rice, steamed legumes and veggies, and a fruit.

LOW INSULIN DOSE & EXERCISE REQUIRED

- Guess insulin dose, inject first shot, eat, exercise 60 min & monitor.
- Your blood glucose level should have been dropped to normal by now!
- Inject second shot to prevent it from rising
  (some people don't need second shot).
- The amount of insulin varies from person to person & from meal to meal.
- Each person needs to determine his/her own insulin dose for a meal.

- Inject 10 units of rapid-acting insulin Humalog just before eating.
- Consume the meal, and start exercising (Treadmill, Biking or Walking)
  for 60 minutes. Or, if you have a bike at home, ride the bike for 60 minutes.
- Monitor blood glucose level, and check if it reached normal.
  - If the blood glucose level is not normal, inject more insulin & monitor.
- This approach would keep your glucose level normal up to 6 hours.
- This experience will help you inject insulin more precisely from next day.

d. Large Meal (High Carbohydrate)

Example: It could be a large high-carbohydrate meal consumed in a restaurant to the fullest satisfaction. Or it could be a large unlimited meal consumed in a buffet-serving restaurant. Refer to Example 2 in which Adam ate lunch (a large meal) in a Thai restaurant, and exercised to lower his after-meal glucose level to normal.

HIGH INSULIN DOSE & EXERCISE REQUIRED

- Guess insulin dose, inject first shot, eat, exercise 30 min & monitor.
- Guess insulin dose, inject second shot, exercise 30 min & monitor.
- Guess insulin dose, inject third shot, no exercise & monitor.
- Your blood glucose level should have been dropped to normal by now!
- This procedure varies from person to person & from meal to meal.
- Each person needs to determine his/her own insulin dose for a meal.

- Inject 10 units of rapid-acting insulin Humalog just before eating.
- Consume the meal, and start exercising (Treadmill, Biking or Walking)
  for 30 minutes. Or, if you have a bike at home, ride the bike for 30 minutes.
- Monitor blood glucose level, and check if it reached normal.
                Normal: 5 mmol/L or 90 mg/dL
- If the glucose level did not reach normal, then inject 5 more units of
  Humalog, and continue exercise for another 30 minutes.
- Monitor blood glucose level. It should be close to normal.
- After 30 minutes, monitor again. You will find the glucose level risen.
- Then inject more insulin (5 to 10 units depending on the glucose level).
- After 30 minutes, monitor again. You will find the glucose level normal.
- This approach would keep your glucose level normal up to 6 hours.
- This experience will help you inject insulin more precisely from next day.

Refer to Example 3 in which Adam consumed a large high-carbohydrate lunch in a restaurant including a cup of white rice and ice cream to his fullest satisfaction, and injected rapid-acting insulin Humalog 2 to 3 times, and brought his after-meal glucose level to normal in 2 hours, just by guessing the insulin dose by trial and error.

Adam injected Humalog 3 times for the large meal he consumed:
20 units + 4 unit + 10 units = 34 units

If Adam did not exercise, he could have needed to inject more than twice that amount (more than 68 units) of rapid-acting insulin to lower his after-meal glucose level to normal. And that excess amount of insulin could have stimulated the Adam's brain to feel hungry, eat more, and could have caused his liver to manufacture fat in the belly, leading to a disastrous performance. Therefore it is obvious that the rapid-acting insulin dose must be optimized by introducing exercise into the diabetes control plan.

TRIAL AND ERROR PROCEDURE: DIABETES CONTROL SOPHISTICATED APPROACH

Please see next page for the flow sheet of trial and error procedure.

Rapid-acting insulin dose for any given meal can be precisely determined by following the trial and error procedure steps described in the following flow sheet. The amount of insulin determined through this trial and error procedure varies from person to person & from meal to meal. Every diabetic person needs to determine his/her own optimal insulin dose for a given meal.

WHY ARE AFTER-MEAL BLOOD GLUCOSE LEVELS NOT TOO HIGH? AN IMPORTANT CLARIFICATION

By examining the self-blood glucose monitoring results in Method 1, Method 2, Method 3, a reader might wonder and raise a question such as "why are the after-meal blood glucose levels not significantly high enough?". Most of the data showed in these examples have after meal-glucose levels under 13 mmol/L or 234 mg/dL.

To understand this, please refer to Method 3 where "Ketones Formation" and "Ketoacidosis" are explained. A diabetic person should be cautious beforehand and should not exercise when the after-meal glucose levels are higher than 13 mmol/L or 234 mg/dL, unless the exercise suits his/her body without forming ketones. A diabetic person should inject the correct amount of insulin just before consuming a major meal to lower his/her blood glucose level close to 13 mmol/L or 234 mg/dL, and then exercise in order to lower his/her after-meal blood glucose level to perfectly normal (5 mmol/L or 90 mg/dL). That is why in all the self-blood glucose monitoring data, you will find the after-meal blood glucose levels below 13 mmol/L or 234 mg/dL.

TRIAL AND ERROR PROCEDURE: DIABETES CONTROL
HOW TO DETERMINE THE INSULIN DOSE TO LOWER AFTER-MEAL GLUCOE LEVEL TO NORMAL
Developed by Rao Konduru, PhD

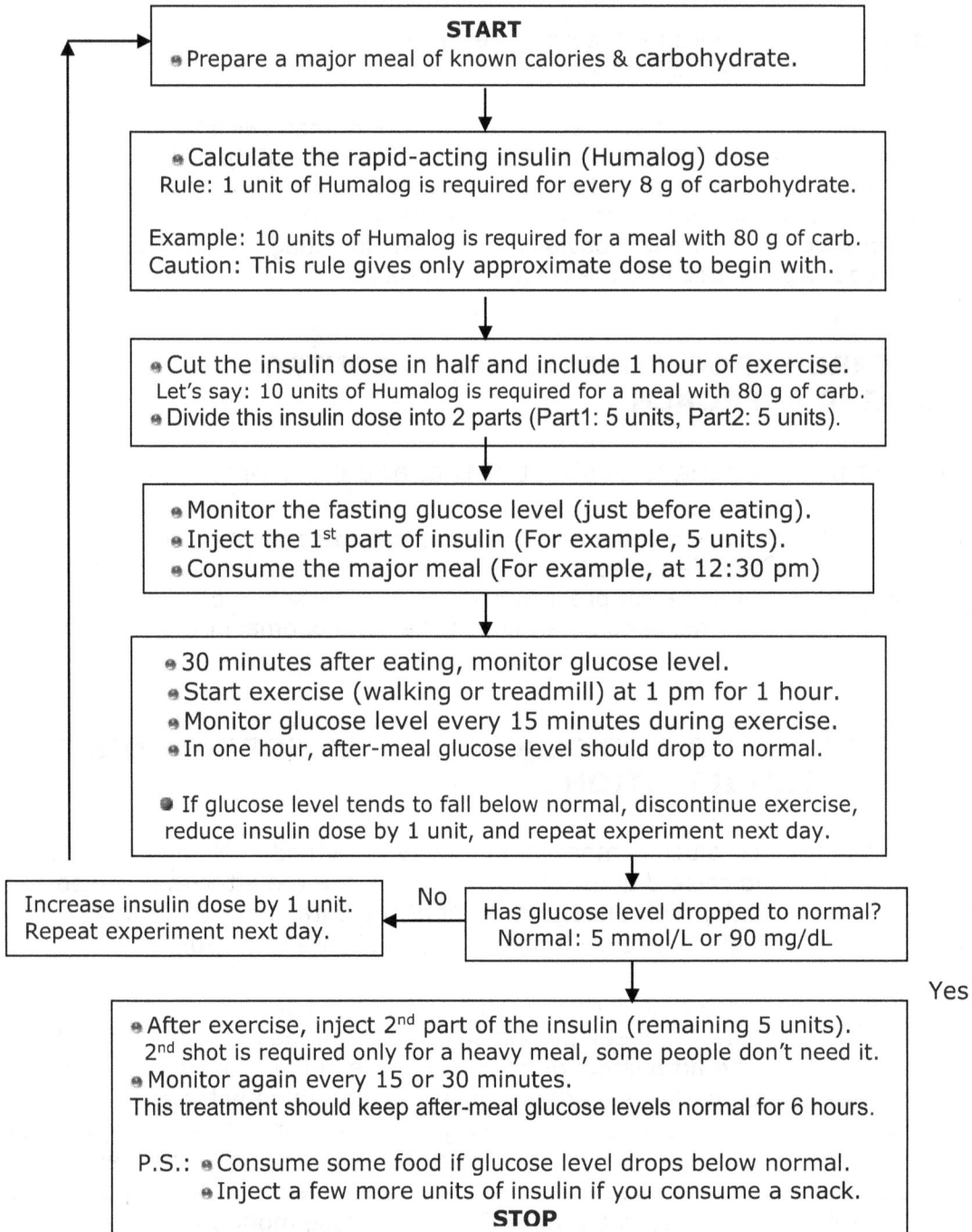

START
- Prepare a major meal of known calories & carbohydrate.

- Calculate the rapid-acting insulin (Humalog) dose
Rule: 1 unit of Humalog is required for every 8 g of carbohydrate.

Example: 10 units of Humalog is required for a meal with 80 g of carb.
Caution: This rule gives only approximate dose to begin with.

- Cut the insulin dose in half and include 1 hour of exercise.
Let's say: 10 units of Humalog is required for a meal with 80 g of carb.
- Divide this insulin dose into 2 parts (Part1: 5 units, Part2: 5 units).

- Monitor the fasting glucose level (just before eating).
- Inject the 1st part of insulin (For example, 5 units).
- Consume the major meal (For example, at 12:30 pm)

- 30 minutes after eating, monitor glucose level.
- Start exercise (walking or treadmill) at 1 pm for 1 hour.
- Monitor glucose level every 15 minutes during exercise.
- In one hour, after-meal glucose level should drop to normal.

- If glucose level tends to fall below normal, discontinue exercise, reduce insulin dose by 1 unit, and repeat experiment next day.

Increase insulin dose by 1 unit.
Repeat experiment next day.

No

Has glucose level dropped to normal?
Normal: 5 mmol/L or 90 mg/dL

Yes

- After exercise, inject 2nd part of the insulin (remaining 5 units).
2nd shot is required only for a heavy meal, some people don't need it.
- Monitor again every 15 or 30 minutes.
This treatment should keep after-meal glucose levels normal for 6 hours.

P.S.: - Consume some food if glucose level drops below normal.
- Inject a few more units of insulin if you consume a snack.
STOP

Dr. RK'S DIABETES HAS BEEN PERMANENTLY CONTROLLED

After suffering from a sudden heart attack in 1998, even though his left artery was 75% clogged and he could not walk a block due to severe angina pain, Dr. RK said "NO" to bypass surgery. He did what none of us would even think of doing. He simply relied on his natural self-prevention diet and exercise, and with it "reversed his critical diabetic heart disease in a matter of months", and developed a method to accomplish Permanent Diabetes Control. He proved to the medical community that a bypass surgery is unnecessary in most cases. He also came up with a trial and error procedure to determine the optimal insulin dose that would tightly control diabetes in 90 days, and would allow a diabetic person to live like a normal person for the rest of his/her life.

Please see his official blood test results below, and notice that his hemoglobin A1c level dropped from a high-risk 12% to a stunning 6.2%, 5.5%, 5.2%, 5.0%, and has been under 6% consistently for many years. His personal best hemoglobin A1c level of 5% is an extraordinary result any diabetic person would hope to accomplish in a lifetime. In spite of being seriously diabetic person and highly insulin-dependent, Dr. RK accomplished Permanent Diabetes Control with his own diligence and expert knowledge on diabetes. Perhaps he is the only diabetic person living in this world with Permanent Diabetes Control!

Official Blood Text Results of Controlled Diabetes

Listed below are the official blood test results of Dr. RK, performed with a physician's requisition, by BC Biomedical Laboratories (Currently Life Labs), Vancouver, British Columbia, Canada. http://www.mydiabetescontrol.com/diabetic-research.html

Table 3.15

Date	Fasting Glucose	Fasting Glucose	Hemoglobin A1c
Units	mmol/L	mg/dL	g/g Hgb (%)
Normal	(3.6 - 6.1)	(65 – 110)	4.5% - 6.2%
11-Jun-1997			**12.0%**
18-Mar-1998	Suffered Heart Attack (not controlled until 1998)!		
21-Apr-1998	9.2	165.6	9.6%
26-Oct-1998	5.7	102.6	8.0%
22-Jan-1999	6.0	108.0	8.4%
05-May-1999	5.1	91.8	8.1%
07-Jan-2000	7.0	126.0	10.2%
07-Jun-2000	Started controlling diabetes seriously!		
01-Aug-2000	6.0	108.0	8.2%
19-Sep-2000	5.6	100.8	7.4%
19-Jan-2001	4.9	88.2	6.6%
29-Non-2001	5.2	93.6	6.5%
05-Mar-2002	5.2	93.6	6.6%
06-May-2002	4.9	88.2	6.5%
26-Jun-2002	4.4	79.2	6.6%
02-Oct-2002	4.0	72.0	6.3%
30-Jan-2003	5.1	91.8	6.2%
08-Apr-2003	4.7	84.6	6.2%

Date	Fasting Glucose	Fasting Glucose	Hemoglobin A1c
Units	mmol/L	mg/dL	g/g Hgb (%)
Normal	(3.6 - 6.1)	(65 – 110)	4.5% - 6.2%
03-Aug-2011	4.9	88.2	6.0%
01-Nov-2011	3.9	70.2	5.8%
01-Feb-2012	3.9	70.2	5.5%
01-May-2012	4.4	79.2	5.5%
01-Aug-2012	3.7	66.7	5.5%
23-Oct-2012	4.1	73.8	5.5%
17-Jan-2013	4.3	77.4	5.3%
01-May-2013	2.9	52.2	5.6%
21-Aug-2013	5.1	91.8	5.5%
02-Jan-2014	4.2	75.8	5.8%
01-Apr-2014	4.0	72.0	5.9%
02-Jul-2014	4.7	84.8	5.7%
01-Oct-2014	3.6	64.8	5.5%
02-Jan-2015	4.9	88.2	5.4%
01-Apr-2015	4.7	84.8	5.4%
03-Jul-2015	5.3	84.8	5.6%
01-Oct-2015	4.1	73.8	5.8%
02-Jan-2016	5.7	102.6	5.8%
01-Apr-2016	4.4	79.2	5.6%
02-Jul-2016	5.5	99.0	5.9%
01-Oct-2016	5.3	95.4	5.0%
			Personal Best
05-Jan-2017	5.1	91.8	5.6%
02-Apr-2017	5.5	99.0	5.4%
02-Jul-2017	4.5	81.0	5.6%
02-Jan-2018	4.2	75.6	5.7%
03-Apr-2018	4.8	86.4	5.9%
02-Jul-2018	4.6	82.8	5.7%
01-Oct-2018	3.4	61.2	5.7%
02-Jan-2019	4.7	84.8	5.5%
01-Apr-2019	3.9	70.2	5.6%
30-Jun-2019	4.2	85.6	5.5%
01-Oct-2019	4.8	86.4	5.6%

Date	Fasting Glucose	Fasting Glucose	Hemoglobin A1c
Units	mmol/L	mg/dL	g/g Hgb (%)
Normal	(3.6 - 6.1)	(65 – 110)	4.5% - 6.2%
01-Apr-2020	5.4	97.2	5.7%
30-Jun-2020	3.6	64.8	5.8%
25-Sep-2020	4.6	82.8	5.5%

CLOSING REMARKS

◉ If you master the concept of injecting rapid-acting insulin along with exercise, you can go easy on the dietary guidelines, and enjoy a high-carbohydrate meal including dessert (your favorite meal in a restaurant) once or twice a week. Some diabetic people with expert knowledge go easy on the dietary guidelines, still manage to control diabetes with insulin shots, and keep their hemoglobin A1c perfectly normal. These people with expert knowledge know how to inject the right dosage of rapid-acting insulin and exercise, and lower after-meal blood glucose spike quickly to normal, and know how to achieve normal A1c.
Did you know "knowledge is power"?

◉ With experience, over time, it becomes very easy to control diabetes with insulin! You cannot do that with oral medications. If you are type 2 diabetic, and currently on pills, and living with uncontrolled diabetes, you need to evaluate your situation. It is strongly recommended to switch to insulin shots. An insulin-dependent type 2 diabetic can control his/her diabetes easily and achieve the perfect normal A1c level in a short period of time, and can keep it controlled forever!

What is "Permanent Diabetes Control"?

◉ When a highly knowledgeable diabetic person is living with tightly controlled diabetes for an extended period of time, and is determined to control diabetes forever, his/her diabetes is said to be permanently controlled.

◉ The author of this book (Dr. RK) accomplished "Permanent Diabetes Control" after conducting very many diligent experiments related to diabetic research. He has researched on his own body with chronic diabetes, and studied extensively the combined influence of healthy diet, rapid-acting insulin (Humalog) and after-meal exercise on after-meal blood glucose levels. All that diabetic research information of "Real-Life Case Study" is explained in the next chapter titled "Permanent Diabetes Control".

REFERENCES

1. Permanent Diabetes Control (Book), Subtitle: The Complete Guide to Living Like A Normal Person Forever, Authored by Rao Konduru, MS, PhD, Reviewed and Endorsed by Dr. Marshal Dahl, MD, PhD., Endocrinologist, Faculty of Medicine, University of British Columbia, Vancouver, British Columbia, Canada, First Published in 2003.
www.mydiabetescontrol.com

2. The Secret to Controlling Type 2 Diabetes, Subtitle: Addendum to Permanent Diabetes Control, Authored by Rao Konduru, Published in 2019, ISBN # 9780973112054, Available on Amazon.com, www.mydiabetescontrol.com

3. Krall, L.P, MD, and Beaser, R.S, MD, Joslin Diabetes Manual, Philadelphia, Lea and Febiger, Pages 3-6, 135, 138, 1989.

4. Glucose Ranges in People Without Diabetes, Lifescan's One Touch Profile Blood Glucose Monitoring Manual, Table on Page 51, Lifescan, Printed in USA, 1996.

5. Do I Need a Longer Insulin Needle? This question was answered by Christy L. Parkin, MSN, RN, CDE, Diabetes Forecast, The Healthy Living Magazine, 2019.
http://www.diabetesforecast.org/2013/dec/do-i-need-a-longer-insulin.html

CHAPTER 4 PERMANENT DIABETES CONTROL

REAL-LIFE CASE STUDY
▶ **Permanent Diabetes Control Accomplished!**
▶ **Rapid Acting Insulin (Humalog) Dose Cut By 60%!**
▶ **Hemoglobin A1c Dropped From A High-Risk 12%** **To a Stunning 6.2%, 5.5%, 5.3%, 5.0%, Etc!**
▶ **Reversed Critical Heart Disease Without Surgery!**

TABLE OF CONTENTS

PLEASE NOTE: If you don't have scientific background or college degree, please skip this Chapter 4. You don't need this Chapter 4 to learn how to control diabetes. Just read and learn all contents in Chapter 3. Anybody can control diabetes by reading and learning the contents in Chapter 3.

CHAPTER 4 PERMANENT DIABETES CONTROL
DIABETIC RESEARCH: REAL-LIFE CASE STUDY

INTRODUCTION

The author of this book, having been an insulin-dependent diabetic for 20 years, has personally participated in this study, collected all the self-blood glucose monitoring data and interpreted the results. The goal of this study was to determine the combined influence of insulin and after-meal exercise on after-meal blood glucose levels in an attempt to lower them to normal and keep them normal for 6 hours every day (7 days a week). The optimal insulin dose for a given meal (of known calories) was determined by trial and error. The detailed case study of the diabetic research is reported with fingerstick blood glucose monitoring data and interpretation with graphs, along with the nutritional information of 4 major meals (chicken meal, tofu meal, fish meal and turkey meal) studied.

INSULIN

Rapid-acting insulin Humalog has been the highlight of this study, injected to lower after-meal glucose levels. The trial and error procedure began with 1 unit of Humalog for every 8 gm of carbohydrate, or 10 units of Humalog for 500 calories of food consumed when exercise is not included. Actual dose was determined by trial and error. Humalog was increased by 1 unit whenever glucose level during exercise was high, and decreased by 1 unit whenever glucose level was too low, and the whole experiment was repeated next day. The body's response was understood with experience and the appropriate insulin dose figured out. Humalog was injected 10 minutes before meal.The action of Humalog ceased in about two and half hours. Intermediate-acting insulin Humulin-N was injected twice a day, 15 units each time, at 7 am and midnight in order to meet the body's minor insulin needs throughout the day (24 hours). The focus here is on the rapid-acting insulin Humalog.

FOOD

Refer to Tables 4.31 to 4.35 for the nutritional information of several meals (chicken meal, tofu meal, fish meal & turkey meal) in the Appendix 4A of this chapter. The major meal (supper) was prepared around 5 pm with a Turbo-cooker. All items were weighed precisely with an electronic balance before cooked. It took 25 minutes to cook brown rice. Vegetables & tofu were steamed for 2 minutes in the same Turbo cooker while cooking brown rice. Chicken, turkey or fish was cooked in a microwave for 2 minutes whenever needed. Cooked brown rice, chicken/tofu/fish, steamed vegetables, diced tomatoes, soymilk were mixed along with diced garlic, salt, cayenne pepper & spices. Udo's oil was sprinkled on the final meal. No item was fried with oil.

EXERCISE

The major purpose of this exercise was to bring after-meal glucose levels to normal values within 1 or 2 hours after a major meal consumption. Exercise was started 45 minutes after the major meal consumption (supper). Either treadmill or regular walk was used as exercise and the intended goal was accomplished successfully.

ROTATION OF INJECTION SITES

Diabetic people should monitor blood glucose levels as many times as possible to control diabetes. When you do "Diabetic Research" on your own body, you may have to poke your finger 10 times or even more than 10 times a day in order to collect data, analyse and interpret the results. Each time you monitor, if the blood glucose level in not normal, you should inject insulin and exercise (walking or treadmill) so that the blood glucose level would drop to normal. Very specifically, you should monitor and inject the appropriate dose of rapid-acting insulin every day in order to slash after-meal glucose spikes. Frequent monitoring is also extremely important because only in that way you can take action, and inject insulin if needed, and achieve normal hemoglobin A1c and perfect diabetes control. Remember a healthy pancreas monitors 500 times a day and automatically adjusts insulin secretion! A systematic procedure therefore is crucial to protect from developing abdominal lumps (what is know as lipohypertrophy!).

In the current Diabetic Research Study, while collecting extensive data (10 times or more than 10 times a day), the abdomen part of the human body was chosen for the injection sites. The abdomen area was known to be the convenient and the most effective spot to inject insulin. It is known that the insulin can be best absorbed and drawn into the bloodstream from the abdomen area, which is around the belly button. For each meal studied (chicken meal, tofu meal, fish meal & turkey meal), insulin was injected more than 5 times a day. For each meal studied, it took about 4 weeks (approximately 1 month) to collect sufficient data. Dividing the abdomen area into 4 equal quadrants, every week a different quadrant was used systematically with the aid of a calendar as shown in the picture below. With this kind of self-organization, each injected site has some 3 to 4 weeks to heal and restore. This kind of approach was found to be safe and successful in injecting insulin as many times as needed every day throughout the research.

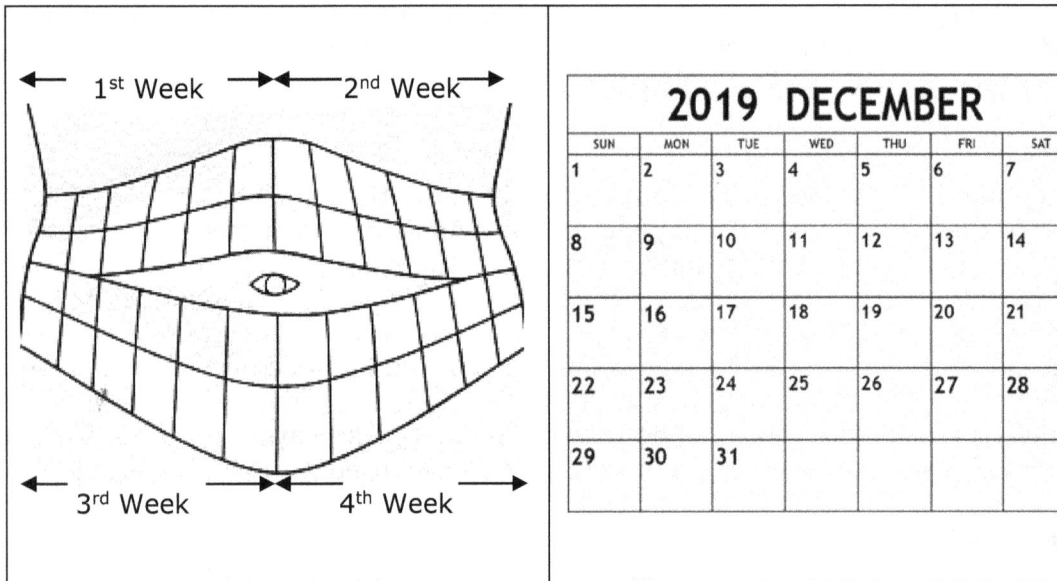

Figure 4.1 Rotation of injection sites on abdomen area.

FINGER-POKING STRATEGY

Fingerstick blood glucose monitoring was performed using the Elite Glucometer. In the current study, while researching, extensive data were collected and the fingers were poked in a systematic way as shown in the picture below. Fingers could get ragged if proper care is not taken. It is possible to poke more than 10 times on each finger by properly selecting and organizing poking sites. Each hand has 5 fingers, and there are 10 fingers in total available for poking. For each set of data collected, there were 10 or more self-blood glucose tests performed in a day, and only one finger was poked 10 or more times in one day. The first finger was used on the first day of data collection, the 2nd finger was used on the 2nd day of data collection, and so on. Data were not collected every single day in order that there could be one or two days rest after each day of data collection. For each meal studied, the data were collected for at least 10 days and each finger was poked 10 or more times each day. In general, it took about a month's time to finish using all 10 fingers. Then the cycle was repeated (finger 1, finger 2, and so on). Therefore there was sufficient time (about 3 to 4 weeks) for each finger to heal and restore the skin. By following this systematic procedure, one can protect the fingers from getting ragged.

Day 1	Day 2	Day 3	Day 4	Day 5	Day 6	Day 7	Day 8	Day 9	Day 10
Finger 1	Finger 2	Finger 3	Finger 4	Finger 5	Finger 6	Finger 7	Finger 8	Finger 9	Finger 10

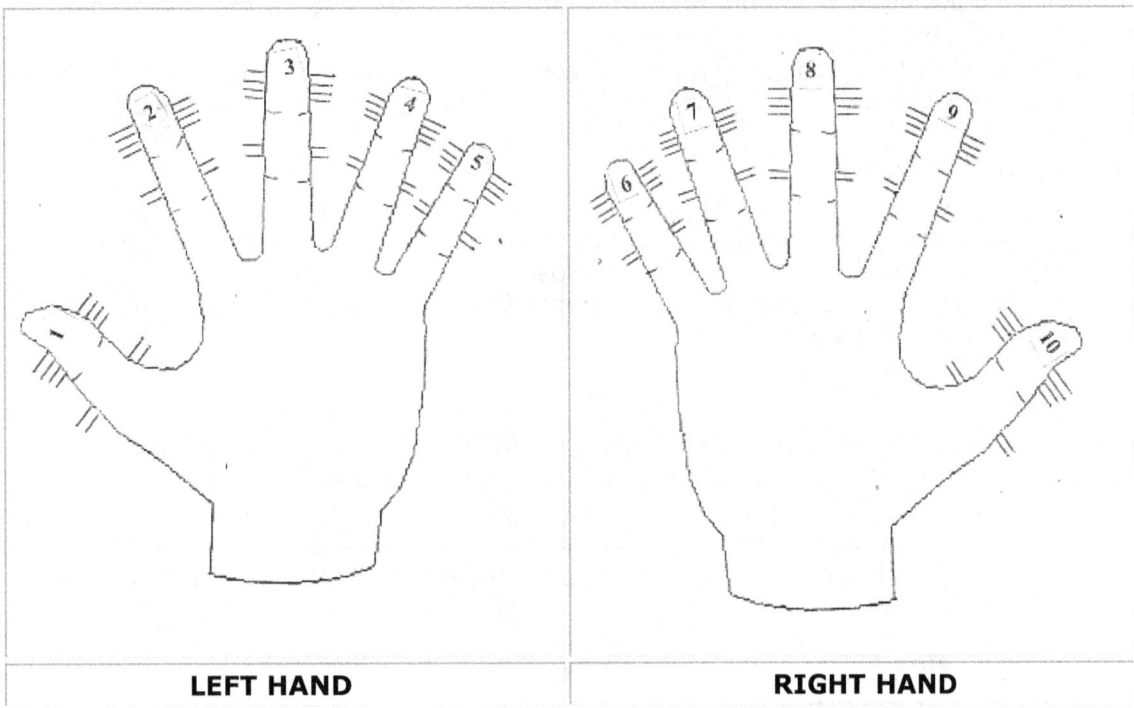

LEFT HAND   **RIGHT HAND**

Figure 4.2 Each Finger with 12 Poking Spots.

DATA COLLECTION AND RESEARCH

INFLUENCE OF INSULIN AND EXERCISE ON AFTER-MEAL GLUCOSE LEVELS

Data were collected in a strictly disciplined manner and no other food was consumed except the one listed. While the study is focused on the major meal supper the data for the entire day (24 hours) are shown in the tables and figures. Experiments with several meals were performed with a keen attention towards maintaining timings as consistently as possible to obtain comparable data.

Insulin Dose Calculated

Rule 1: 1 Unit of Humalog per every 8 gm of carbohydrate in the meal.
Rule 2: 10 Units of Humalog for every 500 calories of the meal.
Refer to Tables 4.32 to 4.34 for nutritional composition of several meals studied.

Table 4.1

Meal	Calories	Carbohydrate (gm)	Insulin Dose Calculated (units) Rule 1	Insulin Dose Calculated (units) Rule 2	Insulin Dose Actual (units)
Chicken Meal	966	135	17	19	17
Tofu Meal	843	139	17	17	25
Fish Meal	955	135	17	19	25

This calculation gave only a rough estimation (the actual dose may vary from one individual to the other). This insulin dose should be further adjusted depending on the fasting glucose level just before the meal. In the current study, the actual insulin dose was determined by trial and error as shown in the last column. These results were shown in detail in Tables 4.11, 4.12. 4.18, 4.19, 4.24, 4.25, and in Figures 4.10, 4.11, 4.14, 4.15, 4.18 and 4.19.

Insulin Dose Cut in Half

Although the general rule suggests that insulin dose should be cut by 50% to include exercise, the actual insulin dose was determined by trial and error procedure. It was shown through conducting experiments that the insulin dose was cut in half for the chicken meal and the fish meal, and 60% for the tofu meal whenever one hour of exercise was included (Refer to conclusions, Table 4.3).

Data Collection

At around 5:45 pm, blood glucose was monitored with the Elite Glucometer just before eating supper. The appropriate dose of Humalog insulin was injected, and supper was consumed in 10 minutes. Blood glucose was monitored again 45 minutes after the meal consumption, and exercise was begun (either treadmill or regular walk). Exercise was continued for a period of 1 hour. Exercise was interrupted every 15 minutes, and glucose level monitored. Data were recorded.

Meals	Tables	Figures
Nutritional Composition	Tables 4.31 to 4.35	
Chicken Meal	Tables 4.10 to 4.16	Figures 4.10 to 4.13
Tofu Meal	Tables 4.17 to 4.22	Figures 4.14 to 4.17
Fish Meal	Tables 4.23 to 4.30	Figures 4.18 to 4.21

INTERPRETATION OF DIABETIC RESEARCH RESULTS

For diabetic people, the general range of fasting glucose levels before meals is:

	Glucose (mmol/L)	Glucose (mg/dL)
Before All Meals	Between 4 and 7	Between 72 and 126

Normal blood glucose levels, for healthy (non-diabetic) people, as published in Joslin Diabetes Manual and in the One Touch Meter Manual are shown below.

Table 4.2 Normal Blood Glucose Levels of Healthy (Non-Diabetic) People
[Courtesy of Joslin Diabetes Center, Adapted from One Touch Meter Manual]

	Glucose (mmol/L)	Glucose (mg/dL)
Between 2 am and 4 am	> 3.9	> 70
Before breakfast (fasting)	3.9 to 5.8	70 to 105
Before lunch or supper	3.9 to 6.1	70 to 110
1 hour after meals	< 8.9	< 160
2 hours after meals	< 6.7	< 120

The above-mentioned normal blood glucose ranges for a non-diabetic person were used as guidelines to strictly control after-meal glucose levels by adjusting insulin and after-meal exercise. Study showed that in most cases, the after-meal blood glucose level reached the peak in 45 minutes. Exercise was commenced 45 minutes after the meal consumption so that the blood glucose level could possibly be brought to normal (less than 8.9 mmol/L or 160 mg/dL) in 1 hour. Whenever this goal became difficult to attain, the blood glucose level was brought to normal in 90 minutes to 2 hours. Two hours after the meal consumption, if the after-meal glucose level dropped to less than 7 mmol/L or 126 mg/dL and remained normal for a few more hours consistently on a daily basis, that would be an excellent accomplishment. Rigorous attention on lowering after-meal glucose levels is very essential for a diabetic person in order to lower the hemoglobin A1c level close to normal.

No Insulin and No Exercise
The data are recorded in Tables 4.10, 4.17 and 4.23 and Figures 4.10 to 4.21.

When no insulin was injected and no exercise was performed, data were collected to see upper levels. After-meal glucose levels were found to be very high for 6 hours, suggesting the fact that the person should take insulin and should exercise to lower after-meal blood glucose levels. If the diabetic person continues to live like that without insulin/medication and without exercise, these elevated glucose levels would contribute to the establishment of a very high average glucose level in 90 days, thereby contributing to high-risk range of hemoglobin A1c. Any such high hemoglobin A1c level over a long time warns that a diabetic person could encounter all kinds of complications such as heart attack, coronary artery disease (CAD), kidney disease or failure, blindness, neuropathy, and others.

Insulin Shot But No Exercise

Refer to Tables 4.11, 4.12. 4.18, 4.19, 4.24, 4.25.
Refer to Figures 4.10, 4.11, 4.14, 4.15, 4.18 and 4.19.

The influence of the rapid-acting insulin Humalog was studied at several doses (10 units, 15 units, 17 units, 20 units, 25 units and so on). After-meal glucose levels were monitored every 15 minutes for 6 hours and the same experiment repeated. The right amount of insulin to lower blood glucose levels to the normal range was determined by trial and error. The following are the final results of insulin doses determined by trial and error for three different meals:

Chicken Meal	17 Units of Humalog
Tofu Meal	25 Units of Humalog
Fish Meal	25 Units of Humalog

These results reveal that too much insulin is required to keep up normal blood glucose levels after a major meal. It is known that too much insulin causes hypoglycemia and constricts arteries, leading to heart attack, stroke and other risk factors. Too much insulin also stimulates the brain and makes the person feel hungry, tempts the person to eat more, and causes the liver to manufacture fat in the belly. This suggests that these mega doses of insulin should be slashed through introducing after-meal exercise.

Exercise But No Insulin Shot

Refer to Tables 4.29 and 4.30.
To see the influence of exercise, data were collected without injecting any insulin but exercising for 1 hour. As can be seen in Table 4.29, there was no significant change in the after-meal glucose levels. Humulin-N was discontinued in the previous night and in the morning to make sure there would be no Humulin-N in the body for at least 24 hours, and data were collected without injecting any insulin but with exercise. As can be seen in Table 4.30, there was no significant change in the after-meal glucose levels during exercise. Exercise alone did not help lower the after-meal glucose levels. The levels remained unchanged even after one hour of exercise. These experiments suggest the desperate need of a rapid-acting insulin such as Humalog.

COMBINED INFLUENCE OF INSULIN AND EXERCISE

The most successful results were obtained when the insulin shot and exercise were combined. The optimum insulin dose for a heavy meal, with 1 hour of exercise, was determined by trial and error procedure (see next page).

Single Shot and Double Shot with Exercise

See Tables 4.13, 4.14, 4.15 and 4.16; Figures 4.12 and 4.13 for **chicken meal**
    Tables 4.20, 4.21 and 4.22; Figures 4.16 and 4.17 for **tofu meal**
    Tables 4.26, 4.27 and 4.28; Figures 4.20 and 4.21 for **fish meal**

TRIAL AND ERROR PROCEDURE: DIABETES CONTROL
HOW TO DETERMINE THE INSULIN DOSE TO LOWER AFTER-MEAL GLUCOE LEVEL TO NORMAL
Developed by Rao Konduru, PhD

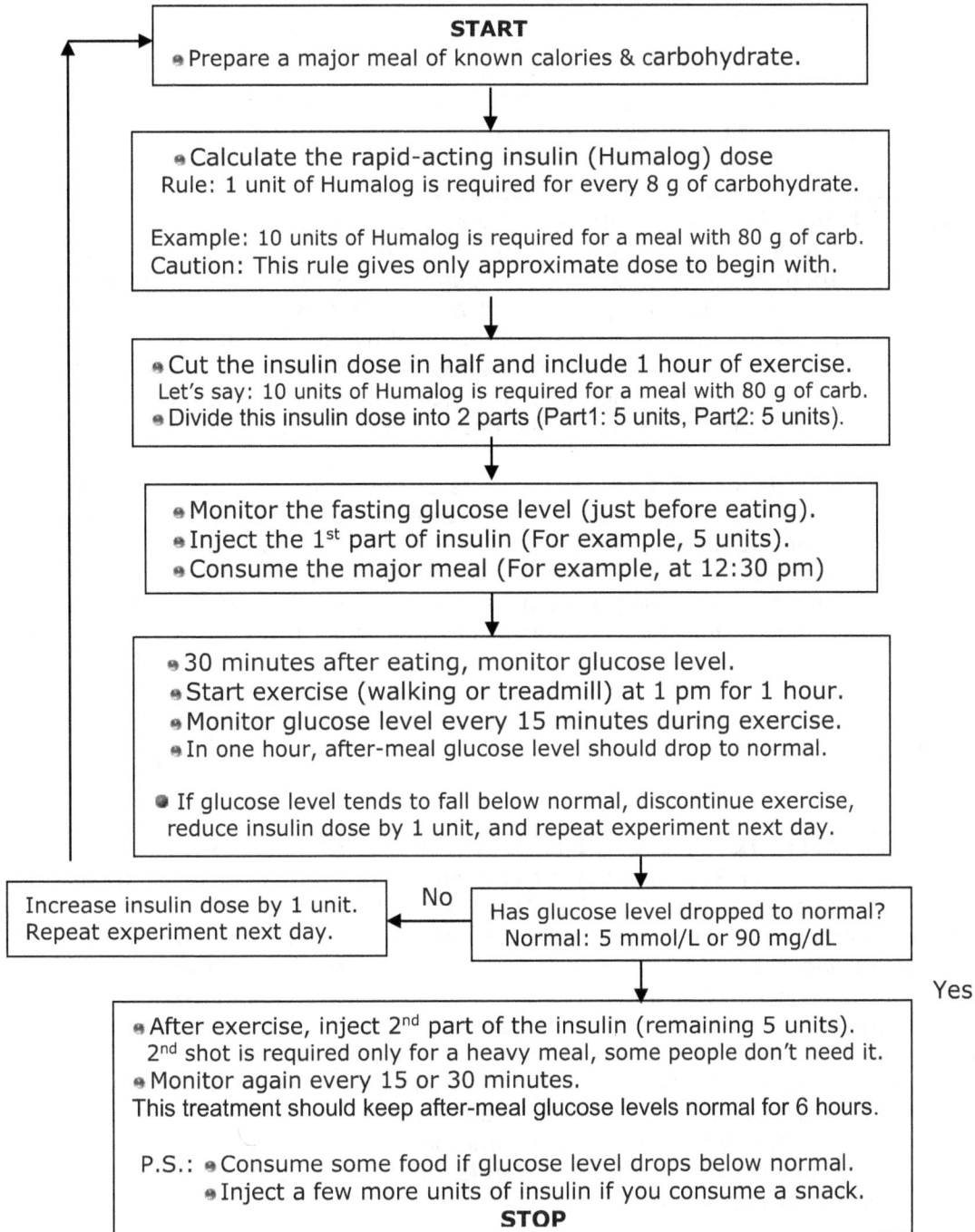

START
- Prepare a major meal of known calories & carbohydrate.

- Calculate the rapid-acting insulin (Humalog) dose
Rule: 1 unit of Humalog is required for every 8 g of carbohydrate.

Example: 10 units of Humalog is required for a meal with 80 g of carb.
Caution: This rule gives only approximate dose to begin with.

- Cut the insulin dose in half and include 1 hour of exercise.
Let's say: 10 units of Humalog is required for a meal with 80 g of carb.
- Divide this insulin dose into 2 parts (Part1: 5 units, Part2: 5 units).

- Monitor the fasting glucose level (just before eating).
- Inject the 1st part of insulin (For example, 5 units).
- Consume the major meal (For example, at 12:30 pm)

- 30 minutes after eating, monitor glucose level.
- Start exercise (walking or treadmill) at 1 pm for 1 hour.
- Monitor glucose level every 15 minutes during exercise.
- In one hour, after-meal glucose level should drop to normal.

- If glucose level tends to fall below normal, discontinue exercise, reduce insulin dose by 1 unit, and repeat experiment next day.

Has glucose level dropped to normal?
Normal: 5 mmol/L or 90 mg/dL

No → Increase insulin dose by 1 unit. Repeat experiment next day.

Yes

- After exercise, inject 2nd part of the insulin (remaining 5 units).
  2nd shot is required only for a heavy meal, some people don't need it.
- Monitor again every 15 or 30 minutes.
This treatment should keep after-meal glucose levels normal for 6 hours.

P.S.: - Consume some food if glucose level drops below normal.
- Inject a few more units of insulin if you consume a snack.
STOP

When 10 units of Humalog were injected before the chicken meal and after-meal exercise was carried out, either treadmill or walking, blood glucose levels dropped too quickly below 4 mol/L (72 mg/dL), giving warning of hypoglycemia. Exercise was discontinued whenever such signs occurred. The goal here is to introduce one hour of exercise after the meal. Then the insulin dose was reduced and the experiment repeated by trial and error with 9 units, 7 units, 5 units of Humalog, and so on. When 4 or 5 units of Humalog were injected just before meals, exercise was allowed to continue for 1 hour and glucose levels dropped gradually to normal. This trial was called **Single Shot**. However, after finishing the exercise, glucose levels rose back above 7 mmol/L (126 mg/dL) indicating that the experiment was unsuccessful (Refer to Table 4.13). It was believed to be unsuccessful because lowering after-meal glucose levels to normal and keeping them normal for 4 to 6 hours after meal consumption was the goal. Experiments were repeated very many times to resolve this problem. After puzzling with this predicament for a number weeks or months without knowing what to do, thoughts came to the mind suggesting the injection of another 5 units of Humalog (2nd shot) a few minutes after the exercise, which was proved to be a wonderful idea to keep the after-meal blood glucose levels normal for a period of 6 hours. This trial was called **Double Shot**. This made sense because the total amount of insulin injected (9 units) when exercise included was close to half of the insulin dose calculated. Refer to Table 4.1 to see insulin dose calculated.

It is expected that the little insulin dose (4 or 5 units of Humalog) had been used up during exercise and there was no more rapid-acting insulin available to control blood glucose. More important reason is that the action of Humalog ceased in 2 and half hours. The pancreas was not producing sufficient insulin nor was the injected insulin available in the body. Therefore a second shot of Humalog insulin (another 5 units) was injected after the exercise, followed by the resting and monitoring blood glucose levels as shown in Tables 4.14 and 4.16.

Similar experiments were conducted with tofu meal and fish meal and the above-mentioned idea of using **Double Shot** of Humalog insulin was confirmed.

DIABETES TREATMENT PLAN SUMMARIZED

Prepared a major meal (over 800 calories). Calculated insulin (Humalog) dose. Insulin dose was cut in half to include 1 hour of exercise. This insulin dose was further divided into two parts (they may not be equal parts but close to equal). Injected the first part (about 50%) of the insulin dose and consumed the major meal. Began exercise, ran on a treadmill or walked, within an hour (say, after 45 min) after the major meal. Continued exercise for 1 hour (one full hour of exercise was required, no exceptions). Monitored the blood glucose level every 15 minutes. About 15 minutes after exercise, injected the second part (the other 50%) of the insulin dose and monitored again the blood glucose level until midnight. This treatment kept the blood glucose levels within the normal range for about 6 hours (from 6 pm to midnight)—which otherwise is the critical time period for accumulating unusually high glucose levels in the bloodstream and **high levels of hemoglobin A1c.** Elevated blood glucose levels over a long time are dangerous as they damage blood vessels.

When blood glucose levels are elevated, glucose sticks to the surface of the cells for a long time and is then converted to a poison called "sorbitol" which damages the cells and causes long-term side effects such as heart attack, coronary heart disease, stroke, kidney disease, kidney failure, amputations, blindness, burning foot syndrome, neuropathy, and other complications.

With this treatment plan, the peak levels of elevated blood glucose levels were not only slashed but also brought to normal. It was concluded that consistent, serious and rigorous efforts with this treatment for 3 to 6 months lowers the average glucose level to normal—thereby lowering hemoglobin A1c level to normal (less than 7%). It was finally concluded after conducting experiments that a steady normal value of hemoglobin A1c for more than a year can be maintained and *permanent diabetes control* can be accomplished.

HUMALOG VERSUS HUMULIN-R

Data were also collected to see and compare the actions of Humalog and Humulin-R. Experiments revealed that Humulin-R is as good as Humalog while exercising (either treadmill or regular walk). However, Humulin-R did not work as efficiently as Humalog during rest periods without exercise. The best insulin currently available is Humalog as it is absorbed quickly and starts acting effectively right away within minutes. Eli Lilly and Company says that Humalog acts like baby's own insulin at mealtime. Humulin-R has to be injected 30 to 45 minutes before the meal posing organizational inconvenience. Therefore the focus was only on Humalog insulin. Visit the Eli Lilly's site for further information regarding Humalog insulin.

www.lillydiabetes.com/Products/Humalog.cfm

CONCLUSIONS AND OBSERVATIONS

The combined influence of the rapid-acting insulin Humalog and exercise (either treadmill or regular walk) on after-meal glucose levels was studied through extensive data collection and research. The following conclusions were drawn.

1. To calculate the insulin dose, Rule 1 (1 unit of Humalog for every 8 gm of carbohydrate) and Rule 2 (10 units of Humalog for every 500 calories of meal) provided only a rough estimation to begin with. The actual dose was determined through trial and error by studying the body's response and by self-monitoring after-meal glucose levels for up to 6 hours. The actual dose was significantly different.

2. Insulin requirement is tabulated below. From this research, it is evident that the insulin dose was cut by up to 60% by incorporating one hour of exercise (either treadmill or regular walk) after the meal.

Table 4.3

| | | | Insulin Requirement | | |
| MEAL Studied | Calories | Carbohydrate | Without | With | |
	(Kcal)	(gm)	Exercise	Exercise	% Cut
Chicken Meal	966	135	17 units	9 units	47%
Tofu Meal	843	139	25 units	10 units	60%
Fish Meal	955	135	25 units	13 units	48%

3. When compared to tofu meal and fish meal, chicken meal consumed a few units less insulin. Even though neither fish nor chicken has carbohydrate, fish meal required a few units more insulin than chicken meal did to lower after-meal glucose levels to normal. While both chicken meal and fish meal contained almost the same amount of calories and carbohydrate, fish meal required more than 45% more Humalog with or without exercise.

4. Daily average glucose levels were computed as shown below. Average glucose level dropped significantly whenever exercise was introduced after the meal.

Table 4.4

| | Daily Average Glucose Level in 24 Hours | | | | |
| MEAL Studied | Without Exercise | | With Exercise | | Glucose Level |
	mmol/L	mg/dL	mmol/L	mg/dL	% Lowered
Chicken Meal	9.4	169.2	5.8	104.4	38.30%
Tofu Meal	10.4	187.2	5.9	106.2	43.30%
Fish Meal	10.9	196.2	6.1	109.8	44.04%

From this research, it is crystal clear that after-meal exercise has multiple benefits. The following are the benefits derived from the data and results.

    a. After-meal exercise cut the insulin dose up to 60%,
    b. Lowered the daily average glucose level by up to 44%, and
    c. Lowered the daily average glucose level from abnormal to normal.

When the daily average glucose level is lowered to normal for 90 days, the hemoglobin A1c will automatically be lowered to normal. Hence the after-meal exercise is proved to be of paramount importance in diabetes control.

5. Either regular walk or treadmill produced almost the same results with the Humalog insulin **Double Shot**. Walking sometimes produced even more favorable results than treadmill. So those people who do not feel comfortable with treadmill can walk and lower after-meal glucose levels and can maintain normal levels for 5 to 6 hours after the major meal consumption.

6. All that has to be done is: "introduce an exercise for 1 hour after every major meal consumed with an appropriate rapid-acting insulin shot."

RECOMMENDATIONS AND FURTHER STUDY

♦ Double shot, before and after exercise, whenever a heavy meal is consumed, helps control diabetes precisely. For a light meal, single shot is enough to accomplish good control. Getting accustomed to a double shot would result in the best overall glucose-level control for an extended period of time. Every individual has to research with a variety of heavy meals and conclude accordingly.

♦ Further experiments are to be conducted to test the method with a large group of diabetics including adults (males and females), children, elderly and disabled. Different people react differently with a rapid-acting insulin such as Humalog and exercise after consuming a variety of heavy meals. Handling and troubleshooting any specific problems or questions that may arise can be an enjoyable task.

WHY DO WE HAVE TO DO IT THIS WAY?

Evening meal or any major meal causes the highest blood sugars in diabetics. Elevated glucose levels are accumulated in the bloodstream soon after the major meal consumption. These elevated glucose levels dominate in and largely contribute to establishing the average glucose level in 90 days. Elevated after-meal glucose levels therefore must be slashed as quickly as possible and brought to normal within 1 or 2 hour of the major meal (supper) consumption in order to bring hemoglobin A1c close to its normal value and control diabetes.

At the same time, the insulin dose must be minimized because too much insulin causes hypoglycemia and constricts arteries leading to heart attack and coronary heart disease. Too much insulin also stimulates the brain so that a person feels hungry and eats more and causes the liver to manufacture fat in the belly. Too little insulin on the other hand is not enough to cover the entire meal and to maintain normal glucose levels. **An optimum insulin dose is therefore crucial.** Insulin is synthesized in such a way that it acts a lot more quickly and much more effectively with exercise. A continuous exercise, either treadmill or regular walk, should be introduced into the diabetes control plan in order to burn fat, lose calories, and optimize both insulin dose and insulin action. If this exercise is introduced after every heavy meal, it not only minimizes the insulin dose but in addition maximizes insulin action and prevents after-meal glucose levels from rising too high, thereby keeping the diabetes under tight control.

Consistent, serious and rigorous efforts at lowering after-meal glucose levels for a period of 3 to 6 months gradually lowers the hemoglobin A1c to its normal value, even if the diabetes had been poorly controlled in the past. Thereafter, continued efforts with reasonable attention to **insulin, food and exercise** are necessary to keep diabetes under tight control. Serious efforts are required only in the beginning in order to do research, and to find out the optimal insulin dose and to understand the body's response for a given meal. The experience gained in one's own research would guide the individual on how to inject appropriate insulin shots and do exercise, and reward the individual by allowing the fingerstick self-blood glucose tests only a few times a day, still producing outstanding results.

REAL-LIFE CASE STUDY OF THE PARTICIPANT (SUMMARIZED)

The author of this book has personally participated in this case study.

Brief History of the Diabetic Person

1980
First diagnosed with diabetes in 1980. Probably he has been suffering from diabetes when he was much younger, but was not diagnosed.

1980 – 1986
On pills. Never heard about insulin and his doctor never recommended. Never controlled diabetes. Never self-monitored glucose levels except a few blood tests taken by his doctor.

1986
Hospitalized after becoming ill with frequent urination problems. Diagnosed with insulin-dependant diabetes, Brussels Hospital, Belgium. Tested with insulin shots for 1 to 2 weeks in the hospital. Responded positively to insulin. Since then on insulin every day.

1988
Participated in training at Diabetes Education Center, Toronto. Started taking insulin shots both Humulin-N and Humulin-R.

1988 – 1998
Still not controlling diabetes. Just took insulin shots every day. Self-monitored fasting glucose some mornings only. Never thought about controlling hemoglobin A1c. Diabetes got totally out of control. Hemoglobin A1c level rose up to 12% (see table below).

March 1998
Suffered heart attack. Hospitalized in Royal Columbian Hospital, Canada. Underwent 2 angioplasties. Still no attention was given to diabetes.

1998 – 1999
Suffered serious heart disease, angina and debilitating chest pains. Could not walk even a block due to severe angina pain. Angiogram done; Diagnosed with Coronary Artery Disease (CAD). Left artery 75% clogged. Used Nitro spray even for a short walk. Cardiologist recommended heart surgery, but said "NO" to surgery.

1999
Realized the past mistakes concerning diabetes and poor control. Awakened the giant within him. Committed to control heart disease. Read books on heart disease and diabetes. By following the prevention diet plan, lost weight, brought cholesterols to normal, and successfully avoided heart surgery. Rigorous self-prevention diet has helped.

July 1999
Started working seriously with treadmill exercise to control after-meal glucose levels with appropriate insulin dose and specially cooked meal. Applied the method outlined in this book, and brought hemoglobin A1c level to normal in 6 months. **Since then A1c remained steady.**

2000
Reversed Critical Heart Disease through self-prevention diet and exercise. No more heart disease/angina pain. No need of Nitro spray anymore.

2001 - 2002
He is now living with tightly controlled diabetes. No more risk factors. He is confident that he will live forever with "permanent diabetes control".

2003
He wrote and published the book "Permanent Diabetes Control". The book earned an immense respect and appreciation.

Official Blood Test Results: Fasting Glucose & Hemoglobin A1c

Listed below are the official blood test results performed, with physician's requisition, by BC Biomedical Laboratories, Vancouver, BC, Canada. This table shows the evidence of how the diabetes has been controlled.

Table 4.5   Official Blood Test Results of Hemoglobin A1c.

Date	Fasting Glucose	Fasting Glucose	Hemoglobin A1c
Units	mmol/L	mg/dL	g/g Hgb (%)
Normal	(3.6 - 6.1)	(65 – 110)	Less than 7%
11-Jun-97			12.0%
18-Mar-1998	Suffered Heart Attack		
21-Apr-1998	9.2	165.6	9.6%
26-Oct-1998	5.7	102.6	8.0%
22-Jan-1999	6.0	108.0	8.4%
5-May-1999	5.1	91.8	8.1%
7-Jun-2000	7.0	126.0	10.2%
7-Jun-2000	**Started controlling diabetes seriously**		
1-Aug-2000	6.0	108.0	8.2%
19-Sep-2000	5.6	100.8	7.4%
19-Jan-2001			6.6%
29-Nov-2001	5.2	93.6	6.5%
5-Mar-2002	5.2	93.6	6.6%
6-May-2002			6.5%
26-Jun-2002	4.4	79.2	6.6%
2-Oct-2002	4.0	72.0	6.3%
30-Jan-2003			6.2%
08-Apr-2003	4.7	84.6	6.2%

For non-diabetic people, the normal range of hemoglobin A1c is from 4.8% to 6.2%. American Diabetic Association recommended that the goal of a diabetic person should be a value of hemoglobin A1c less than 7% (2). Studies showed that the average hemoglobin A1c level among the Type 2 diabetics in the USA is estimated to be about 9.4% (2).

In the current study hemoglobin A1c level dropped from a very high-risk 12% to 10% and from 10% to 6.5%, and then remained normal and steady for a period of more than a year—indicating that the diabetes has been permanently controlled. The **treatment method** proposed in this book was seriously applied beginning June 2000. In 6 months time, amazingly the hemoglobin A1c dropped from 10% to 6.5% and remained normal since then.

Lowering hemoglobin A1c from very high value 12% to target value, below 7%, involved a great deal of self-discipline, diligence and continuous fine-tuning efforts on a daily basis by means of after-meal exercise. It is clear from the above-mentioned official blood test results of hemoglobin A1c that *permanent diabetes control* can be successfully accomplished.

Official Blood Test Results of Cholesterols (mmol/L)

Listed below are the official blood test results performed, with physician's requisition, by BC Biomedical Laboratories, Vancouver, BC, Canada. This table shows the evidence of how cholesterols were brought to normal.

Table 4.6 Official Blood Test Results of Cholesterols in mmol/L.
(Refer to **Table 4.7** for Cholesterols in mg/dL)

Date	Chol	LDL	HDL	HDL Ratio	TriGly	(1mmol/L = 38.67 mg/dL)		
Units	mmol/L	mmol/L	mmol/L	**Ratio**	mmol/L			
Normal	(2.0 - 5.2)	(1.5 - 3.4)	(>0.9)	(< 5.0)	(< 2.3)			
1-Jan-97	10.3							
11-Jun-97	8.1	5.9	1.5	5.4	1.6			
18-Mar-98						Suffered Heart Attack		
19-Mar-98						1st Angioplasty Done		
26-Mar-98						2nd Angiplasty Done		
21-Apr-98	5.8					Severe Angina Pain Started		
						Heart Disease (diagnosed)		
26-Jun-98						Angiogram Done		
						Left Artery 75% Blocked		
						Surviving with Nitro Spray		
1-Jul-98						Prevention Diet Started		
4-Aug-98	5.1					(Dr. Dean Ornish)		
26-Oct-98	6.3	4.1	0.9	7.0	2.8			
3-Dec-98						Self-Prevention Diet Started		
22-Jan-99	3.9	2.3	1.0	3.9	1.3	Mild Angina Pain		
5-May-99	4.6	2.9	1.2	3.8	1.2	Angina Pain is Gone		
7-Jun-00	5.4	3.3	1.2	4.5	2.0	No More Angina Pain		
						No More Nitro Spray		
29-Jun-00	4.2	2.4	1.1	3.8	1.5	Reversed Heart Disease		
19-Jan-01	4.3	2.6	1.2	3.6	1.0			
11-Jun-01	4.8	2.9	1.2	4.0	1.6			
29-Nov-01	5.1	3.2	1.2	4.2	1.5			
16-Jan-02	4.9	2.9	1.1	4.5	1.9			
2-Oct-02	4.8	2.9	1.1	4.4	1.8			

Official Blood Test Results of Cholesterols (mg/dL)

Listed below are the official blood test results performed, with physician's requisition, by BC Biomedical Laboratories, Vancouver, BC, Canada. This table shows the evidence of how cholesterols were brought to normal.

Table 4.7   Official Blood Test Results of Cholesterols in mg/dL
(Refer to **Table 4.6** for Cholesterols in mmol/L)

Date	Chol	LDL	HDL	HDL Ratio	TriGly	(1mmol/L = 38.67 mg/dL)		
Units	mg/dL	mg/dL	mg/dL	Ratio	mg/dL			
Normal	(77 - 201)	(58 - 131)	(>34.8)	(< 5.0)	(< 89)			
1-Jan-97	398.30							
11-Jun-97	313.23	228.15	58.01	5.4	61.87			
18-Mar-98						Suffered Heart Attack		
19-Mar-98						1st Angioplasty Done		
26-Mar-98						2nd Angiplasty Done		
21-Apr-98	224.29					Severe Angina Pain Started		
						Heart Disease (diagnosed)		
26-Jun-98						Angiogram Done		
						Left Artery 75% Blocked		
						Surviving with Nitro Spray		
1-Jul-98						Prevention Diet Started		
4-Aug-98	197.22					(Dr. Dean Ornish)		
26-Oct-98	243.62	158.55	34.80	7.0	108.28			
3-Dec-98						Self-Prevention Diet Started		
22-Jan-99	150.81	88.94	38.67	3.9	50.27	Mild Angina Pain		
5-May-99	177.88	112.14	46.40	3.8	46.40	Angina Pain is Gone		
7-Jun-00	208.82	127.61	46.40	4.5	77.34	No More Angina Pain		
							No more Nitro Spray		
29-Jun-00	162.41	92.81	42.54	3.8	58.01	Reversed Heart Disease		
19-Jan-01	166.28	100.54	46.40	3.6	38.67			
11-Jun-01	185.62	112.14	46.40	4.0	61.87			
29-Nov-01	197.22	123.74	46.40	4.2	58.01			
16-Jan-02	189.48	112.14	42.54	4.5	73.47			
2-Oct-02	185.62	112.14	42.54	4.4	69.61			

Table 4.8 **Up-To-Date Official Blood Test Results of Dr. RK**

Date	Fasting Glucose	Fasting Glucose	Hemoglobin A1c
Units	mmol/L	mg/dL	g/g Hgb (%)
Normal	(3.6 - 6.1)	(65 – 110)	4.5% - 6.2%
03-Aug-2011	4.9	88.2	6.0%
01-Nov-2011	3.9	70.2	5.8%
01-Feb-2012	3.9	70.2	5.5%
01-May-2012	4.4	79.2	5.5%
01-Aug-2012	3.7	66.7	5.5%
23-Oct-2012	4.1	73.8	5.5%
17-Jan-2013	4.3	77.4	5.3%
01-May-2013	2.9	52.2	5.6%
21-Aug-2013	5.1	91.8	5.5%
02-Jan-2014	4.2	75.8	5.8%
01-Apr-2014	4.0	72.0	5.9%
02-Jul-2014	4.7	84.8	5.7%
01-Oct-2014	3.6	64.8	5.5%
02-Jan-2015	4.9	88.2	5.4%
01-Apr-2015	4.7	84.8	5.4%
03-Jul-2015	5.3	84.8	5.6%
01-Oct-2015	4.1	73.8	5.8%
02-Jan-2016	5.7	102.6	5.8%
01-Apr-2016	4.4	79.2	5.6%
02-Jul-2016	5.5	99.0	5.9%
01-Oct-2016	5.3	95.4	5.0%
			Personal Best
05-Jan-2017	5.1	91.8	5.6%
02-Apr-2017	5.5	99.0	5.4%
02-Jul-2017	4.5	81.0	5.6%
02-Jan-2018	4.2	75.6	5.7%
03-Apr-2018	4.8	86.4	5.9%
02-Jul-2018	4.6	82.8	5.7%
01-Oct-2018	3.4	61.2	5.7%
02-Jan-2019	4.7	84.8	5.5%
01-Apr-2019	3.9	70.2	5.6%
30-Jun-2019	4.2	85.6	5.5%
01-Oct-2019	4.8	86.4	5.6%

FREQUENTLY ASKED QUESTIONS
1. How would a diabetic person know that his/her diabetes is controlled?

Answer: Hemoglobin A1c is the indicator of diabetes control. When the value of hemoglobin A1c from a recent blood test has been found to be normal, below 7%, that means the average blood glucose level for the last 90 days has been below 8.3 mmol/L or below 150 mg/dL (**See Table 5.1, chapter5**). This indicates that the diabetes has been controlled for the last 3 months. If the hemoglobin A1c has been kept normal (below 7%) for an extended period of time (1 year or more), then the diabetes is said to be tightly controlled. When a highly knowledgeable diabetic person is living with tightly controlled diabetes for an extended period of time, and is determined to control diabetes for the rest of his/her life, his/her diabetes is said to be permanently controlled.

2. a. How diabetics can benefit from the current research findings?
b. Can this treatment be used for both Type 1 and Type 2 diabetes?

Goal: The goal of a diabetic person should be to lower after-meal glucose levels to normal within one or two hours and keep them normal for an extended period of time, up to 6 hours. Lowering after-meal glucose levels would bring the hemoglobin A1c close to its normal value and as a result control diabetes effectively. A consistent hemoglobin A1c value (below 7%) for long periods (1 year or more) means the diabetes has been permanently controlled. It can remain controlled forever with a reasonable attention to insulin, food and after-meal exercise. The research usually takes 3 to 6 months with good organizational skills. This goal can be accomplished by both Type 1 or Type 2 diabetics.

This book however does not recommend any specific treatment that is commonly applicable to all diabetics. The current research findings reveal the fact that every diabetic person, after an extensive research phase of 3 to 6 months similar to the one outlined in this book, can develop and accomplish his/her own method of diabetes control. This book provides with a step-by-step procedure to research and accomplish healthy lifestyle on an individual basis.

The individual has to do research first and find out how high the blood glucose levels are and how long they remain high soon after a major meal (usually an evening dinner) is consumed. If he/she finds that the glucose levels are too high for a significant period of time (3 to 6 hours), then immediate action is required. This research should be continued diligently for 3 to 6 months through consuming a variety of heavy meals of his/her choice in an attempt to optimize insulin dose through introducing one hour of after-meal exercise. By doing so, a diabetic can not only lower the after-meal glucose level quickly to normal but in addition can keep them normal for an extended period of time, up to 6 hours.

Insulin-dependent diabetics (Both Type 1 and Type 2)
a. A diabetic person should learn how to take a rapid-acting insulin shot such as Humalog. Through frequent fingerstick blood glucose monitoring data, he/she should try to lower after-meal glucose levels and keep them normal for a significant period of time (up to 6 hours).
b. Use the trial and error procedure, described in a flow sheet, in page 99, and learn how to cut insulin dose up to 60%.
c. Read and understand thoroughly all examples of Chapter 3.

Non-insulin-dependent diabetics (Type 2)

a. A Type 2 diabetic person who takes oral medications should do exercise (either treadmill or walking) to lower the after-meal glucose levels as described in Chapter 3. Exercise alone may help lower after-meal glucose levels for some diabetics whose pancreas is active and producing insulin.

b. The individual should research diligently for 3 to 6 months through consuming a variety of heavy meals and figure out his/her own steps to control after-meal glucose levels. Lowering after-meal glucose levels would bring the hemoglobin A1c close to its normal value and as a result control diabetes. When the oral medications do not keep the diabetes under tight control, a Type 2 diabetic should switch to insulin shots with an attempt to lower after-meal glucose levels.

c. Read and understand thoroughly all examples of Chapter 3.

3. It seems the treatment procedure is extensive and could consume a lot of time and effort every day to control diabetes. How can a person find that much time to devote to diabetes care?

Answer: It takes a lot of time only while doing research for 3 to 6 months. However, health is more important than anything else. The person who works hard in doing research will be rewarded for the rest of his/her life. He/she can live in the near future without diabetes complications. To implement the current treatment, a diabetic person must first commit to healing diabetes, then work with determination for 3 to 6 months to collect all the necessary fingerstick blood glucose data in order to find out the optimal insulin dose for several meals of his/her own interest. Once the research is completed, the person can manage the diabetes with only a few fingerstick blood tests per day while producing outstanding results. Through rigorous control, hemoglobin A1c levels will gradually drop to normal in 3 to 6 months, glucose levels will be stabilized, and the individual will become motivated, get used to the treatment and will indeed realize that **controlling diabetes is an interesting and enjoyable task**.

4. Why don't we do exercise some other time and rest after meals?

Answer: For an insulin-dependent diabetic person, exercise should not be performed on an empty stomach because glucose levels could go too low and could lead to the dilemma of hypoglycemia. If the person decides to skip exercise after the meals, then the rapid-acting insulin (Humalog) dose has to be more than doubled to bring glucose levels to normal, which is not a good practice in diabetes control. Too much insulin constricts arteries leading to heart attack and heart disease. Too much insulin also stimulates the brain, makes the person feel hungry, tempts the person to eat more and causes the liver to manufacture fat in the belly. Exercise cuts the insulin dose by 50%, 60% or more, maximizes the insulin action and lowers after-meal glucose levels quickly to normal. More importantly, exercise should be introduced soon after the meal because only by lowering after-meal glucose levels can hemoglobin A1c and thereby the total diabetes be tightly controlled, as is proved to be the most effective and trustworthy treatment in the current "case study."

5. Are the recipes (meals) in this book recommended to other diabetics?

Answer: The purpose of this book is not to teach recipes that help maintain lower blood glucose levels. The goal here is not to consume low-sugar foods in order to avoid high blood glucose levels. Maybe those lower glucose levels with low-sugar foods are better than higher glucose levels, but they may not be the normal glucose levels. The goal here is to precisely bring after-meal glucose levels to normal through an adequate insulin dose and after-meal exercise. **Diabetics are allowed to eat any kind of food they enjoy.** <u>They can eat even in restaurants including high carbohydrate meals and desserts as long as they assume responsibility to inject adequate insulin dose and do after-meal exercise in order to bring after-meal glucose levels to normal within one or two hours.</u> There is no need to worry about recipes. However, some diabetics who experience high cholesterol and cardiovascular problems should follow the guidelines described in chapter 3 to keep their cholesterols normal. To follow the treatment plan described in this book, and to do research in the first 3 to 6 months, diabetics are advised to prepare their own recipes (meals) of their liking, learn how to calculate the calories and carbohydrate of the prepared meal, learn how to calculate the required rapid-acting insulin dose and understand thoroughly the trial and error procedure develope. **This kind of approach will enable diabetics to eat whatever food they like**.

6. How does a diabetic person manage when eating in a restaurant?

Answer: There are 3 methods being recommended.

First Method: Before going to a restaurant, call ahead and ask the restaurant manager or chef for nutritional information on menus (meals) they serve. Most famous restaurants have already published such information in their web sites. From that information, figure out the total calories and/or carbohydrate of a menu item of interest. Refer to chapter 3 where this aspect is discussed.

Then calculate the appropriate insulin (Humalog) dose as explained in this book. Carry an insulin pen (Humalog pen) to the restaurant and then inject the insulin just before consuming the meal. After coming home, monitor the glucose level after 1 hour and/or 2 hours, and take a second shot depending on how high the glucose level is. The second shot can be calculated from the difference between the current glucose level and normal glucose level. The very basic rule is that approximately 1 to 2 units of Humalog is required to lower 1 mmol/L (18 mg/dL) of glucose level. This rule can change and does not apply to insulin pump users. Frequent monitoring data gives many clues to find out exact dosage. Or, the person can divide the insulin dose into two parts. Inject the first part just before the meal in the restaurant, do the exercise 45 minutes or 1 hour after the meal is consumed, monitor the glucose level and then inject a second shot of Humalog as explained in this book (double shot experiments). This can keep the glucose levels normal up to 6 hours. Whenever exercise is planned, the first shot of insulin dose in the restaurant should be cut in half.

Second Method: If the nutritional information is not available beforehand, order the meal of interest to take home in the first attempt. After bringing it home, try to separate all items of the meal (meat, chicken or fish, starches, vegetables, soup, salad, fruit, drink, etc). Take the weight of each item and find out roughly the total calories, carbohydrate, fat and protein following the procedure explained in chapter 3. A lot of guesswork and approximation while weighing food items is required in this attempt. From this information, it is possible to determine the approximate insulin dose either including or excluding the exercise. Once this information is gathered, on the next attempt, the person can go in person and sit and eat in the restaurant. Again blood glucose should be monitored after 1 hour and/or 2 hours, and a second shot should be injected if needed. Whenever exercise is planned, the first shot of insulin dose should be cut in half.

Example (Fictitious): Elza is 64-year-old female. She has been Type 2 diabetic for 15 years and switched to insulin shots 6 months ago. She lives in New Westminster, BC, Canada, where she knew a restaurant called "Old Spaghetti Factory." She is cautious with her health and is practicing **diabetes control**. She ordered and brought her evening meal home at 5:15 pm. She separated all the meal items: baked chicken, spaghetti, soup, garlic bread, lettuce, tomatoes, and measured the weight of each item. From the calorie-counter table, she calculated approximately 1150 as the total calories. She calculated her insulin dose as 23 units (1150/500 * 10 = 23). Because she planned to exercise, her insulin dose required was 11.5 units (half of 23 units). She took 5.8 units of Humalog (half of 11.5 units) before she ate at 5:30 pm. Her level rose to 12.6 mmol/L or 226.8 mg/dL one hour after the meal. She walked for 1 hour in her neighborhood. She monitored her levels every half an hour. After 1 hour of walking, her blood glucose level dropped to 5.5 mmol/L or 102.6 mg/dL. She then injected a second shot, about 5.8 units of Humalog. Her levels remained normal until midnight. She then took 15 units of Humulin-N, ate one Savory Garlic Matzo (fat free and cholesterol free) and baby carrots as her bedtime snack, and went to sleep. By next morning, her level was 4.6 mmol/L or 82.8 mg/dL (perfect normal).

Next time when she goes to the same restaurant (Old Spaghetti Factory), she can sit and eat in the restaurant without panic. She can order the same meal and inject 5.8 units of Humalog twice (before meal and after exercise). Or she can inject 23 units of Humalog (11.5 units before meal and 11.5 units after one or two hours) if she is not planning to exercise. Her diabetes will remain controlled.

Third Method: A trial and error procedure can be applied if the person is stuck outside somewhere and is unable to know about total calories or carbohydrate content in order to pre-determine the insulin dose. If the meal to be consumed is heavy, the person can inject about 10 units of Humalog (which is guessed to be approximately half of the total actual insulin dose required) with an insulin pen just before the meal is consumed in the restaurant. After coming home from the restaurant, the person can monitor the glucose 1 hour and/or 2 hours after the meal is consumed. Depending on the level of glucose, the person can inject a second shot of insulin, or even a third shot, to further lower the glucose level to normal. Or the person can do the exercise first, monitor the glucose level and then inject a second shot of Humalog after the exercise as explained in this book in order bring the glucose levels to normal within 2 hours of the meal. Again whenever exercise is planned, the first insulin dose should be cut in half.

Example (Fictitious): Raymond, a 52-year-old athletic person, used to be a very active football player and wrestler. Three years ago, he was diagnosed with Type-2 diabetes. Raymond chose to take insulin shots to control his diabetes effectively. Raymond was on his way home driving from Seattle, WA, United States to Vancouver, BC, Canada. It was 5:30 pm. It would take another hour to get home. He was hungry and decided to eat. He drove into a highway restaurant in Bellingham and ate a lot of food from the buffet (salad bar, pasta, chicken, sushi, tempura, fruit salad, dessert and beer). He injected 10 units of Humalog with his insulin pen just before the meal. He finished his meal by 6 pm. He got home at 7 pm, and monitored his blood glucose level. It was very high: 15.5 mmol/L or 279 mg/dL. He wanted to go to the gym and do treadmill. But he had already read the book *Permanent Diabetes Control* in which **he learned that he should not do exercise if his blood glucose level is above 13 mmol/L or 234 mg/dL because ketones would accumulate**. He therefore injected another shot of Humalog, about 4 units, and drove to the gym in half an hour (7:30 pm), where he monitored his level again as 12.5 mmol/L or 225 mg/dL. He then exercised (ran on treadmill at high speed) for 1 hour, and found his glucose level dropped to 4.9 mmol/L or 88.2 mg/dL by 8:30 pm. He got home by 9 pm and monitored his level again. The level had risen to 8.1 mmol/L or 151.2 mg/dL. He injected another shot, 4 more units of Humalog, and watched TV. By 9:30 am his level had dropped to 5.3 mmol/L or 95 mg/dL and remained normal till 11:45 pm. He then injected 15 units of intermediate-acting insulin Humalog-N, ate fresh carrots and a few dried apricots (bedtime snack), and went to sleep. By 7 am the next morning, his level was 5.5 mmol/L or 98 mg/dL.

Raymond made clear notes on items he consumed in the restaurant and all insulin shots injected so that next time he can consume the same meal and manage his insulin shots comfortably. Raymond eats in the restaurant to his fullest satisfaction twice a week, and his diabetes is still tightly controlled.

7. Can the athletes benefit from this treatment plan?

Answer: Most certainly! Athletes are most likely to benefit from this treatment plan. Athletes are stronger and are easily adaptable to exercise. They can consume any kind of food they like. All they need to do is exercise soon after the meal in order to precisely bring their blood glucose level to normal and to keep it normal for an extended period of time. They do not even have to worry about fingerstick blood glucose monitoring so many times. Read the following:

During the research phase of 3 to 6 months, the participant (the author of this book) monitored his fingerstick blood glucose levels 10 or more times a day in order to find out his own optimal parameters. He successfully brought down his hemoglobin A1c level from a very high-risk 12% to a stunning 6.5% and since then the level has remained normal for more than a year—indicating that his diabetes has been permanently controlled. His A1c level is now 6.2%.
After the completion of his research phase, as he was rewarded by his own monitoring and researching experience, the same participant skillfully monitors his fingerstick blood glucose levels only a few times a day, still his diabetes is tightly controlled. He is confident that his diabetes will surely remain tightly controlled forever. This is what the *permanent diabetes control* is all about.

8. Is this treatment applicable to older and disabled people?
Answer: The answer is "yes." The concept of lowering after-meal glucose levels will work for any diabetic person of any age. If the person is not capable of running on a treadmill, he/she can walk or do other exercises of interest. For example, swimming is also an excellent exercise. If the person is unable to walk or exercise at all (totally disabled), he/she can then adjust the insulin dose as explained in this case study. For example in this study, for tofu meal or fish meal, with treadmill exercise or walking about 10 units of Humalog was enough to lower after-meal glucose levels. Without exercise or walking, about 25 units of Humalog were needed to lower after-meal glucose levels for the same meal consumed. Even the totally disabled people can do exercise by rotating the upper arm on which insulin

was injected in order to stimulate the insulin action. Again, this has to be determined through an extensive research (monitoring and recording with several doses for a given meal). If the person is seriously ill or more severely disabled, low-fat and low-calorie diet should be consumed. Lower calories of the meal means lower insulin dose. In this way, the insulin dose can be reduced and/or minimized.

9. Can diabetes be cured permanently with this treatment?

Answer: The straight answer is "no." There is no permanent cure thus far for diabetes. However the experience gained through the extensive research that is unavoidably required in applying the treatment presented in this book, will certainly guide the individual to manage and control diabetes forever. This treatment is even better than a so-called permanent cure through a surgery because the surgical results do not last forever and the side effects of the drugs prescribed immediately after a surgery are unbearably painful.

10. Without following this extensive treatment, can a diabetic person achieve results by taking some insulin dose recommended by his doctor or nurse?

Answer: In most cases the results are not achievable. Diabetes requires self-controlling skills. The doctor or nurse would not know what kind of junk food the diabetic person consumes now and then. Elevated glucose levels even for short periods on a daily basis contribute to an abnormal value of hemoglobin A1c.

Preparing or ordering an appropriate meal of known calories or carbohydrate content, the ability to guess or calculate and adjust the insulin doses, self-blood testing skills, record keeping, after-meal exercise, researching the recorded glucose levels and ability to take prompt decisions on "insulin, food and exercise" are the most important habits required in implementing the treatment outlined in this book.

APPENDIX-4A

REAL-LIFE CASE STUDY
▶ **SELF-BLOOD GLUCOSE MONITORING TABLES**
▶ **SELF-BLOOD GLUCOSE MONITORING GRAPHS**
▶ **NUTRITIONAL COMPOSITION OF MEALS** (Chicken Meal, Tofu Meal, Fish Meal, Turkey Meal)

WHY ARE AFTER-MEAL BLOOD GLUCOSE LEVELS NOT TOO HIGH? AN IMPORTANT CLARIFICATION

By examining the self-blood glucose monitoring data in Chapter 4 (Real-Life Case Study), a reader might wonder and raise a question such as "why are the after-meal blood glucose levels not significantly high enough in the collected glucose data?". Most of the data showed in this book have after meal-glucose levels under 13 mmol/L or 234 mg/dL.

HERE IS THE EXPLANATION

(i) All the fingerstick blood glucose data were collected after consuming the healthy diet (low carbohydrate diet) so the collected glucose levels were not too high, but however they are high enough to significantly raise or elevate hemoglobin A1c level.

(ii) In order to prevent the ketones formation, a diabetic person should not exercise when the blood glucose level is over 13 mmol/L or 234 mg/dL unless the exercise suits a person without forming ketones. Each person is different so each person should find out if exercise is causing ketones formation or not by doing the ketones test. To understand this, please refer to Chapter 3 (Method 3) where "Ketones Formation" and "Ketoacidosis" are explained. A diabetic person should be cautious beforehand and should not exercise when the after-meal glucose levels are higher than 13 mmol/L or 234 mg/dL, unless the exercise suits his/her body without forming ketones. A diabetic person should inject the correct amount of insulin just before consuming a major meal so that the after-meal glucose spike would be close to or below 13 mmol/L or 234 mg/dL, and then exercise in order to lower his/her after-meal blood glucose level to perfectly normal (5 mmol/L or 90 mg/dL). That is why in all the self-blood glucose monitoring data, you will find the after-meal blood glucose levels below 13 mmol/L or 234 mg/dL.

AN EXAMPLE OF EATING WHITE RICE

● When a diabetic person eats white rice with starchy vegetables, 30 minutes after the meal consumption, the after-meal blood glucose level could reach 20 mmol/L or 360 mg/dL, or even more. With brown rice and starchy vegetables, the after-meal blood glucose level could reach up to 15 mmol/L or 270 mg/dL. Therefore a diabetic person should never eat white rice. Brown rice is okay, but it still needs serious glucose control with appropriate amount of insulin and exercise.

● However, if you have expert knowledge on diabetes control, you can knowingly eat white rice, desserts, or any high-carbohydrate meal, can perfectly control diabetes with insulin and exercise, and can live like a normal person forever.

SELF-BLOOD GLUCOSE MONITORING TABLES

CHICKEN MEAL Tables 4.10 To 4.16

Table 4.10   No Insulin and No Exercise.
Glucose levels remained too high for 5 hours.
At 23:00, 7 units of Humalog injected to lower glucose levels.

Breakfast	7:15		Time	7:15	12:00	17:50	23:00	23.55
Lunch	12:10		Insulin (Units)	15 N	4 H		7 H	15 N
Supper	18:00			N = Humulin-N		H = Humalog		

Time	7:15	12:00	17:45	18:45	19:05	19:25	19:45	20:05
Glucose (mmol/L)	5.8	5.6	4.6	11.9	12.5	12.1	11.6	10.8
Glucose (mg/dL)	104.4	100.8	82.8	214.2	225.0	217.8	208.8	194.4
Time	20:30	21:30	22:00	23:30	24:00			Ave
Glucose (mmol/L)	11.0	10.8	10.9	7.9	6.3			9.4
Glucose (mg/dL)	198.0	194.4	196.2	142.2	113.4			168.6

Ave = Average glucose level in 24 hours

Table 4.11   10 Units of Humalog and No Exercise.
Glucose levels remained high; not enough insulin.
At 23:30 walked to lower the glucose level.

Breakfast	7:15		Time	7:15	12:00	17:50	20.30	23.50
Lunch	12:00		Insulin (Units)	15 N	4 H	6 H	4 H	15 N
Supper	18:00			N = Humulin-N		H = Humalog		

Time	7:10	12:00	17:45	18:45	19:05	19:25	19:45	20:05
Glucose (mmol/L)	5.0	5.6	5.5	8.3	8.8	8.9	8.5	7.9
Glucose (mg/dL)	90.0	100.8	99.0	149.4	158.4	160.2	153.0	142.2
Time	20:30	21:30	22:00	23:30	24:00			Ave
Glucose (mmol/L)	6.6	7.1	7.5	7.2	5.0			6.7
Glucose (mg/dL)	118.8	127.8	135.0	129.6	90.0			120.3

Table 4.12   17 Units of Humalog and No Exercise.
Glucose levels remained normal for 6 hours, but too much insulin.
At 23:00 food was consumed to prevent any hypoglycemia.

Breakfast	7:20		Time	7:15	12:00	17:55	20.30	23.50
Lunch	12:00		Insulin (Units)	15 N	4 H	13 H	4 H	15 N
Supper	18:00			N = Humulin-N H = Humalog				

Time	7:15	12:00	17:50	18:45	19:05	19:25	19:45	20:05
Glucose (mmol/L)	5.5	4.8	5.2	7.1	6.1	5.3	5.6	5.5
Glucose (mg/dL)	99.0	86.4	93.6	127.8	109.8	95.4	100.8	99.0

Time	22:00	22:30	23:00	24:00				Ave
Glucose (mmol/L)	4.9	5.4	4.9					5.5
Glucose (mg/dL)	88.2	97.2	88.2					98.7

Table 4.13   4 Units of Humalog Plus Treadmill Exercise (Single Shot).
Glucose levels lowered to normal but rose after the exercise.
At 23:30, 4 units of Humalog injected to lower the glucose level.

Breakfast	7:20		Time	7:15	12:00	17:50	23:30	23.45
Lunch	12:10		Insulin (Units)	15 N	4 H	4 H	4 H	15 N
Supper	18:00			N = Humulin-N H = Humalog				

Speed: 3.3 mph; Calories Lost: 270

◄———————— Treadmill ————————►

Time	7:15	12:00	17:45	18:45	19:05	19:25	19:45	20:05
Glucose (mmol/L)	5.8	5.5	5.8	10.5	8.6	6.6	5.2	4.9
Glucose (mg/dL)	104.4	99.0	104.4	189.0	154.8	118.8	93.6	88.2

Time	20:30	21:30	22:30	23:30				Ave
Glucose (mmol/L)	6.9	8.8	9.2	6.9				7.1
Glucose (mg/dL)	124.2	158.4	165.6	124.2				127.1

Table 4.14   9 Units of Humalog Plus Treadmill Exercise (Double Shot).
Glucose levels remained normal for 6 hours.

Breakfast	7:15		Time	7:10	12:00	17:50	20:35	23.45
Lunch	12:10		Insulin (Units)	15 N	4 H	4 H	5 H	15 N
Supper	18:00			N = Humulin-N H = Humalog				

Speed: 3.3 mph; Calories Lost: 270

◄──────── Treadmill ────────►

Time	7:10	12:00	17:50	18:45	19:05	19:25	19:45	20:05
Glucose (mmol/L)	5.9	4.9	5.0	10.9	8.2	6.3	4.9	5.1
Glucose (mg/dL)	106.2	88.2	90.0	196.2	147.6	113.4	88.2	91.8

Time	20:30	21:30	22:30	23:30				Ave
Glucose (mmol/L)	7.1	6.2	5.4	5.1				6.3
Glucose (mg/dL)	127.8	111.6	97.2	91.8				112.5

Table 4.15   4 Units of Humalog plus Regular Walk (Single Shot).
Glucose levels lowered to normal but rose after 2 hours.
At 23:00, 4 units of Humalog injected to lower the glucose level.

Breakfast	7:15		Time	7:10	12:00	17:55	23:00	23.45
Lunch	12:05		Insulin (Units)	15 N	4 H	4 H	4H	15 N
Supper	18:00			N = Humulin-N H = Humalog				

Speed: 3.3 mph; Calories Lost: 270

◄──────── Walked ────────►

Time	7:10	12:00	17:50	18:45	19:05	19:25	19:45	20:05
Glucose (mmol/L)	4.1	5.0	5.5	10.9	8.4	6.8	5.4	5.2
Glucose (mg/dL)	73.8	90.0	99.0	196.2	151.2	122.4	97.2	93.6

Time	21:00	22:00	23:00	23:45				Ave
Glucose(mmol/L)	6.8	8.8	9.7	7.4				7.0
Glucose(mg/dL)	122.4	158.4	174.6	133.2				126.0

120

Table 4.16   9 Units of Humalog Plus Regular Walk (Double Shot).
Glucose levels remained normal for 6 hours.

Breakfast	7:20		Time	7:15	12:00	17:50	20:30	23.45
Lunch	12:00		Insulin (Units)	15 N	4 H	4 H	5 H	15 N
Supper	18:00			N = Humulin-N		H = Humalog		

Speed: 3.3 mph; Calories Lost: 270

←——— Walked ———→

Time	7:15	12:00	17:50	18:45	19:05	19:25	19:45	20:05
Glucose (mmol/L)	4.9	4.6	5.2	10.4	7.9	6.0	4.7	4.4
Glucose (mg/dL)	88.2	82.8	93.6	187.2	142.2	108.0	84.6	79.2

Time	20:30	21:30	22:30	23:30				Ave
Glucose (mmol/L)	6.6	5.4	4.9	5.0				5.8
Glucose (mg/dL)	118.8	97.2	88.2	90.0				105.0

TOFU MEAL   Tables 4.17 To 4.22

Table 4.17   No Insulin and No Exercise.
Glucose levels remained too high for 5 hours.
At 23:00, 8 units of Humalog injected to lower glucose levels.

Breakfast	7:25		Time	7:15	12:00	17:50	23.30	11.50
Lunch	12:00		Insulin(Units)	15 N	4 H		6H	15 N
Supper	18:00			N = Humulin-N		H = Humalog		

Time	7:15	12:00	17:50	18:45	19:05	19:25	19:45	20:05
Glucose (mmol/L)	5.0	5.6	5.5	12.7	13.5	13.2	12.5	12.6
Glucose (mg/dL)	90.0	100.8	99.0	228.6	243	237.6	225.0	226.8

Time	20:30	21:30	22:30	23:30				Ave
Glucose (mmol/L)	12.5	11.1	10.0	10.2				10.4
Glucose (mg/dL)	225.0	199.8	180.0	183.6				186.6

Ave = Average glucose level in 24 hours

Table 4.18   15 Units of Humalog and No Exercise.
Glucose levels remained high; Not enough insulin.
At 20:30, 5 units of Humalog injected to lower glucose levels.

Breakfast	7:20		Time	7:15	12:00	17:50	20.30	23.50
Lunch	12:00		Insulin(Units)	15 N	4 H	10 H	5 H	15 N
Supper	18:00			N = Humulin-N		H = Humalog		

Time	7:10	12:00	17:50	18:45	19:05	19:25	19:45	20:05
Glucose (mmol/L)	5.0	5.6	5.5	8.9	8.8	9.0	8.6	7.9
Glucose (mg/dL)	90.0	100.8	99.0	160.2	158.4	162.0	154.8	142.2

Time	20:30	21:30	22:30					Ave
Glucose(mmol/L)	8.2	8.6	7.5					7.6
Glucose(mg/dL)	147.6	154.8	135.0					136.8

Table 4.19   25 Units of Humalog and No Exercise.
Glucose levels remained normal for 6 hours, but too much insulin.
At 22:30, food was consumed to prevent any hypoglycemia.

Breakfast	7:20		Time	7:15	12:00	17:50	20.30	23.50
Lunch	12:00		Insulin(Units)	15 N	4 H	15 H	10 H	15 N
Supper	18:00			N = Humulin-N		H = Humalog		

Time	7:20	12:00	17:50	18:45	19:05	19:25	19:45	20:05
Glucose (mmol/L)	5.5	4.8	5.2	7.3	6.6	6.3	6.6	5.1
Glucose (mg/dL)	99.0	86.4	93.6	131.4	118.8	113.4	118.8	91.8
Time	20:30	21:30	22:30					Ave
Glucose (mmol/L)	4.7	5.1	4.2					5.6
Glucose (mg/dL)	84.6	91.8	75.6					100.5

Table 4.20   5 Units of Humalog Plus Treadmill Exercise (Single Shot).
Glucose levels lowered to normal but rose after the exercise.
At 23:00, 4 units of Humalog injected to lower the glucose level.

Breakfast	7:10		Time	7:10	12:00	17:50	23:00	23.45
Lunch	12:00		Insulin(Units)	15 N	4 H	5 H	4H	15 N
Supper	18:00			N = Humulin-N		H = Humalog		

Speed: 3.3 mph; Calories Lost: 270

←——————— Treadmill ——————→

Time	7:10	12:00	17:50	18:45	19:05	19:25	19:45	20:05
Glucose (mmol/L)	5.6	4.4	5.0	10.8	7.2	6.4	5.8	5.0
Glucose (mg/dL)	100.8	79.2	90.0	194.4	129.6	115.2	104.4	90.0
Time	20:30	21:30	22:30	23:30	23:45			Ave
Glucose (mmol/L)	8.0	10.8	9.9	7.9	7.0			7.2
Glucose (mg/dL)	144.0	194.4	178.2	142.2	126			129.9

Table 4.21   11 Units of Humalog Plus Treadmill Exercise (Double Shot).
Glucose levels remained normal for 6 hours.

Breakfast	7:15		Time	7:15	12:00	17:55	20:05	23.45
Lunch	12:10		Insulin(Units)	15 N	4 H	5 H	6 H	15 N
Supper	18:00			N = Humulin-N		H = Humalog		

Speed: 3.3 mph; Calories Lost: 270

◄———— Treadmill ————►

Time	7:15	12:00	17:50	18:45	19:05	19:25	19:45	20:05
Glucose (mmol/L)	5.6	4.9	5.2	10.4	7.5	6.1	5.5	5.1
Glucose (mg/dL)	100.8	88.2	93.6	187.2	135	109.8	99.0	91.8

Time	20:30	21:30	22:30	23:00				Ave
Glucose (mmol/L)	5.2	5.0	5.4	4.8				5.9
Glucose (mg/dL)	93.6	90.0	97.2	86.4				106.1

Table 4.22   11 Units of Humalog Plus Regular Walk (Double Shot).
Glucose levels remained normal for 6 hours.

Breakfast	7:15		Time	7:10	12:15	17:50	20:05	23.45
Lunch	12:20		Insulin(Units)	15 N	4 H	5 H	6 H	15 N
Supper	18:00			N = Humulin-N		H = Humalog		

Speed: 3.3 mph; Calories Lost: 270

◄———— Walked ————►

Time	7:10	12:00	17:50	18:45	19:05	19:25	19:45	20:05
Glucose (mmol/L)	5.8	4.8	5.2	10.9	7.9	6.8	5.6	5.1
Glucose (mg/dL)	104.4	86.4	93.6	196.2	142.2	122.4	100.8	91.8

Time	20:30	21:30	22:30	23:00				Ave
Glucose (mmol/L)	5.5	5.0	4.2	4.0				5.9
Glucose (mg/dL)	99.0	90.0	75.6	72.0				106.2

FISH MEAL   Tables 4.23 To 4.30

Table 4.23   No Insulin and No Exercise.
Glucose levels remained too high for 5 hours.
At 23:00, 8 units of Humalog injected to lower glucose levels.

Breakfast	7:15		Time	7:15	12:00	17:50	23:30	23.55
Lunch	12:10		Insulin(Units)	15 N	4 H		8 H	15 N
Supper	18:00			N = Humulin-N		H = Humalog		

Time	7:15	12:00	17:45	18:45	19:05	19:25	19:45	20:05
Glucose (mmol/L)	5.8	5.3	5.7	14.9	12.9	13.4	14.5	14.1
Glucose (mg/dL)	104.4	95.4	102.6	268.2	232.2	241.2	261.0	253.8
Time	20:30	21:30	22:00	23:30	24:00			Ave
Glucose (mmol/L)	12.9	12.8	12.6	10.2	6.5			10.9
Glucose (mg/dL)	232.2	230.4	226.8	183.6	117.0			196.1

Ave = Average glucose level in 24 hours

Table 4.24   15 Units of Humalog and No Exercise.
Glucose levels remained high; Not enough insulin.

Breakfast	7:20		Time	7:15	12:00	17:55	20.30	11.50
Lunch	12:00		Insulin(Units)	15 N	4 H	10 H	5 H	15 N
Supper	18:00			N = Humulin-N		H = Humalog		

Time	7:10	12:00	17:50	18:45	19:05	19:25	19:45	20:05
Glucose (mmol/L)	4.3	5.4	6.1	9.5	8.8	7.9	8.0	8.5
Glucose (mg/dL)	77.4	97.2	109.8	171.0	158.4	142.2	144.0	153.0
Time	20:30	21:30	22:30	23:30				Ave
Glucose (mmol/L)	8.2	8.8	7.9	7.7				7.6
Glucose (mg/dL)	147.6	158.4	142.2	138.6				136.7

Table 4.25   25 Units of Humalog and No Exercise.
Glucose levels remained normal for 6 hours, but too much insulin.

Breakfast	7:20		Time	7:15	12:00	17:55	21.00	11.50
Lunch	12:00		Insulin(Units)	15 N	4 H	15 H	10 H	15 N
Supper	18:00			N = Humulin-N		H = Humalog		

Time	7:20	12:00	17:50	18:45	19:05	19:25	19:45	20:05
Glucose (mmol/L)	5.8	5.5	4.9	8.8	7.1	5.3	6.2	6.1
Glucose (mg/dL)	104.4	99.0	88.2	158.4	127.8	95.4	111.6	109.8
Time	20:30	21:30	22:30	23:30				Ave
Glucose (mmol/L)	6.0	5.5	5.3	6.1				6.1
Glucose (mg/dL)	108.0	99.0	95.4	109.8				108.9

Ave = Average glucose level in 24 hours

Table 4.26   5 Units of Humalog Plus Treadmill Exercise (Single Shot).
Glucose levels lowered to normal but rose after the exercise.
At 23:30, 4 units of Humalog injected to lower the glucose level.

Breakfast	7:10		Time	7:10	12:00	17:55	20:30	23.45
Lunch	12:00		Insulin(Units)	15 N	4 H	6 H	4 H	15 N
Supper	18:00			N = Humulin-N		H = Humalog		

Speed: 3.3 mph; Calories Lost: 270
◄─────────── Treadmill ───────────►

Time	7:10	12:00	17:50	18:45	19:05	19:25	19:45	20:05
Glucose (mmol/L)	5.9	4.4	5.3	11.4	8.8	6.8	5.9	5.6
Glucose (mg/dL)	106.2	79.2	95.4	205.2	158.4	122.4	106.2	100.8
Time	20:30	21:30	22:30	23:30	23:45			Ave
Glucose (mmol/L)	8.8	10.4	11.6	10.8	9.9			8.1
Glucose (mg/dL)	158.4	187.2	208.8	194.4	178.2			146.2

Table 4.27   11 Units of Humalog Plus Treadmill Exercise (Double Shot).
Glucose levels remained normal for 6 hours.

Breakfast	7:15		Time	7:15	12:00	17:50	20:05	23.45
Lunch	12:10		Insulin(Units)	15 N	4 H	6 H	7 H	15 N
Supper	18:00			N = Humulin-N		H = Humalog		

Speed: 3.3 mph; Calories Lost: 270

◄──────── Treadmill ────────►

Time	7:15	12:00	17:45	18:45	19:05	19:25	19:45	20:05
Glucose (mmol/L)	5.6	4.9	5.2	11.2	8.9	7.2	6.0	5.4
Glucose (mg/dL)	100.8	88.2	93.6	201.6	160.2	129.6	108	97.2
Time	20:30	21:30	22:30	23:30				Ave
Glucose (mmol/L)	5.2	5.0	5.4	5.2				6.3
Glucose (mg/dL)	93.6	90.0	97.2	93.6				112.8

Table 4.28   11 Units of Humalog Plus Regular Walk (Double Shot).
Glucose levels remained normal for 6 hours.

Breakfast	7:15		Time	7:10	12:15	17:50	20:05	23.45
Lunch	12:20		Insulin(Units)	15 N	4 H	6 H	7 H	15 N
Supper	18:00			N = Humulin-N		H = Humalog		

Speed: 3.3 mph; Calories Lost: 270

◄──────── Walked ────────►

Time	7:10	12:00	17:45	18:45	19:05	19:25	19:45	20:05
Glucose (mmol/L)	5.3	4.4	5.5	10.6	8.3	6.2	5.6	5.3
Glucose (mg/dL)	95.4	79.2	99.0	190.8	149.4	111.6	100.8	95.4
Time	20:30	21:30	22:30	23:30				Ave
Glucose (mmol/L)	6.0	5.5	5.6	4.9				6.1
Glucose (mg/dL)	108.0	99.0	100.8	88.2				109.8

Table 4.29   No Insulin Injected. Treadmill Exercise for 1 Hour.
                      Glucose levels remained high; No significant drop in levels.
                      At 20:05, 7 units of Humalog injected to lower the glucose level.

Breakfast	7:15		Time	7:10	12:15	17:55	20:05	23.45
Lunch	12:20		Insulin(Units)	15 N	4 H	0 H	7 H	15N
Supper	17:55			N = Humulin-N		H = Humalog		

Speed: 3.3 mph; Calories Lost: 270

←———————— Treadmill ————————→

Time	7:10	12:00	17:45	18:45	19:05	19:25	19:45	20:05
Glucose (mmol/L)	5.2	4.4	5.7	11.9	11.6	10.7	10.6	10.0
Glucose (mg/dL)	93.6	79.2	102.6	214.2	208.8	192.6	190.8	180

Time	20:30	21:00	22:00	23:00				Ave
Glucose (mmol/L)	5.7	5.5	5.6	5.3				7.7
Glucose (mg/dL)	102.6	99.0	100.8	95.4				138.3

Table 4.30   No Insulin Injected. Treadmill Exercise for 1 Hour.
                      Humulin-N was discontinued for 24 hours (previous day).
                      Glucose levels remained high; No significant drop in levels.
                      At 20:05, 7 units of Humalog injected to lower the glucose level.

Breakfast	7:15		Time	7:10	12:15	17:50	20:05	23.45
Lunch	12:20		Insulin(Units)	0 N	0 H	0 H	7 H	15 N
Supper	18:00			N = Humulin-N		H = Humalog		

Speed: 3.3 mph; Calories Lost: 270

←———————— Treadmill ————————→

Time	7:10	12:00	17:45	18:45	19:05	19:20	19:50	20:05
Glucose (mmol/L)	6.6	7.7	9.4	12.7	12.4	11.5	10.6	9.9
Glucose (mg/dL)	118.8	138.6	169.2	228.6	223.2	207	190.8	178.2

Time	20:30	21:00	22:00	23:00				Ave
Glucose (mmol/L)	6.0	5.5	5.6	4.9				8.6
Glucose (mg/dL)	108.0	99.0	100.8	88.2				154.2

SELF-BLOOD GLUCOSE MONITORING GRAPHS
The data collected by the diabetic person were plotted and the results interpreted.

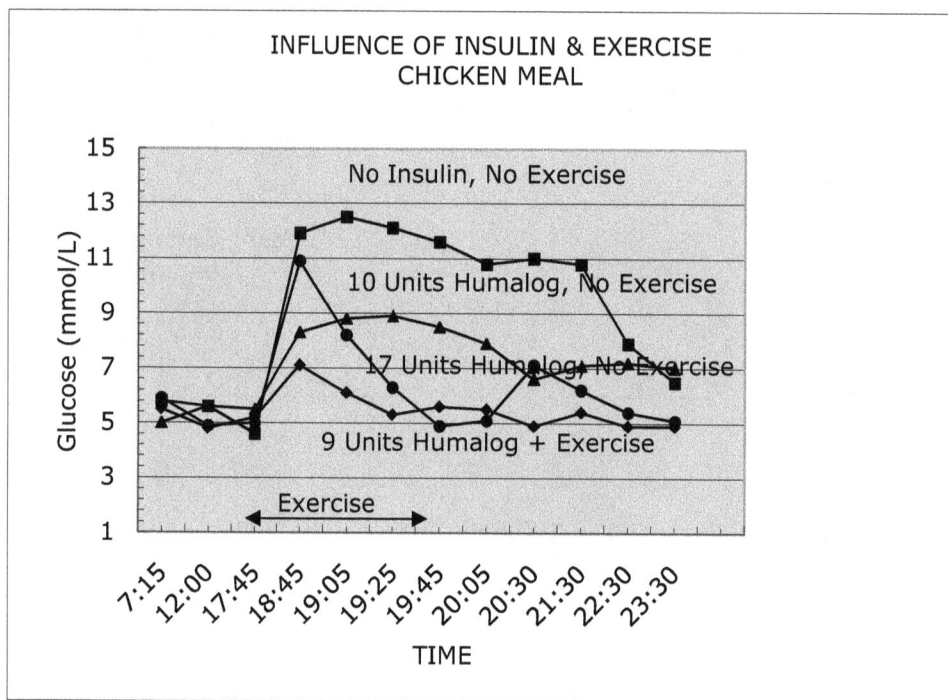

Figure 4.10 Treadmill or regular walk cut the insulin dose almost in half.
And maintained the after-meal glucose levels normal for 6 hours.

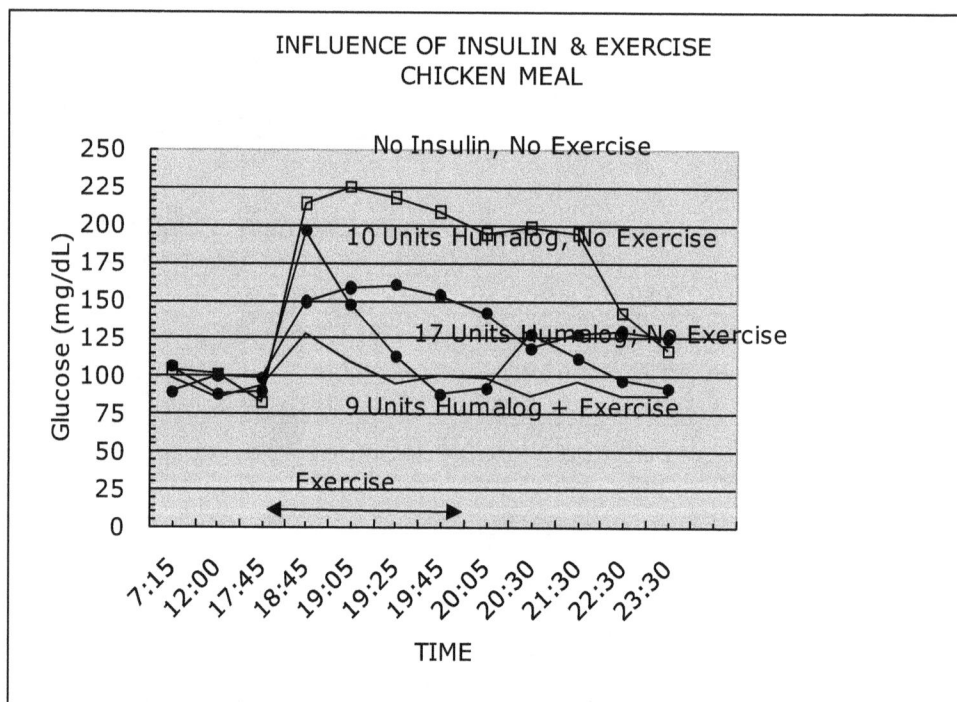

Figure 4.11   Treadmill or regular walk cut the insulin dose almost in half.
And maintained the after-meal glucose levels normal for 6 hours.

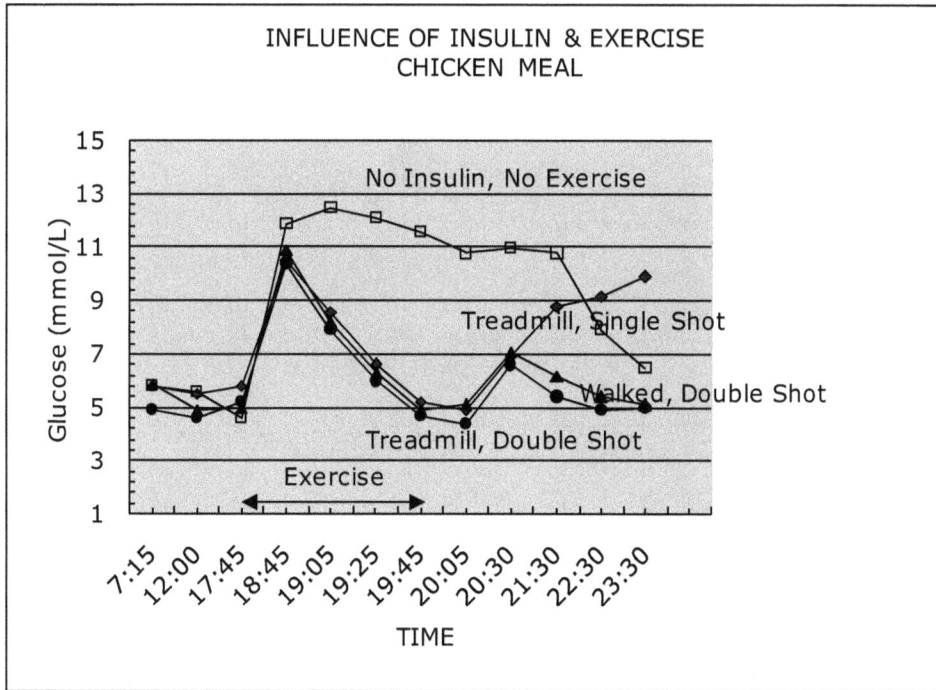

INFLUENCE OF INSULIN & EXERCISE
CHICKEN MEAL

Figure 4.12   Treadmill or regular walk with double shot was proved to be the best.
Lowered the after-meal glucose levels to normal for 6 hours.

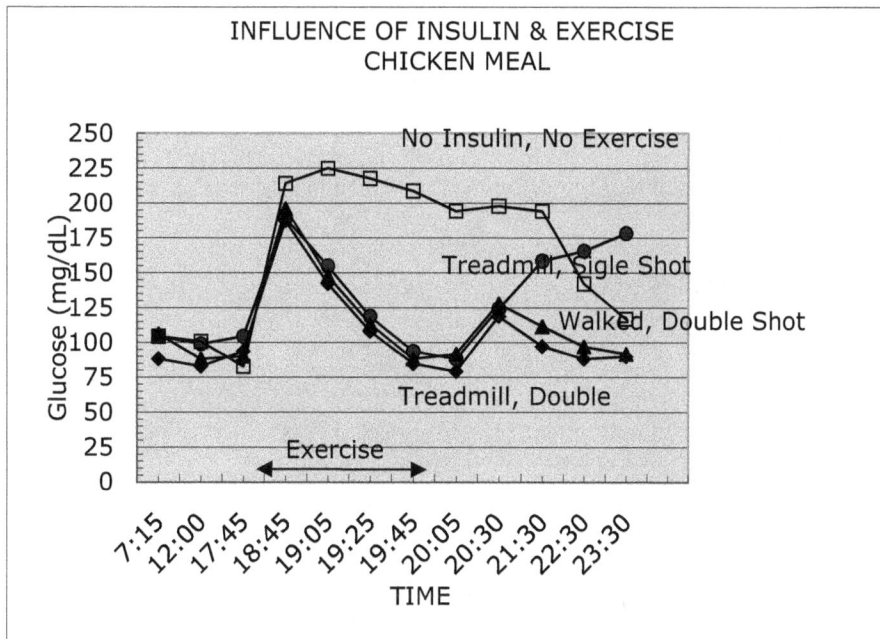

INFLUENCE OF INSULIN & EXERCISE
CHICKEN MEAL

Figure 4.13   Treadmill or regular walk with double shot was proved to be the best.
Lowered the after-meal glucose levels to normal for 6 hours.

130

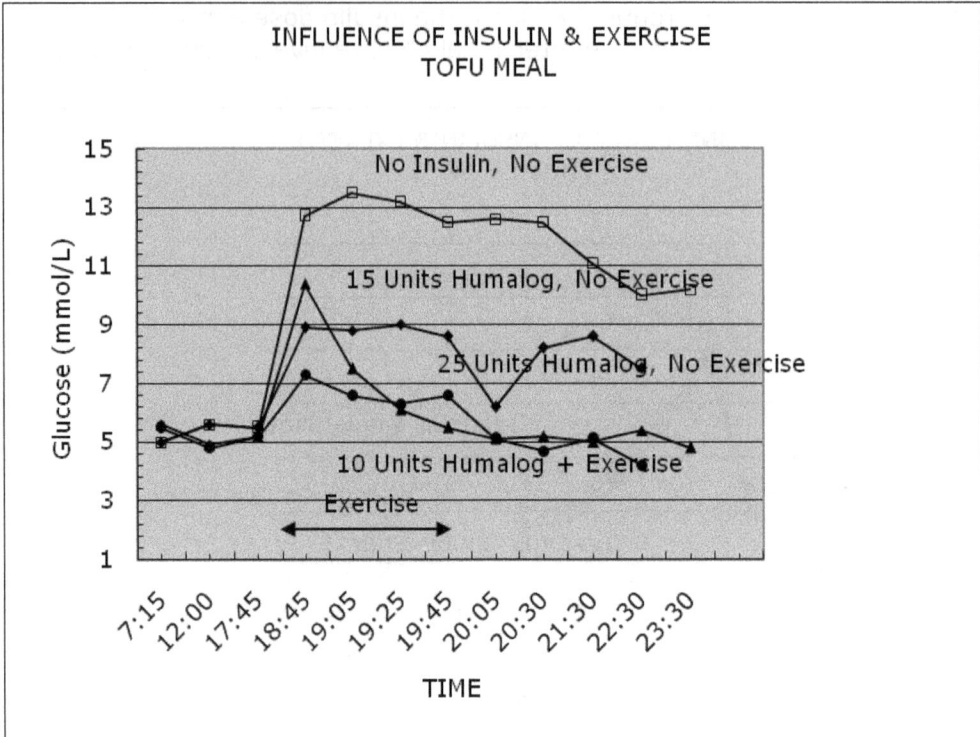

Figure 4.14   Treadmill or regular walk cut the insulin dose by 60%.
             And maintained the after-meal glucose levels normal for 6 hours.

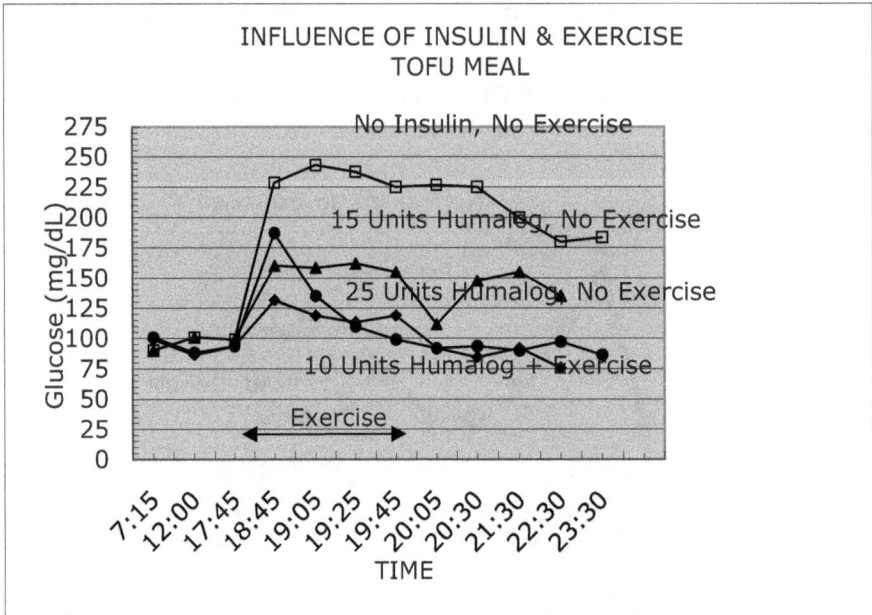

Figure 4.15   Treadmill or regular walk cut the insulin dose by 60%.
             And maintained the after-meal glucose levels normal for 6 hours.

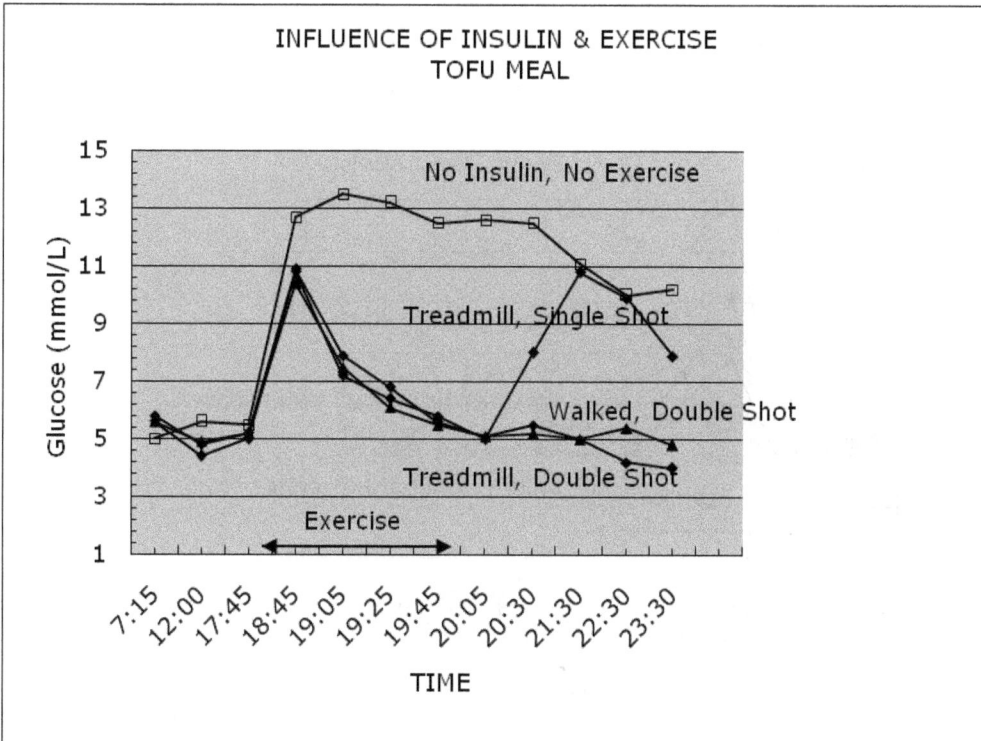

Figure 4.16 Treadmill or regular walk with double shot was proved to be the best. Lowered the after-meal glucose levels to normal for 6 hours.

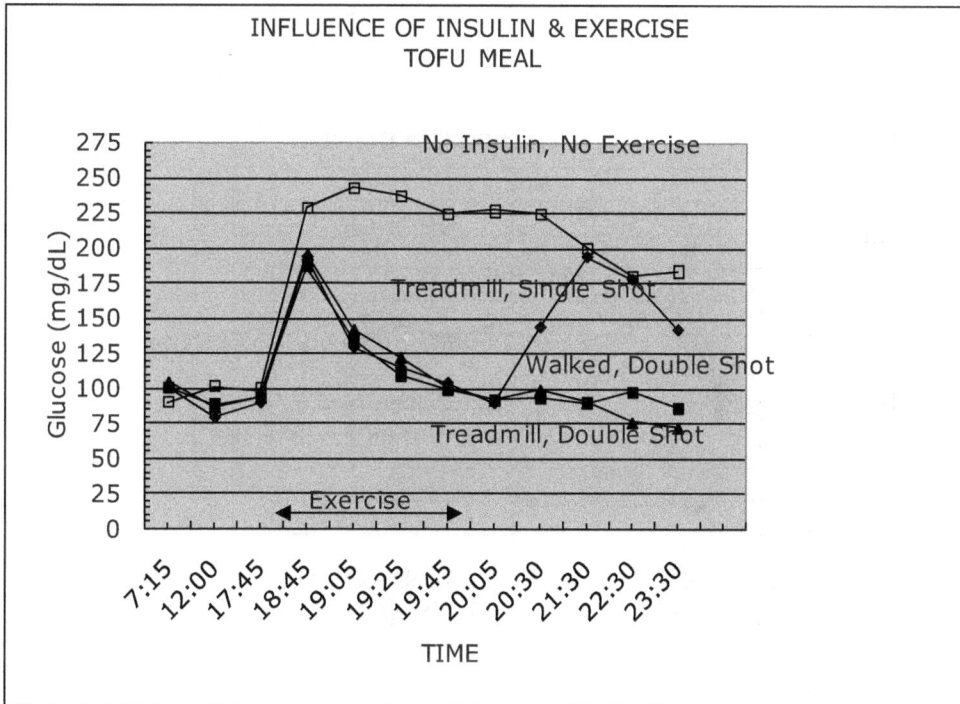

Figure 4.17 Treadmill or regular walk with double shot was proved to be the best. Lowered the after-meal glucose levels to normal for 6 hours.

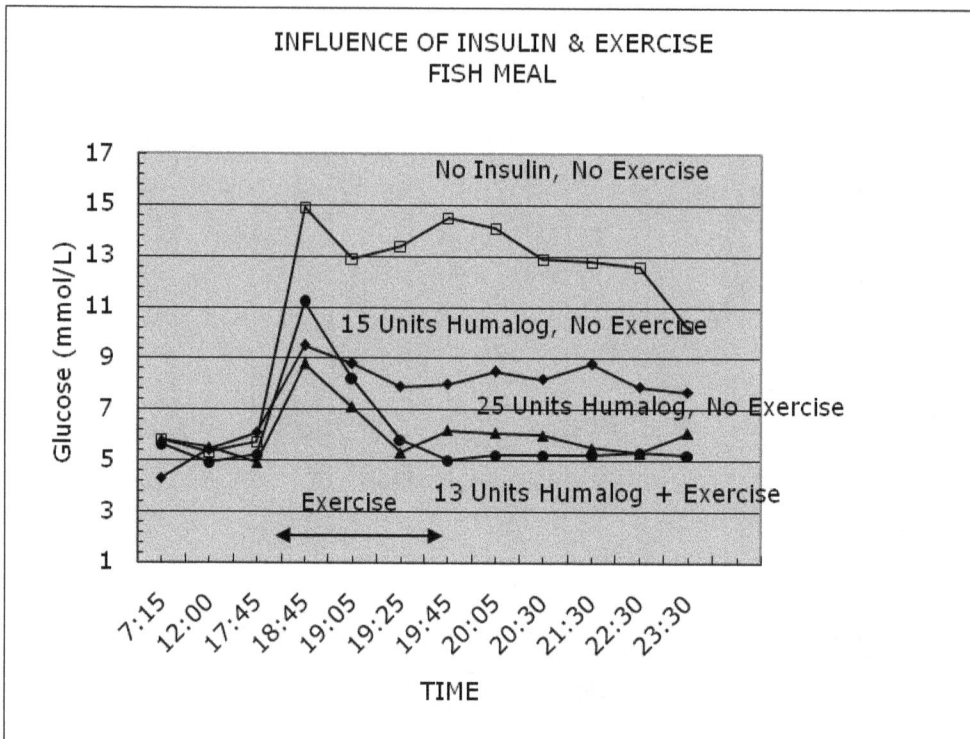

Figure 4.18   Treadmill or regular walk cut the insulin dose almost in half, and maintained the after-meal glucose levels normal for 6 hours.

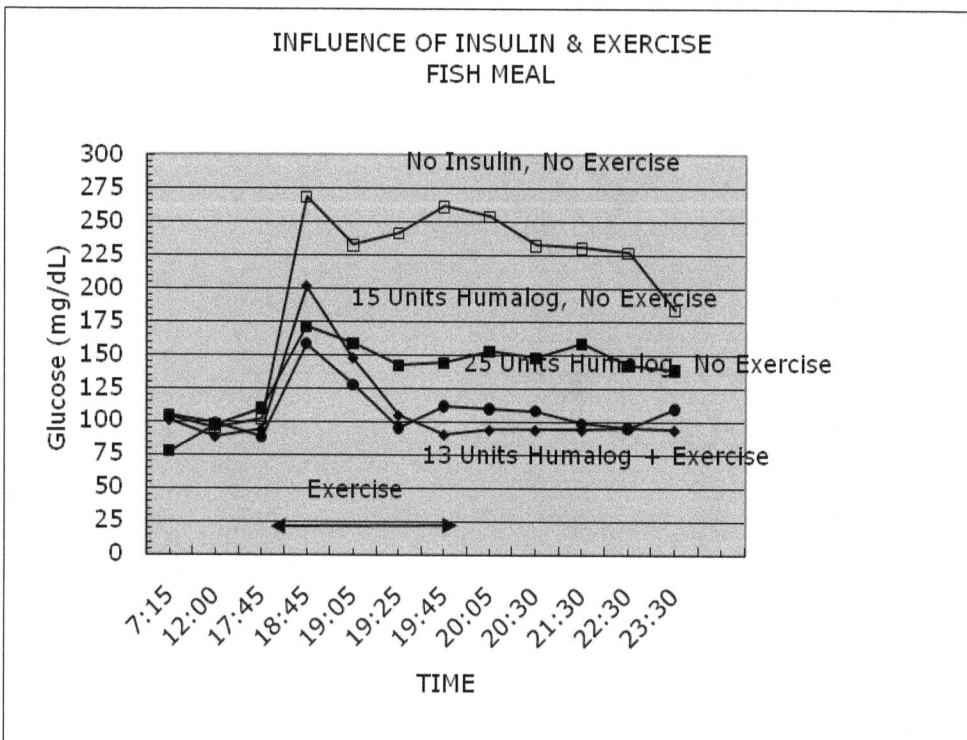

Figure 4.19   Treadmill or regular walk cut the insulin dose almost in half, and maintained the after-meal glucose levels normal for 6 hours.

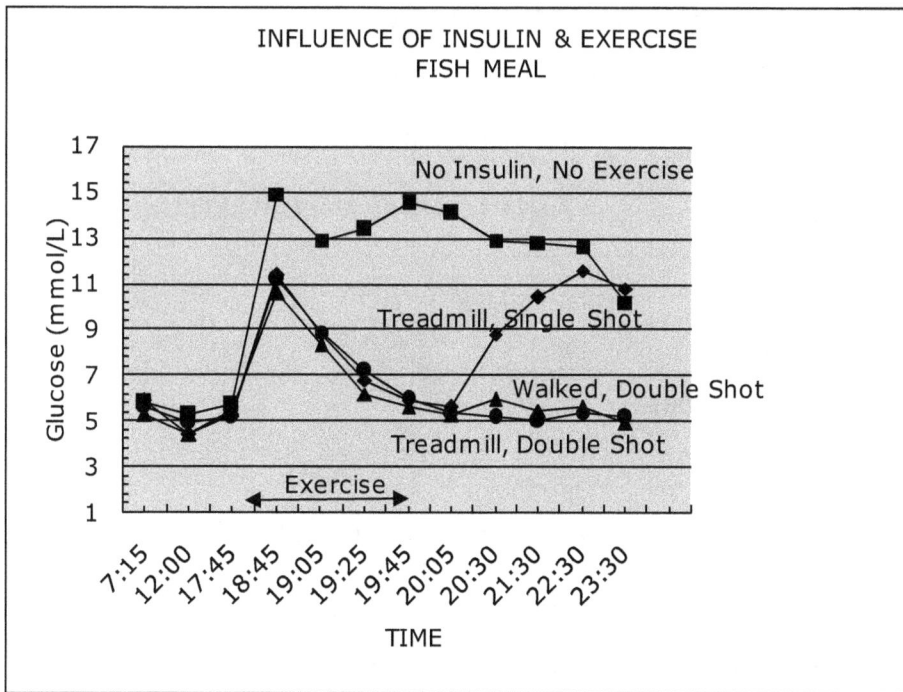

Figure 4.20   Treadmill or regular walk with double shot was proved to be the best. Lowered the after-meal glucose levels to normal for 6 hours.

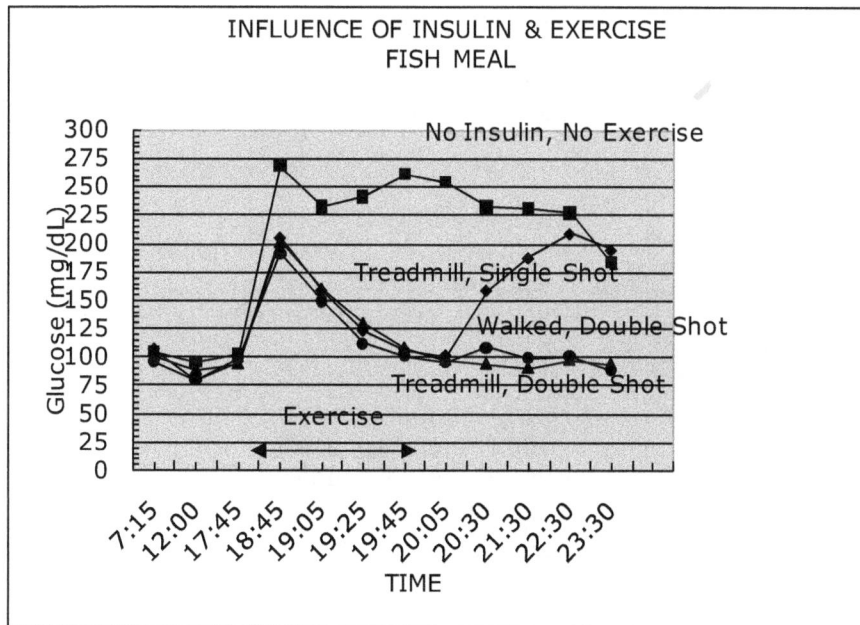

Figure 4.21   Treadmill or regular walk with double shot was proved to be the best. Lowered the after-meal glucose levels to normal for 6 hours.

RECIPES AND NUTRITIONAL COMPOSITION OF MEALS
Chicken Meal, Tofu Meal, Fish Meal, Turkey Meal

Table 4.31   Sources of the nutritional composition for all foods studied.

FOOD ITEM	NUTRITIONAL INFORMATION SOURCE
Chicken (skinless) Fish (salmon) Turkey (skinless) Broccoli, Mushrooms, Onion, Tomato, Lemon Juice	Dean Ornish, MD Program For Reversing Heart Disease, Ivy Books Pages: 555-585, 1996, ISBN: 0-8041-1038-7.
Garlic	Lynn Sonberg, The Complete Nutrition Counter, Berkley Books, Page 204, New York, 1993.
Brown Rice (Long Grain)	Purchased in Safeway http://www.safeway.com/ Produced by Western Rice Mills 8599 Fraser St, Vancouver, BC, Canada Tel: 604-321-0338 or 1-877-321-7423
Tofu (Firm Tofu)	Jayone Foods, Inc., Paramount, CA-90723
Soy Milk (Fat Free)	Soya World Inc., Vancouver, BC, Canada, V6B-3X5 1-888-401-0019 www.sogoodbeverage.com
Udo's Oil (Udo's Choice) Ultimate Oil Blend	Flora Manufacturing 7400 Fraser Park Drive Burnaby, BC, Canada, V5J-5B9 1-888-436-6697 www.florahealth.com
Turbo Cooker	Turbo Cooker™ Customer Service 12 Commercial St., Hicksville, NY-11801 Tel: 1-516-433-9143 www.turbocooker.com/ContUS.htm

RECIPES AND NUTRITIONAL COMPOSITION OF MEALS
Chicken Meal, Tofu Meal, Fish Meal & Turkey Meal

Table 4.32 Chicken Meal - Nutritional Composition
All items were weighed with an electronic balance before cooked.

Food Item	Weight (gm)	Calories	Protein (gm)	Fat (gm)	Carbo (gm)
Chicken (skinless, boneless)	100	182.14	32.86	5.0	0
Brown Rice (long grain)	125	452.5	7.68	3.46	94.88
Mushrooms	100	28.57	2.71	0.29	4.43
Broccoli	100	34	4	0.36	5.85
Onion (fresh)	100	38	1.53	0.12	8.71
Garlic (fresh)	30	32	0	0	8
Tomato (medium-sized)	150	30	1.5	0.3	6.5
Soymilk (fat free) 1/4 cup	62.5	25.5	2.13	0.063	4.0
Salt	2	0	0	0	0
Cayenne Pepper	2	0	0	0	0
Udo's Oil (1 tsp)	15	135	0.2	14.5	0
Lemon Juice (2 tsp) + water	30	8	0.2	0	2.4
Total →	816.50	965.71	52.81	24.09	134.77
Calories calculated →		967.13	211.22	216.83	539.08
Percentage (%) →			22%	22%	56%

Table 4.33   Tofu Meal - Nutritional Composition
All items were weighed with an electronic balance before cooked.

Food Item	Weight (gm)	Calories	Protein (gm)	Fat (gm)	Carbo (gm)
Tofu (firm)	100	59.65	7.02	1.75	4.21
Brown Rice (long grain)	125	452.5	7.68	3.46	94.88
Mushrooms	100	28.57	2.71	0.29	4.43
Broccoli	100	34	4	0.36	5.85
Onion (fresh)	100	38	1.53	0.12	8.7
Garlic (fresh)	30	32	0	0	8
Tomato (medium-sized)	150	30	1.5	0.3	6.5
Soymilk (fat free) 1/4 cup	62.5	25.5	2.13	0.063	4.0
Salt	2	0	0	0	0
Cayenne Pepper	2	0	0	0	0
Udo's Oil (1 tsp)	15	135	0	14.5	0
Lemon Juice(2 tsp) + water	30	8	0.2	0	2.4
Total →	816.5	843.22	26.765	20.84	138.97
Calories calculated →		850.52	107.06	187.58	555.88
Percentage (%) →			13%	22%	65%

Table 4.34   Fish Meal - Nutritional Composition
All items were weighed with an electronic balance before cooked.

Food Item	Weight (gm)	Calories	Protein (gm)	Fat (gm)	Carbo (gm)
Fish (salmon fillet)	100	171.43	27.50	5.71	0
Brown Rice (long grain)	125	452.5	7.68	3.46	94.88
Mushrooms	100	28.57	2.71	0.29	4.43
Broccoli	100	34	4	0.36	5.85
Onion (fresh)	100	38	1.53	0.12	8.71
Garlic (fresh)	30	32	0	0	8
Tomato (medium-sized)	150	30	1.5	0.3	6.5
Soymilk (fat free) 1/4 cup	62.5	25.5	2.13	0.063	4.0
Salt	2	0	0	0	0
Cayenne Pepper	2	0	0	0	0
Udo's Oil (1 tsp)	15	135	0	14.5	0
Lemon Juice (2 tsp) + water	30	8	0.2	0	2.4
Total →	816.5	955	47.245	24.80	134.77
Calories calculated →		951.28	188.98	223.22	539.08
Percentage (%) →			20%	23%	57%

Table 4.35   Turkey Meal - Nutritional Composition
All items were weighed with an electronic balance before cooked

Food Item	Weight (gm)	Calories	Protein (gm)	Fat (gm)	Carbo (gm)
Turkey (skinless)	100	160.71	33.21	2.5	0
Brown Rice (long grain)	125	452.5	7.68	3.46	94.88
Mushrooms	100	28.57	2.71	0.29	4.43
Broccoli	100	34	4	0.36	5.85
Onion (fresh)	100	38	1.53	0.12	8.7
Garlic (fresh)	30	32	0	0	8
Tomato (medium-sized)	150	30	1.5	0.3	6.5
Soymilk (fat free) 1/4 cup	62.5	25.5	2.13	0.063	4.0
Salt	2	0	0	0	0
Cayenne Pepper	2	0	0	0	0
Udo's Oil 1 tsp	15	135	0	14.5	0
Lemon Juice (2 tsp) + water	30	8	0.2	0	2.4
Total →	816.5	944.28	52.96	21.59	134.76
Calories calculated →		945.19	211.82	194.33	539.04
Percentage (%) →			22%	21%	57%

REFERENCE

1. Permanent Diabetes Control (Book), Subtitle: The Complete Guide to Living Like A Normal Person Forever, Authored by Rao Konduru, MS, PhD, Reviewed and Endorsed by Dr. Marshal Dahl, MD, PhD., Endocrinologist, Faculty of Medicine, University of British Columbia, Vancouver, British Columbia, Canada, First Published in 2003. www.mydiabetescontrol.com

2nd Part of the Book Begins Here!
2nd Part of the Book Contains Very Important Information!

A Person With Diabetes Must Understand Thoroughly
(i) FOOD CONSUMPTION AND NUTRITIONAL CONTROL
(ii) ORAL MEDICATIONS AND INSULIN SHOTS
(iii) DAILY EXERCISE
2nd Part of the Book Is Designed to Help You Understand All About It!

2nd Part of the Book Contains 6 Chapters	
The Following 6 Chapters Will Give You All the Tools Necessary to Fight and Control Diabetes Permanently!	
CHAPTER 5	**HUMAN DIGESTIVE SYSTEM & KIDNEYS: HOW DO THEY FUNCTION?**
CHAPTER 6	**HOW TO READ LABELS AND COUNT CALORIES?**
CHAPTER 7	**a. WHAT ARE FATS AND CHOLESTEROL?** **b. HOW TO PREVENT HIGH CHOLESTEROLS & HEART DISEASE?**
CHAPTER 8	**a. EAT WHOLE FOODS ONLY!** **b. AVOID PROCESSED FOODS AND REFINED FOODS!** **c. LEARN HOW TO LOSE WEIGHT!** **d. LOWER YOUR BODY MASS INDEX TO NORMAL!**
CHAPTER 9	**DIABETES MEDICATIONS** **a. Oral Medications (for Type 2 Diabetes)** **b. Insulin (for Type 2 Diabetes & Type 1 Diabetes)**
CHAPTER 10	**EXERCISE WITH DIABETES** **[Exercise is the Invisible Insulin for Diabetic People]**

2nd Part of the Book Begins Here!
2nd Part of the Book Contains Very Important Information!

A Person With Diabetes Must Understand Thoroughly
(i) FOOD CONSUMPTION AND NUTRITIONAL CONTROL
(ii) ORAL MEDICATIONS AND INSULIN SHOTS
(iii) DAILY EXERCISE
2nd Part of the Book Is Designed to Help You Understand All About It!

CHAPTER 5 HUMAN DIGESTIVE SYSTEM & KIDNEYS

TABLE OF CONTENTS

INTRODUCTION [1]

Food is a wonder medicine. In ancient times, until the discovery of insulin in 1921 diabetes was controlled by means of a diet plan. The foods we eat give us the energy and scope based on which we survive on the planet Earth today. A diabetic person should be more knowledgeable about food than a non-diabetic person. Knowing the effects, both good and bad, that various foods have on one's health from one's own research is an essential part of diabetes care. Only through a thorough understanding of the influence of various foods on blood glucose levels and self-disciplined daily eating habits, can diabetes be reasonably controlled. A diabetic person should at first educate himself/herself and understand what the human digestive system is all about.

THE HUMAN DIGESTIVE SYSTEM [1]

The amazing human body is composed of roughly 206 bones, 600 muscles, 10,000 nerve fibers, 2 million optic nerve fibers, 100 billion nerve cells, 30 trillion blood cells, 62,000 miles in total length of blood vessels, capillaries and arteries, and so on.[1] All body parts, which work together round the clock (24 hours a day 7 days a week), need energy to survive. The food along with water that humans consume on a daily basis is transformed into gruel, a thin liquid formed with the help of enzymes by the wonderfully structured and beautifully designed digestive system. The role of the human digestive system is to produce nutrients from any food being consumed.

Please refer to Figure 3.1. The human digestive system is comprised of main organs and accessory organs. Main organs include the mouth, esophagus, stomach, small intestine, large intestine, rectum and anus. Accessory organs are the tongue, salivary glands, liver, gall bladder and pancreas. Each organ participates in the digestion process, releasing necessary enzymes for digestion and each organ performs its function individually and in conjunction with other organs.

The raw or cooked food consumed first enters the alimentary canal, which is simply a one-way tube with the entrance being the mouth and the exit being the anus. The mechanical digestion of food, chewing and crushing with teeth, takes place in the mouth. The crushed food is then mixed with the enzyme called saliva produced by 3 pairs of salivary glands located in the mouth. The chemical digestion of carbohydrate begins in the mouth. The food then enters the stomach by passing through the esophagus. Within the stomach linings, there are several types of cells performing various functions. The parietal cells produce hydrochloric acid, which kills most bacteria and promotes protein digestion. The gastric glands produce an important enzyme called gastric juice that stimulates the secretion of hydrochloric acid. The stomach functions like a naturally equipped pressure vessel or reactor with thorough agitation and mixing. Further mechanical digestion takes place in the stomach and gruel (a thin liquid) is formed. This gruel from the stomach enters the small intestine where most of the digestion takes place. An adult small intestine is about 7 meters (23 feet) long. The gruel mixes with more enzymes such as pancreatic juice produced by the pancreas. The gruel also mixes with the bile produced by the liver. The acids contained in the bile are responsible for digesting fats. The gall bladder stores bile and releases it into the small intestine where chemical digestion of carbohydrates, proteins and lipids takes place and sugars, amino acids and fatty acids are separated.

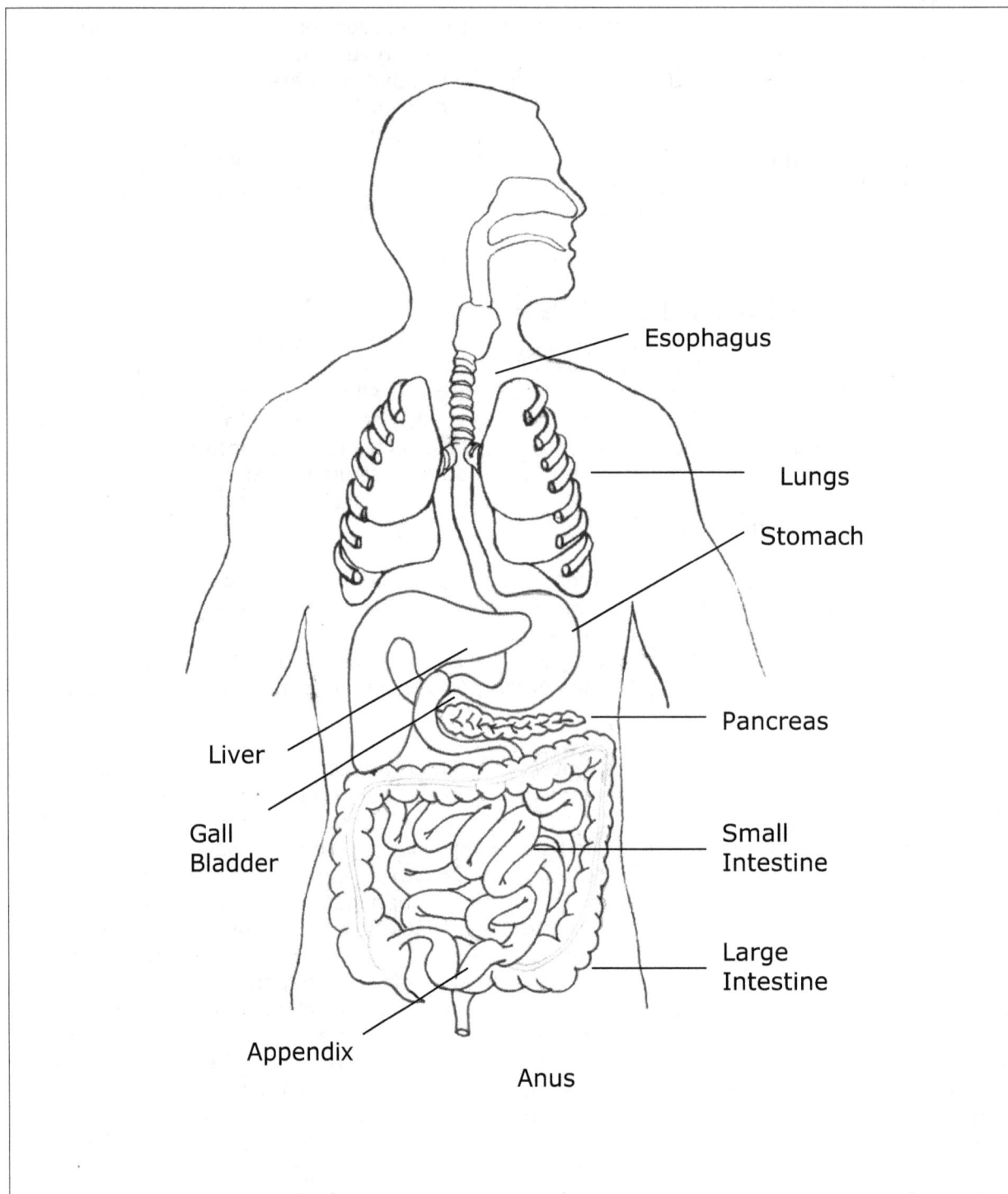

Figure 5.1 Human Digestive System.

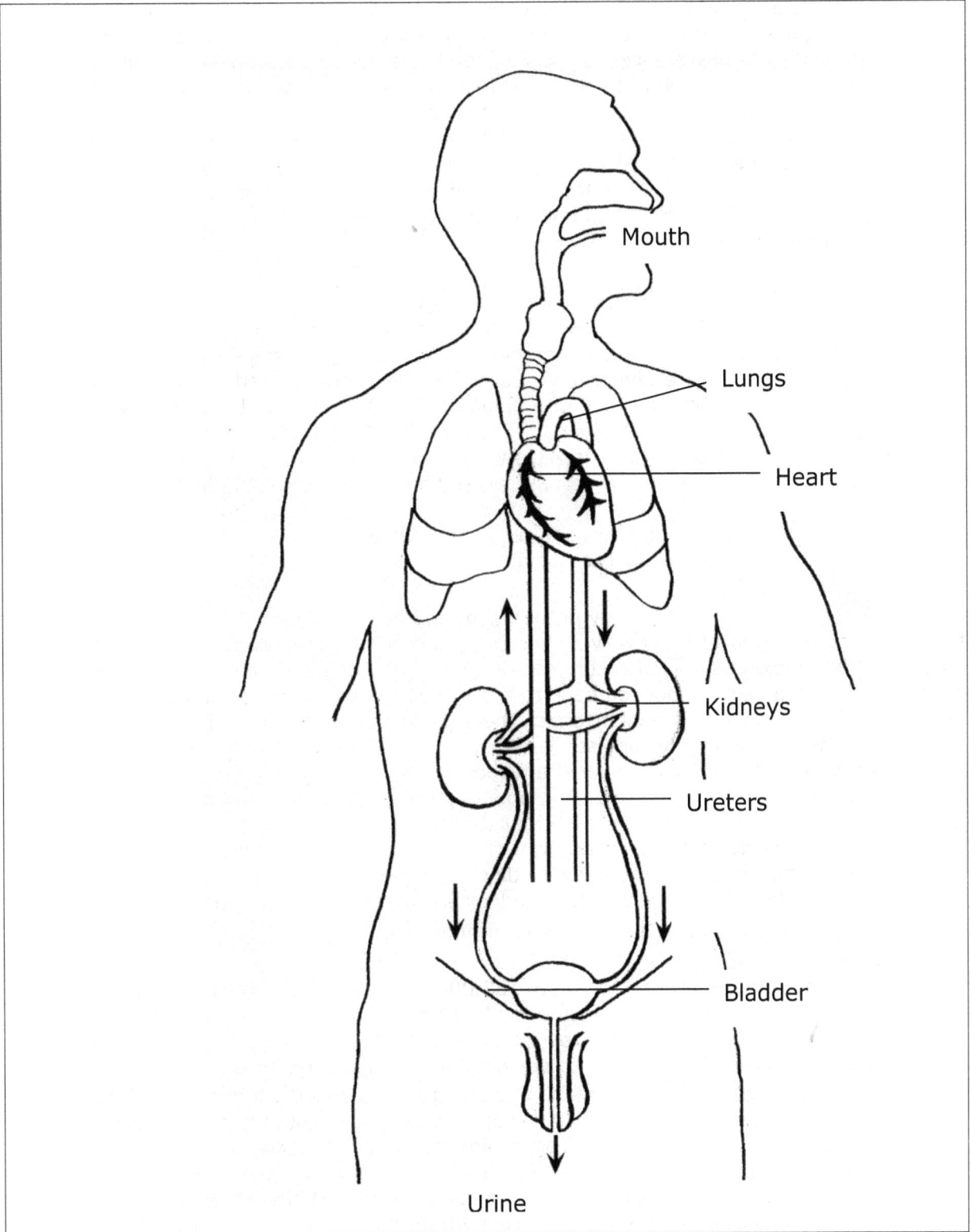

Figure 5.2 Kidneys and the Urinary System.

The final product, consisting of nutritious elements, thus obtained by the digestive system is absorbed into the small intestinal walls and transported by means of a vein to the liver which processes and converts it into energy, and supplies it to the cells of the human body as nourishment. The undigested food and spare water are then pushed into the large intestine that consists of the ascending colon, the transverse colon, the descending colon, the rectum and the anus. The large intestine is about 5 feet in length and 3 inches in diameter. The large intestine absorbs the water and sends it back to the bloodstream. The filtered gruel is then squeezed further, solidified and propelled into the colon. The solid waste (feces) is pushed further along. The feces are temporarily stored in the rectum and later sent into the anus from where they are evacuated. The food after consumption spends about 10 hours in the small intestine and 20 hours in the large intestine before the waste is evacuated through the anus.

KIDNEYS AND THE URINARY SYSTEM [1]

The human body is 55% to 60% water by weight, and this water in the body must be purified 60 times a day and replaced once every 5 to 10 days. Kidneys do this job. Kidneys filter about 180 liters of water every day. Water is the essential ingredient in every process that is required to transform the food into blood. Kidneys are one of the two major sets of paired organs, the other pair being lungs. The architect of the human body purposely planned lungs and kidneys as pairs perhaps with one goal in mind, that is the "backup system." If one organ fails the other organ can still function to keep the body alive.

The kidneys are two bean-shaped organs reddish brown in color the size of a fist located in the middle of the back just below the ribcage.

Blood carries the nutrients of energy produced by the human digestive system and oxygen from the lungs in order to fuel every body's cells, and picks up metabolic waste products such as carbon dioxide and lactic acid, including dead and damaged cells, pollutants, microbes, etcetera being deposited back to the bloodstream. The heart pumps the dirty blood to the kidneys via the renal arteries. The kidneys purify the dirty blood miraculously by means of millions of highly sophisticated tiny built-in filters called "nephrons" and returns about 80% of the clean water back to the bloodstream. The purified blood is thus returned back to the heart via veins. The heart distributes purified blood all around the body via the arteries. It takes one to two minutes to circulate purified blood all around the body. Two ureters carry the waste material called urine from the kidneys to the bladder. Up to 1.5 liters of urine finally leaves the body every day. The bladder is like an expandable bag with thin spongy muscle walls. Whenever the bladder is emptied by passing urine through a tube called the urethra, the bladder shrinks to its original size.

The purified blood travels around the body 168,000 miles per day in order to supply about 60 trillion cells of the human body. Inside the heart are four chambers and each chamber acts like a pump. The heart pumps blood about 103,000 times a day. In the hands and feet, the blood is transferred from arteries to veins before it is returned to the heart.
Here it is important to note, for the diabetic person's information, that partly digested food in the small intestine consists of nutrients such as glucose obtained from carbohydrate digestion, amino acids obtained from protein digestion and fatty acids obtained from fat digestion, all of which are carried to the liver. The liver then converts these nutrients into glucose, and most of this glucose (about 90%) comes from carbohydrate. This is why, immediately after consumption of a high carbohydrate meal, the blood glucose level rises dramatically.

DIGESTION TIMES: The following table shows the digestion times (approximate time spent in stomach) of generally classified foods. This table gives a rough idea of relative digestion times when comparing one class of foods to another. The actual digestion times vary significantly from person to person and also depending on whether the food is eaten individually or in combination with other items. [60] Any improper combination could delay digestion several more hours. Digestion time can be accelerated by exercise.

Table 5.1 Digestion Times.

Fruit properly combined	15 min to 2 hours
Fruit improperly combined	Up to 4 hours to leave stomach
Fresh Salad (no dressing)	1 to 2 hours
Fresh Salad (dressed with oil)	Up to 4 hours
Starch Meal	Up to 4 hours
Protein Meal	Up to 4 hours

NUTRITIONAL BREAKDOWN OF FOODS [1]

Despite the fact that food is a wonder medicine, if the diabetic person does not know how to control food intake and how to eat in the appropriate proportions, his/her diabetes worsen. Controlling food intake involves understanding the body's function as a result of each combination of food consumed. To be more specific, the response and performance of a diabetic person's blood glucose levels depend on the consumption of each type of food. Some diabetic people live with a misconception believing that diabetes is controlled as long as fasting glucose levels are normal every morning. The fact is that the average of all blood glucose levels of the entire day (24 hours) is the factor that determines the diabetic person's performance and reveals directly whether or not the diabetes is controlled.

Emphasis must be focused, as is the sole object of this book, on the after-meal glucose levels but not simply on the fasting glucose level. If the diabetic person understands and controls the after-meal glucose levels up to certain extent, if not to perfection, he/she has done a good or fair job in controlling the diabetes. This can be accomplished through monitoring and researching after-meal glucose levels as frequently as possible with an intention to lower them close to the normal range.

All foods contain 7 basic components such as protein, fat and carbohydrate in major quantities, and vitamins, minerals, fiber and water in minor quantities. If we know the quantities of protein, fat and carbohydrate in a meal, we can calculate the total calories offered by that meal. Enzymes are not present in the food, but the body's organs produce enzymes. Vitamins stimulate living tissues in order to produce enzymes. Calories counting is discussed below in detail.

REFERENCE

1. Permanent Diabetes Control (Book), Subtitle: The Complete Guide to Living Like A Normal Person Forever, Authored by Rao Konduru, MS, PhD, Reviewed and Endorsed by Dr. Marshal Dahl, MD, PhD., Endocrinologist, Faculty of Medicine, University of British Columbia, Vancouver, British Columbia, Canada, First Published in 2003. www.mydiabetescontrol.com

CHAPTER 6 HOW TO COUNT FOOD CALORIES?

A Person With Diabetes Must Understand
a. How to Read Labels While Shopping
b. How to Count Calories While Cooking
C. How to Adjust Protein, Fat & Carbohydrate in a Given Meal

If You Practice On Counting Calories, Then You Will Be A Winner!

TABLE OF CONTENTS

IMPORTANT NOTE

Many people with diabetes eat high-meat meals without consuming carbohydrate to keep low blood sugars, which is not recommended at all. Research showed that early death comes if you don't consume enough carbohydrate every day. You must eat enough carbohydrate every day, and learn how to lower after-meal glucose levels.

This book teaches you how to lower after-meal glucose levels, even if you consume high carbohydrate meals.

HOW TO COUNT CALORIES?

CONCEPT OF CALORIES [1, 2]

Energy offered by any food item is expressed in "calories." A calorie is the unit of heat in the international system (SI) of units. Heat is the kinetic energy transfer from one medium to another. A calorie is defined as the amount of energy transfer required to raise the temperature of one cubic centimeter of pure water (provided the water temperature is above the freezing point and below the boiling point) by one degree centigrade. Water is said to be pure if its density is perfectly 1 gm/cm^3. All foods have calories. A calorie is a small unit. In all the labels of all foor packages, calories always imply kilocalories.

Food scientists refer to and count food calories in "Kilocalories." One Kilocalorie is equivalent to 1000 calories. For example, one tablespoon of granulated sugar weighing 12 grams has 46 Kcal. That means 12 grams of granulated sugar offers 46 Kilocalories of energy. In calorie counter tables, it is usually listed as "46 cal" instead of 46 Kcal. "Calories or Cal" is a slang word being used in the food industry to represent Kcal. So the confusion between calories and kilocalories has to be clarified. In some other books, food calories are expressed in Kilojoules (KJ). 1 KJ = 0.238 Kcal or 1 Kcal = 4.2 KJ.

So the actual definition is: "One Kilocalorie (Kcal) is the amount of heat necessary to raise the temperature of one kilogram of water by one degree centigrade."

The energy content of a food item can be determined by means of a bomb calorimeter. A food sample of known weight is burned in an atmosphere of pure oxygen in a jacketed bomb calorimeter. The heat released by the burned food is absorbed by the water in the jacket. The amount of energy is then calculated from the rise in water temperature and the weight of the food sample. There are several scientific methods developed and being used by food scientists to experimentally determine the nutritional composition (protein, fat and carbohydrate content) of any food item.

Table 6.1 Standard food calories of nutrients.

Food Calories of the Nutrients

All food items that humans consume comprise carbohydrates, fats and proteins. After thorough research, food scientists have established the following facts:
    ● Carbohydrates have approximately 4 Calories Per Gram.
    ● Fat has approximately 9 Calories Per Gram.
    ● Protein has approximately 4 Calories per Gram.
    ● Alcohol has approximately 7 Calories Per Gram.

READING LABELS AND COUNTING CALORIES

EXAMPLE CALCULATION-I

How to Calculate the Calories (Energy) Offered by a Food Item

By knowing the amounts of carbohydrates, fats and proteins present in a food item, it is possible to calculate the total calories or the energy being offered by that food item. For example, Avalon Dairy posted the nutritional information for 2% organic milk as follows (see the label shown below).

Table 6.2 Avalon Label: Calories and nutritional information of 2% organic milk.

Courtesy of Avalon

3. Avalon Dairy 2% Organic Milk (Nutritional Information)
http://www.avalondairy.com/organic-milk/

I have tabulated the values of calories, carbohydrates, fats and proteins of the Avalon label in the table below:

Table 6.3 Calories and nutritional information of 2% organic milk.

Food Item	Weight (gm)	Calories	Protein (gm)	Fat (gm)	Carbo (gm)
Avalon Dairy 2% Orgaic Milk (1 cup)	250	130	9.0	5.0	12.0

Calories are calculated as follows:
1 cup of 2% organic milk has 12 g of carbohydrates. Therefore 12 x 4 = 48 calories
1 cup of 2% organic milk has 5 g of fats.   Therefore 5 x 9 = 45 calories
1 cup of 2% organic milk has 9 g of proteins.   Therefore 9 x 4 = 36 calories

Therefore 1 Cup of 2% organic milk offers 48 + 45 + 36 = 129 calories of energy.
Avalon Dairy already posted on the label that 1 cup of 2% organic milk has 130 calories. So the 129 calories that I just calculated matched with 130 calories posted.

Which means if you know the amounts of carbohydrates, fats and proteins present in a food item, you can calculate the total calories being offered by that food item.
+++

EXAMPLE CALCULATION-II [2]
HOW TO CALCULATE THE CALORIES OF A MEAL ON A DINNER PLATE DISTRIBUTION OF FAT, PROTEIN AND CARBOHYDRATES

Suppose you recently purchased the oven-baked Rotisserie chicken at Save-On-Foods supermarket, brought it home and dished out a handful of chicken breast from the whole chicken, and placed it on your dinner plate. You also placed 1.5 cups of cooked brown rice, and 1/2 cup of cooked/boiled black beans on your dinner plate along with a pinch of sea salt & Cayenne pepper. So your dinner plate has 3 food items: Rotisserie chicken breast, cooked brown rice and boiled black beans. You want to calculate the total calories and the distribution of fat, protein and carbohydrates in your meal.

THIS IS WHAT YOU SHOULD DO
1. Determine the weight of each food item on your dinner plate using an electronic balance. For example,
a. Rotisserie Chicken Breast On Your Dinner Plate   = 125 g
b. Cooked Brown Rice (1.5 Cups) On Your Dinner Plate   = 67.5 g
c. Cooked Black Beans (1/2 Cup) On Your Dinner Plate   = 85 g

2. Find out the standard nutritional information (calories, fat, protein & carbohydrates) for Rotisserie chicken, cooked brown rice and cooked black beans.
You can find this nutritional information:
a. On the label of the package (with food item) you purchased.
b. In the handbooks of nutritional values/calorie-counting tables
c. By doing a Google search on the internet

By doing a Google search, I found the following values (calories, protein, fat and carbohydrates) for Rotisserie chicken, cooked brown rice and cooked black beans.

Table 6.4 Calories and nutritional information of Rotisserie chicken meal from Google search.

Food Item	Weight (gm)	Calories	Protein (gm)	Fat (gm)	Carbo (gm)
Rotisserie Chicken Breast (1 Cup)	100	148	29	4.00	0
Brown Rice (1/4 Cup Dry, 1 Cup Cooked)	45	150	3	1.5	35
Organic Cooked Black Beans (1 Cup)	172	227	15.2	0.9	40.8

I got the following URLs when I did the Google search:
Google search: calories Rotisserie chicken breast
http://www.myfitnesspal.com/food/calories/kds-rotisserie-chicken-breast-no-skin-387187970

Google search: calories cooked brown rice (short grain)
http://www.lundberg.com/product/organic-brown-short-grain-rice/

Google search: calories cooked black beans
https://draxe.com/black-beans-nutrition/
http://www.calorieking.com/foods/calories-in-fresh-or-dried-legumes-beans-black-boiled_f-ZmlkPTEzMDYwNg.html

3. Now that you know the nutritional breakdown (Protein, Fat & Carbohydrate content) for a given "Serving Size," you can calculate the same for any serving size or for any amount of food item or items on your dinner plate. The calculations are shown below:

Rotisserie Chicken:
For the Serving Size = 100 g, Calories = 148, Protein = 29 g, Fat = 4 g, Carbo = 0 g
For the Dinner Plate Size = 125 g, Calories = (125/100)(148) = 185 g
Protein = (125/100)(29) = 36.25 g
Fat = (125/100)(4) = 5.0 g
Carbohydrates = (125/100)(0) = 0 g

Cooked Brown Rice
For the Serving Size = 45 g, Calories = 150, Protein = 3 g, Fat = 1.5 g, Carbo = 35 g
For the Dinner Plate Size = 67.5 g, Calories = (67.5/45)(150) = 225 g
Protein= (67.5/45)(3) = 4.5 g
Fat = (67.5/45)(1.5) = 2.25 g
Carbohydrates = (67.5/45)(35) = 52.5 g

Cooked Black Beans
For the Serving Size = 172 g, Calories = 227, Protein = 15.2 g, Fat = 0.9 g, Carbo = 40.8 g
For the Dinner Plate Size = 85 g,   Calories = (85/172)(227) = 112.1 g
Protein = (85/172)(15.2) = 7.51 g
Fat = (85/172)(0.9) = 0.44 g
Carbohydrates = (85/172)(40.8) = 20.2 g

4. After calculating the nutritional information for all food items on your dinner plate, arrange the values in a table as shown below, and then calculate the percentage distribution of protein, fat and carbohydrates in your meal.

Table 6.5 Calculations for the nutritional information of Rotisserie chicken meal.

Food Item	Weight	Calories	Protein	Fat	Carbo
	(gm)		(gm)	(gm)	(gm)
Rotisserie Chicken Breast(1 Cup)	125	185	36.25	5.00	0
Brown Rice (1.5 Cups Cooked)	67.5	225	4.5	2.25	52.5
Organic Black Beans Boiled (1/2 Cup)	85	112.1	7.51	0.44	20.2
Total ☐	277.5	522.1	48.26	7.69	72.7
Calories calculated ☐		553.05	193.04	69.21	290.8
Percentage (%) ☐			35%	13%	53%

● Protein has approximately 4 Calories per Gram.
● Fat has approximately 9 Calories Per Gram.
● Carbohydrates have approximately 4 Calories Per Gram.
● Alcohol has approximately 7 Calories Per Gram.

Protein Calories   = 48.26 x 4 = 193.04 calories
Fat Calories   = 7.69 x 9 = 69.21 calories
Carbohydrate Calories =72.7 x 4 = 290.80 calories
% Protein   = 193.0/(193 + 69.21 + 290.8) ≈ 35%
% Fat   = 69.21/(193 + 69.21 + 290.8) ≈ 12%
% Carbohydrates = 290.8/(193 + 69.21 + 290.8) ≈ 53%
TOTAL ≈ 100%

As shown above, you can do your own calculations using a simple hand calculator, and arrange all values in a table manually. Or you can use the Microsoft EXCEL program, and by means of simple formulae (for addition, multiplication and division) do the calculations. By copying and pasting the formulae from one cell to another, you can do the same kind of calculations for any kind of meal.

WHEN YOU CREATE A NEW DIET: You don't put whatever amounts of food items you want in the dinner plate (bowl) and do calorie counting as explained in the aforementioned example. Instead, you place the pre-determined amounts of food items (1 cup, 1/2 cup, 1/4 cup, etc.) and then take their weights using an electronic balance, only on the first day. From second day onwards, you create the same or a similar meal of which you have already done the calorie counting using measuring cups (1 cup, 1/2 cup, 1/4 cup, etc.). You don't have to weigh the items every day. You don't have to do calorie counting every day.

After you have extensive experience, you don't even need the measuring cups. You would be able guess the amount of any food item by simply placing a handful of the food item. So take a handful of that food item (approximately) in a bowl, and cook the whole meal.
IT IS AS EASY AS COOKING REGULAR MEALS WITHOUT CALORIE COUNTING!

NUTRITIONAL INFORMATION OF LIQUID EGG WHITES [2]
The following nutritional information for liquid egg whites is posted by Rabbit River Farms.

4. Calories and Nutritional Information of Liquid Egg Whites, Posted by Rabbit River Farms, Richmond, BC, Canada.
http://www.rabbitriverfarms.com/products/organic-eggs-2/

Table 6.6 Calories and nutritional information of liquid egg whites.

Food Item	Weight (gm)	Calories	Protein (gm)	Fat (gm)	Carbo (gm)
Egg Whites (1/2 cup)	47	25	5	0	0

Table 6.7 Label for the calories and nutritional information of liquid egg whites.

Liquid Egg Whites
per 3 tbsp (47g)

Nutrient	amt	%dv
Calories	25	
Fat	0g	0%
Saturated Fat + Trans Fat	0g +0g	0%
Cholesterol	0mg	
Sodium	80mg	3%
Carbohydrate	0g	0%
Fibre	0g	0%
Sugars	0g	
Protein	5g	
Vitamin A		0%
Vitamin C		0%
Calcium		0%
Iron		0%

Courtesy of Rabbit River Farms

Extra Large Organic Eggs (Rabbit River Farms): I purchased this item in a Whole Foods store. I cracked one extra large whole organic egg in a small metal bowl, and removed 98% to 99% of egg yolk with a large spoon, and then weighed the egg white using an electronic balance.

I found that the weight of the egg white is approximately 47 g, matching the information on the label. Therefore I confirmed the following nutritional information for egg whites.

Table 6.8 Calculations for the calories and nutritional information of liquid egg whites.

Food Item	Weight (gm)	Calories	Protein (gm)	Fat (gm)	Carbo (gm)
Egg White (1 Ex Large Organic Eggs)	47	25	5	0	0
(98% of Egg Yolk is removed with a spoon)					
Egg White (2 Ex Large Organic Eggs)	94	50	10	0	0
(98% of Egg Yolk is removed with a spoon)					

READING LEBELS AND COUNTING CALORIES (Continued) [1]

Several food items such as Pita Bread, Tofu, Black Beans and Seasoned Fillet were purchased from a local supermarket, the nutritional composition was noted down from the labels as shown in the table below. Every food item has calories and nutrients. The purpose of this table is to view and understand the energy content and the nutrients protein, fat, carbohydrate of each food item, and calculate the calories for any desired size.

Table 6.9 Nutritional composition collected from labels.

Pita Bread		Firm Tofu		Black Beans		Seasoned Fillets	
Per 1 Pita, 54 gm		Per 10 Oz, 285 gm		Per 125 mL, 1/2 Cup		Per 100 gm, 2 Fillets	
Energy (cal)	136	Energy (Cal)	170	Energy (Cal)	100	Energy (Cal)	215
Protein (gm)	5.5	Protein (gm)	20	Protein (gm)	4.4	Protein (gm)	11
Fat (gm)	0.8	Fat (gm), 40 cal	5	Fat (gm)	0.3	Fat (gm),	11
Carbohydrate (gm)	29	Carbohydrate (gm)	12	Carbohydrate (gm)	20	Carbohydrate (gm)	18
Sugars (gm)	0.8	Sugars (gm)	0	Dietary Fibre (gm)	9.3	Sodium (mg)	500
Dietary Fibre (gm)	4.9	Dietary Fibre (gm)	0	Sodium (mg)	280	Potassium (mg)	140
Sodium (mg)	232	Sodium (mg)	30	Potassium (mg)	210	Cholesterol (mg)	30
Potassium (mg)	165	Potassium (mg)	0	Cholesterol (mg)	0		
Cholesterol (mg)	0	Cholesterol (mg)	0				

For example, for Pita Bread from the known serving size of 54 grams, we can calculate the nutritional composition for a serving size of 100 gm. The calculations are shown below:

Serving Size = 54 gm (Listed)

Food Item	Weight (gm)	Calories (Kcal)	Protein (gm)	Fat (gm)	Carbo (gm)
Pita Bread	54	136	5.5	0.8	29

It should be understood that calories on food labels always imply kilocalories.

Calories (for 100 gm)	= (100/54)(136)	= 251.9 Kcal
Protein (for 100 gm)	= (100/54)(5.5)	= 10.2 gm
Fat (for 100 gm)	= (100/54)(0.8)	= 1.5 gm
Carbohydrate (for 100 gm)	= (100/54)(29.0)	= 53.7 gm

Serving Size: 100 gm (Calculated)

Food Item	Weight (gm)	Calories(Kcal)	Protein (gm)	Fat (gm)	Carbo (gm)
Pita Bread	100	251.9	10.2	1.5	53.7

Once we have calculated the nutritional composition for 100 gm, we can weigh the Pita Bread and consume exactly 100 gm if needed.

Similarly we can calculate the nutritional composition for any serving size of firm tofu, black beans, seasoned fillets, and for any other food items purchased.

USING CALORIE-COUNTER TABLES [1]

When the purchased food has no label and nutritional information is unavailable, this information can be collected and jotted down from any calorie-counter book.

For example the following information is gathered from the calorie-counter table of Dr. Dean Ornish (Reference 1). The serving size of the nutritional composition listed for Turkey (skinless) is 28 grams. The corresponding calories, protein, fat and carbohydrate are listed as 45 Kcal, 9.3 gm, 0.7 gm and 0 gm respectively.

Serving Size: 28 gm (listed)

Food Item	Weight (gm)	Calories (Kcal)	Protein (gm)	Fat (gm)	Carbo (gm)
Turkey (skinless)	28	45	9.3	0.7	0

Based on this information, we can calculate the "nutritional composition" of any quantity. For example for a serving size of 100 gm:
It should be understood that calories on calorie-counter tables always imply Kcal.
Calories (for 100 gm)   = (100/28)(45)   = 160.7 Kcal
Protein (for 100 gm)   = (100/28)(9.3)   = 33.2 gm
Fat (for 100 gm)   = (100/28)(0.7)   = 2.5 gm
Carbohydrate (for 100 gm) = (100/28)(0)   = 0 gm

Serving Size: 100 gm (calculated)

Food Item	Weight (gm)	Calories (Kcal)	Protein (gm)	Fat (gm)	Carbo (gm)
Turkey (skinless)	100	160.7	33.2	2.5	0

Note: Most animal products such as beef, chicken, turkey, fish and pork do not have carbohydrate unless they are breaded. That is why in the above-cited example the carbohydrate content of turkey is zero.

Similarly the nutritional composition of Chicken, Mushrooms and Tomato is taken from the calorie-counter table of Dr. Dean Ornish (Reference 1) for serving sizes of 28 gm, 70 gm and 200 gm respectively, and calculated for a desired serving sizes of 100 gm, 100 gm and 150 gm respectively as shown in the table below.

Table 6.10 Nutritional composition from calorie-counter tables.

Food Item	Weight (gm)	Calories (Kcal)	Protein (gm)	Fat (gm)	Carbo (gm)
Chicken (skinless)	28	51	9.2	1.4	0
	100	182.14	32.86	5	0
Mushrooms	70	20	1.9	0.2	3.1
	100	28.57	2.71	0.29	4.43
Tomato (raw)	200	40	2	0.4	8.6
	150	30	1.5	0.3	6.45
	100	20	1	0.2	4.3

Conversion Factors: 1 cup = 8 oz (Ounces); 1 oz = 28.3 gm

CALCULATION OF PROTEIN, FAT AND CARBOHYDRATE [1]

> **Protein has approximately 4 kilocalories per gram.**
> **Fat has approximately 9 kilocalories per gram.**
> **Carbohydrate has approximately 4 kilocalories per gram.**
> **Alcohol has approximately 7 kilocalories per gram.**

Table 3.4 shows how to calculate the breakdown of protein, fat and carbohydrate in a meal. From the calorie-counter table, the nutritional composition (the values of calories, protein, fat and carbohydrate) is jotted down for all lunch items (Pita Bread, Baked Potato, Black Beans, Tofu, Onion) separately. Total protein, total fat and total carbohydrate offered by the lunch are calculated as shown in the table below. Calories from protein, calories from fat, and calories from carbohydrate are calculated as shown in the table below:

$$\text{Calories from Protein} = (17.03)(4) = 68.12$$
$$\text{Calories from Fat} = (3.6)(9) = 32.40$$
$$\text{Calories from Carbohydrate} = (74.8)(4) = 299.20$$
$$\text{Total calories} = 68.12 + 32.4 + 299.2 = 399.72$$

The percentage composition of protein, fat and carbohydrate is calculated from the calories of each nutrient and total calories:

$$\text{Protein (\%)} = 68.12/399.72 = 17.04\%$$
$$\text{Fat (\%)} = 32.40/399.72 = 8.11\%$$
$$\text{Carbohydrate (\%)} = 299.20/399.72 = 74.85\%$$

That means the lunch has 17% protein, 8% fat and 75% carbohydrate.

Table 6.11 Lunch – Nutritional Composition.

Food Item	Weight (gm)	Calories (Kcal)	Protein (gm)	Fat (gm)	Carbo (gm)
Pita Bread	55	136	5.5	0.8	29
Baked Potato	100	75	2.1	1.5	15
Black Beans (1/2 Cup)	100	117	4.4	0.3	20
Tofu	50	30	3.5	0.88	2.1
Onion	100	38	1.53	0.12	8.7
Salt & Pepper	2	0	0	0	0
Total	407	396	17.03	3.6	74.8
Calories calculated		399.72	68.12	32.4	299.2
Percentage (%)			17.04%	8.11%	74.85%

P.S.: There is a misconception in food labelling. "Calorie" is a slang word used by people on labels or books. Food calories always imply "kilocalories."

MANIPULATION OF CARBOHYDRATE CONTENT [1]

In the previous example, the carbohydrate content of the lunch was very high (75%). Carbohydrate is the source of sugar (glucose). The term "carbohydrate" is derived from the fact that glucose is made up of carbon and water. All foods, except meat, chicken and fish, contain carbohydrate ranging from very low to very high. A low carbohydrate meal is strongly recommended for diabetic people.

In order to lower the carbohydrate content in the above-cited example, Pita Bread, Black Beans and Onion are removed from the lunch, and Kidney Beans, Tomato and Lettuce are added to the lunch as shown below. Similar calculations are performed. The carbohydrate content is then reduced from 75% to 62%.

Table 6.12 Lunch – Nutritional Composition.

Food Item	Weight (gm)	Calories (Kcal)	Protein (gm)	Fat (gm)	Carbo (gm)
Baked Potato	100	75	2.1	1.5	15
Kidney Beans (canned)	100	117	7.78	0.49	20
Tofu	100	60	7	1.76	4.2
Tomato	100	20	1	0.2	4.3
Lettuce	55	7	0.5	0.1	1.6
Salt & Pepper					
Total	455	279	18.38	4.05	45.1
Calories calculated		290.37	73.52	36.45	180.4
Percentage (%)			25%	13%	62%

Similarly the protein content and fat content can be adjusted in a given meal by choosing appropriate ingredients. This kind of approach to "nutritional control" is always good for diabetic people.

LISTEN TO THE EXPERTS [1, 2]

While low carbohydrate food is strongly recommended for diabetic people, high carbohydrate food would do no harm as long as the person is exercising after the meal in order that the glucose level drops to normal in two hours. The authors of the book "Glucose Revolution" suggested that at least 50% to 60% of total calories should be from carbohydrate. Dr. Andrew Weil in his book "Eating Well for Optimum Health" suggested that protein needs are much lower than most people imagine, and the risk of protein deficiency is negligible. A protein intake of 10% to 20% of total calories would be sufficient. Milk protein and any kind of animal protein should be avoided. A fat content of lower than 30% (5% from saturated fat, 20% from monounsaturated fat and 5% from polyunsaturated fat) is the best choice. Dr. Dean Ornish in his reversal diet and prevention diet plans recommends a fat content of 10% without using any oils. Harvey Diamond in his book "Fit For Life" gives a detailed explanation and interpretation with reasoning on complete diet and health plan.

ACCURATE CARBOHYDRATE COUNTING [2]

The American Diabetes Association, some organizations related to nutrition and diabetes education, dietitians and weight loss experts recommended the following formula, making an effort to further correct the amount of total carbohydrates being printed on food labels:

Amount of Total Carbohydrates Corrected =
Total Carbohydrates (g) on the Label – Dietary Fiber (g) on the Label – 1/2 Sugar Alcohol (g) on the Label

The food manufacturers in some countries are required by law to publish a label on the manufactured item by revealing the total carbohydrates in grams. This total carbohydrates includes the amount of starch, dietary fiber, sugar and sugar alcohol. However dietary fiber does not raise blood-glucose levels. So it does not contribute to the energy content. Therefore the dietary fiber content in grams is to be entirely subtracted from total carbohydrates in grams in order to correct it. Sugar alcohol is a type of reduced-calorie sweetener, such as sorbitol, xylitol, mannitol, etc., added to food items by food manufacturers. But the research showed that sugar alcohols are only half-effective in raising blood-glucose levels. So only half of the sugar alcohol content in grams is to be subtracted from the total carbohydrates in grams in order to correct it.

IT IS IMPORTANT TO NOTE THAT WHOLE FOODS DO NOT CONTAIN SUGAR AND ALCOHOL BUT CONTAIN DIETARY FIBER AND SOME WHOLE FOODS MAY CONTAIN SUGAR. PROCESSED FOODS DO CONTAIN SUGAR ALCOHOL. If you eat only a whole food meal, you don't need to worry about sugar alcohol. Therefore the general rule is that the fiber content in grams and half of the sugar alcohol content in grams are to be subtracted from the total carbohydrates in grams listed on the label to obtain the accurate amount of carbohydrates that indeed represents the energy and contributes to raising blood-glucose levels. The amount of total carbohydrates corrected is to be multiplied by 4 to obtain the calories being offered by the total carbohydrates corrected.

IS CARBOHYDRATE CORRECTION NECESSARY?
IS THE DEDUCTION OF FIBER FROM CARBOHYDRATE NECESSARY?

I decided not to correct the amount of total carbohydrates being printed on the food labels while calculating calories in my weight-loss diet recipes because of the following reasons:
(i) There are two types of dietary fiber: (i) soluble fiber that dissolves in water and is fermented in the colon to produce byproducts and (ii) insoluble fiber that does not dissolve in water and acts like a bulking agent mixed with water in order to sweep the wastes through the colon along with it. Insoluble fiber does not offer any energy so it has no calories. But soluble fiber does offer energy and therefore has calories. Food scientists have conducted research on soluble fiber and reported that the bacteria in the gut reacts with the water-soluble fiber, resulting in the production of short chain fatty acids, which offer some sort of energy.

Some dietitians have reported that soluble fiber offers 1.9 calories per gram. [7, 8] FDA reported that the amount of caloric contribution due to bacterial degradation is about 1.5 calories per gram of fiber. [6] So we cannot ignore the fact that soluble fiber has calories. As the food labels do not reveal how much soluble fiber is there in any food item, there is no way we can correct the amount of carbohydrates based on the fiber content. Dr. Mike Roussell Wrote the Following: Don't worry about improving the accuracy of your calorie-counting by being technically correct about the contribution of fiber. It is simply a wasted effort. If there is a caloric difference due to fiber, it's small enough that it's probably easily obliterated if you walk to work or take your dog for a stroll after dinner.

(ii) If you go by "accuracy," the counting of calories itself is only by approximation and there is no need to worry about the accuracy of the amount of carbohydrates.

As a matter of fact, when counting calories, all the aforementioned educators multiply the amount of carbohydrates by 4 instead of 4.1 or 4.2. If they want to count calories accurately, they should actually multiply the amount of carbohydrate in grams by 4.1 or 4.2 (not by 4). So there was an error generated already by multiplying by 4. Carbohydrates actually offer 4.1 or 4.2 calories per gram (4 calories per gram is an approximation or rounded value). Similarly fat has 9.5 calories per gram (not 9 calories per gram), and protein has 4.1 calories per gram (not 4 calories per gram). Different studies report different calories per gram of carbohydrates, fats and proteins. For example, in the article of Nutrition [11], it was reported that Carbohydrates have 4.2 Calories per gram, Fat has 9.5 Calories per gram and Protein has 4.1 Calories per gram.

And also Sadava, David and Orians, Gordon H. Life reported the following values: Carbohydrates have 4.2 Calories per gram, Fat has 9.5 Calories per gram and Protein has 4.1 Calories per gram.

There was no general consensus reached regarding the energy values being offered by carbohydrates, fats and proteins. All calorie-counting calculations are by approximation as they are not the accurate values. So don't worry about accuracy.

(iii) More than that, when you deduct the amount of dietary fiber from the total carbohydrates and multiply by 4, your total daily calorie intake is going to be lower than that without deduction, which could trick your brain to feel free to eat more because your total calorie intake was lower. As a result, you could gain weight by eating more. If you do not deduct the dietary fiber from total carbohydrates, then you feel satisfied by the total daily calorie instate, and then you could lose weight by eating less.

(iv) In some countries, the food manufacturers don't even list the amount of dietary fiber so you never know how much fiber is to be deducted from the total carbohydrates. So the deduction of dietary fiber from the total carbohydrates is not universally verified and validated when counting calories.

(v) Calorie counting should be used to compare the total daily calorie intake from one day to another. It is the relative calorie counting that is important, not the absolute calorie counting. From the approximate calorie count, you can either lower the total daily calorie intake by eating less or increase it by eating more. The approximate calorie counting, without worrying too much about its accuracy, should be used by keeping in mind that you should eventually eat less in an attempt to lose weight. That can be accomplished by means of the measuring cups, by using the 3/4 cup instead of the 1 cup or by using the 1 cup instead of the 1.5 cup, etc. on your dinner plate. By counting the number of cups you have been eating until today, you can easily lower the amount of food being consumed right from the next day, thereby accomplishing your weight loss goal. Healthy eating habits "such as eating whole foods" would allow you to consume lower calories, and lose weight. Accurate calorie counting is not going to help you lose weight. So don't worry too much about it!

CONCLUSION: The deduction of fiber from carbohydrate is unnecessary while counting calories of a food item or a meal. Approximate calorie-counting would do the job.

REFERENCES

1. Permanent Diabetes Control (Book), Subtitle: The Complete Guide to Living Like A Normal Person Forever, Authored by Rao Konduru, MS, PhD, Reviewed and Endorsed by Dr. Marshal Dahl, MD, PhD., Endocrinologist, Faculty of Medicine, University of British Columbia, Vancouver, British Columbia, Canada, First Published in 2003. www.mydiabetescontrol.com
2. Andrew Weil, MD, Eating Well For Optimum Health, Borzoi Books, Published by Alfred A. Knopf, New York, 2000.

CHAPTER 7 FATS AND CHOLESTEROL

A Person With Diabetes Must Not Eat:
a. Foods That Contain Saturated Fats
b. Foods That Contain Hydrogenated Fats
C. Foods That Contain Partially Hydrogenated Fats or Trans Fats
d. Foods That Contain High Cholesterol
This Chapter Is Designed to Help You Understand About It!

CAUTION: Eating foods that contain saturated fats, hydrogenated fats, partially hydrogenated fats or trans fats could lead to high cholesterols (total cholesterol & LDL cholesterol), hardening of arteries or what is known as atherosclerosis, coronary heart disease, heart attack, heart failure, stroke, and many other diabetes-related complications. Hamburgers, cheeseburgers, deep-fried potatoes (so called fries), all kinds of processed meat, all kinds of bakery items, all kinds of ready-to-eat meals from fast-food restaurants, all kinds of breads, anything made by adding starchy white flour & syrup, all foods with high cholesterol content are typical food items to be avoided.

TABLE OF CONTENTS

FATS AND CHOLESTEROLS [1]
FATS

While fats are high in calories (9 calories per gram), they do not convert to glucose as efficiently and quickly as carbohydrates do. Carbohydrates provide energy to the muscles and brain. Carbohydrates are immediately converted into glucose and unused glucose is stored in the liver as glucagon. Proteins provide amino acids, which are the building material for the body's cells to grow and maintain their structure. About 20% of the human body is protein. Fats provide fatty acids contributing to build-up of cell membranes. Fats act as carriers for fat soluble vitamins and the unused portion of fat is stored in fatty tissues.

Foods contain both saturated and/or unsaturated fats. Total fat is the sum of both saturated and unsaturated fats. The classification of fats is shown below:

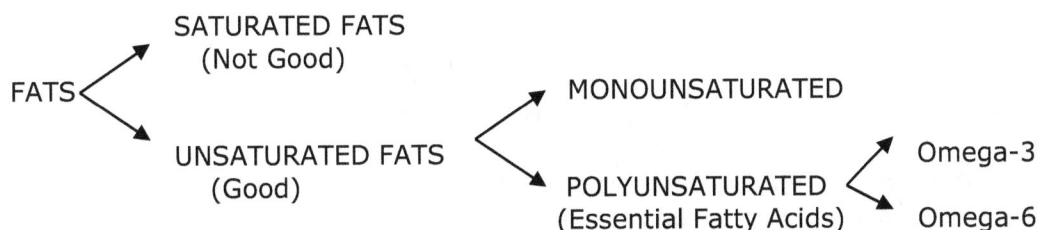

```
                    SATURATED FATS
                    (Not Good)
                                        MONOUNSATURATED
FATS
                    UNSATURATED FATS
                    (Good)                                              Omega-3
                                        POLYUNSATURATED
                                        (Essential Fatty Acids)        Omega-6
```

Saturated fat, cholesterol and essential fatty acids such as omega-3 and omega-6 are very essential for the good functioning of the kidneys. To purify the blood, to maintain proper blood volume and composition and to maintain normal blood pressure, kidneys make use of fats not only as energy but also for their cushioning. Kidney fat contains more saturated fat than any other human body part.

Saturated fat, if consumed in more calories than being burned, could clog arteries and cause heart attack and heart disease. A lot of food items that people buy and eat every day in convenience stores, gas stations, restaurants and supermarkets such as bakery items, snack packs, potato chips, French fries, cakes, cookies, snacks, hamburgers, sandwiches, etc. are cooked with or dressed with oils or oil-based products which contain saturated fats A fat product is made up of fatty acids and glycerol.

A fatty acid is a long hydrocarbon chain (CH_2) with a methyl group (CH_3) on one end attached to a carboxyl group (COOH) on the other end as shown in the picture below (65). It is the COOH group that makes it acid. Each carbon atom in the hydrocarbon chain is attached to one or two hydrogen atoms. When a fatty acid has all the hydrogen atoms it can hold, the acid chain is said to be "saturated." Fatty acids are classified by the length of hydrocarbon chain, by the degree of unsaturation (number of double bonds in a chain) and the location of the double bonds in the hydrocarbon chain.

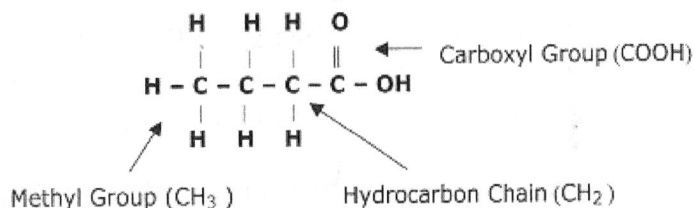

```
        H   H   H   O
        |   |   |   ||       ←── Carboxyl Group (COOH)
    H – C – C – C – C – OH
        |   |   |
        H   H   H

    Methyl Group (CH3)         Hydrocarbon Chain (CH2)
```

Saturated Fats contain saturated fatty acids in which the hydrocarbon chain is fully saturated with hydrogen bonding. Typical examples are palmitic acid and stearic acid in which all carbon atoms are bound with hydrogen. Saturated fatty acids are solid and stable at room temperature and do not react readily with oxygen at room temperature.

Animal Products such as beef, lamb, pork, bacon, lard, poultry with skin, whole milk, even 2% milk, butter & cheese contain saturated fats. Avoid them.

Plant-Based Products such as coconut oil, palm oil, palm kernel oil and cocoa butter, avocados, nuts and seeds also contain saturated fats.

Saturated Fatty Acids	Molecular Formula
Capric Acid	$CH_3(CH2)_8COOH$
Lauric Acid	$CH_3(CH2)_{10}COOH$
Myristic Acid	$CH_3(CH2)_{12}COOH$
Palmitic Acid	$CH_3(CH2)_{14}COOH$
Stearic Acid	$CH_3(CH2)_{16}COOH$

Unsaturated Fats are made up of unsaturated fatty acids and are divided into two types monounsaturated fats and polyunsaturated fats. If the hydrocarbon chain is not saturated (all carbon atoms are not bound with hydrogen atoms) but one or more positions are vacant with a double bond, then the fatty acid is said to be unsaturated. If there is one double bond, then it is called monounsaturated and if there are two or more than two double bonds in the chain, then the fatty acid is said to be polyunsaturated. Unsaturated fatty acids have at least one vacant carbon atom to which hydrogen is not bound. A typical example is oleic acid in which there are two vacant carbon atoms where hydrogen is not bound [66, 67]. Unsaturated fatty acids have lower melting points than saturated fatty acids. Unsaturated fatty acids are usually liquid at room temperature.

Monounsaturated Fats are liquid at room temperature but begin to solidify when placed in a cooler or refrigerator. Examples are plant-based oils such as olive oil, canola oil, peanut oil, etc.

Monounsaturated Fatty Acids	Molecular Formula
Crotonic Acid	$CH_3CH=CHCOOH$
Palmitoleic Acid	$CH_3(CH_2)_5CH=CH(CH_2)_7COOH$
Oleic acid	$CH_3(CH_2)_7CH=CH(CH_2)_7COOH$

Polyunsaturated Fats are liquid at room temperature and also in a cooler or refrigerator but react quickly with oxygen and get rotten or sour. Examples are plant-based oils such as sunflower oil, sesame oil, soy oil, etc.

Polyunsaturated Fatty Acids	Molecular Formula
Linolenic acid (Omega-3)	$CH_3(CH_2CH=CH)3(CH_2)_7COOH$
Linoleic acid (Omega-6)	$CH_3(CH_2)_3(CH_2CH=CH)_2(CH_2)_7COOH$
Arachidonic acid (Omega-6)	$CH_3(CH_2)_3(CH_2CH=CH)_4(CH_2)_3COOH$

Hydrogenated Fats are manufactured from unsaturated fatty acids in which the vacant carbon atoms are artificially bound with hydrogen to make the hydrocarbon chain saturated. In this process of hydrogenation, the liquid oil is solidified. An example is margarine.

In the hydrogenation process, a catalyst metal such as nickel, zinc or copper is mixed with hydrogen gas at high heat and bubbled through the unsaturated fatty acid mixture. The metal catalyses the reaction between carbon and hydrogen in order to transform the double bond attachment into single bond. This process creates a new molecular shape similar to that of saturated fat with increased stiffness and solidification. The process of hydrogenation generates two forms called trans fatty acids and cis fatty acids. If the direction of folding that occurs in the carbon double bond is natural then it is cis fatty acid. On the other hand, if the direction of folding that occurs in the carbon double bond is altered it is trans fatty acid. Partial hydrogenation or brush hydrogenation takes place when the reaction is partly completed. It increases stability for polyunsaturated fatty acids. The commercial salad dressing oil such as soybean oil is partially hydrogenated.

Hydrogenated fats are produced for economical benefits to the manufacturer because the fats last longer before they become rancid, they have creamy consistency with good taste, it costs less to produce them, and they can be sold in greater quantities to consumers at lower price tags. **Hydrogenated fats or partially hydrogenated fats directly cause heart attack and stroke by raising LDL (bad cholesterol) levels.** They also cause diseases and obesity.

Trans Fats are unsaturated fats but partially hydrogenated, derived by adding hydrogen atoms mostly to vegetable oils and are used extensively in fast food restaurants and bakeries.

Partially Hydrogenated Fats or Trans Fats are found in cookies, cakes, french fries, onion rings, muffins, crackers, frozen pizza, bread, potato chips, corn chips, cake mixes, biscuit mixes, pancake mixes, donuts, etc.

Essential Fatty Acids: The human body is able to manufacture most common fatty acids from nutrients available in the human digestive system. Unfortunately the human body does not manufacture essential fatty acids, which are made up of polyunsaturated fatty acids such as omega-3 fatty acids and omega-6 fatty acids where 3 and 6 refer to the first carbon double bond located in the hydrocarbon chain.

Alpha Linolenic acid is Omega-3 Fatty Acid in which the first double bond occurs at the third carbon atom. Omega-3 fatty acids are found in fish oil, flax seed oil, pumpkin seed oil, sardines, mackerel or shell fish, green leafy vegetables, etc.
CH_3-CH_2-**CH=CH**-CH_2-**CH=CH**-CH_2-**CH=CH**-CH_2-CH_2-CH_2-CH_2-CH_2-CH_2-CH_2-COOH

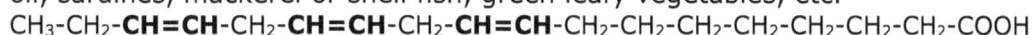

Linoleic acid is Omega-6 Fatty Acid in which the first double bond occurs at the sixth carbon atom. Omega-6 fatty acids are found in corn oil, peanut oil, soybean oil, sunflower oil, safflower oil, cottonseed oil, grape seed oil, etc.

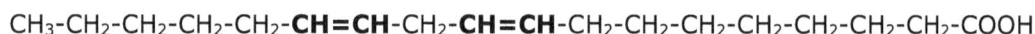

CH_3-CH_2-CH_2-CH_2-CH_2-**CH=CH**-CH_2-**CH=CH**-CH_2-CH_2-CH_2-CH_2-CH_2-CH_2-CH_2-COOH

Omega-3 and omega-6 fatty acids should be balanced with a ratio between 1:1 and 1:2. [33d, 64] Most people in the USA currently maintain ratios from 1:10 to 1:20 because of the habits of eating too many omega-6 products.

CHOLESTEROL [1]

It is important that diabetic people thoroughly understand cholesterol because only by knowing how harmful it is, can high cholesterol be controlled.

What is Cholesterol? Cholesterol is a biochemical, greasy or waxy fat-like substance called "lipid" found in the bloodstream and in all cells. The human body needs normal levels of cholesterol because it is the main source to form cell membranes, some hormones and other essential tissues.

The liver manufactures and delivers about 80% of the cholesterol in the human body and the remaining 20% of cholesterol comes from the food being consumed.

Most of this remaining 20%, which is called dietary cholesterol, comes from animal products such as meats, fish, eggs, poultry, butter, cheese and whole milk. Food from plants such as vegetables, fruits and cereals do not have cholesterol. Both fat and cholesterol belong to a group called "lipids." Cholesterol is used to build cell membranes and brain and nerve tissues. Cholesterol helps produce steroid hormones needed for body regulation, including bile acids for digestion.

LDL AND HDL: Because cholesterol and other fats do not dissolve in the blood, they are transported to and from the cells by special carriers called lipoproteins. There are two types of lipoproteins: Low density lipoprotein (LDL) and high density lipoprotein (HDL). LDL is the bad cholesterol and HDL is the good cholesterol. Up to one-fourth of blood cholesterol is carried by HDL.

Excessive LDL can be harmful as it clogs arteries and causes heart attack and coronary artery disease (CAD). Luckily, the human body makes HDL in order to protect from clogging arteries. Higher levels of HDL significantly reduce the risk of heart attack and heart disease. Total cholesterol consists of LDL, HDL and some other substances not reported in a blood test. HDL is the **good cholesterol** because it carries cholesterol away from the arteries, back to the liver, preventing the build-up on the arteries' walls. LDL is **bad cholesterol** because any excess LDL is deposited on the arteries. There is another type of bad cholesterol called very low density lipoprotein (VLDL) more harmful than LDL.

Total Cholesterol is mostly LDL and HDL plus some other substances.

HDL Ratio is the ratio between Total Cholesterol and HDL. It is an indicator of cardiovascular disease. The perfect normal value is under 3.5. A value of 4.5 is considered to be very good, and a value under 5.0 is also accepted to be normal.

Triglycerides are another form of fat, a small portion of which is found in the bloodstream while the large portion is in fat tissue. The body needs insulin to clean up this type of fat from the blood. Higher levels of triglycerides alone do not contribute to clogging arteries. But lipoproteins that are concentrated with triglycerides are usually mixed with cholesterol, which significantly contributes to the clogging of arteries and heart disease.

NORMAL LEVELS OF CHOLESTEROL [1]

Shown below are the normal levels of cholesterol and triglycerides in both system of units (mmol/L and mg/dL).

Table 7.1 Normal levels of cholesterol.

Cholesterol (mmol/L)	LDL mmol/L	HDL mmol/L	HDL Ratio	Triglycerides mmol/L
2.0 - 5.2	1.5 - 3.4	>0.9	< 5.0	< 2.3
Cholesterol mg/dL	LDL mg/dL	HDL mg/dL	HDL Ratio	Triglycerides mg/dL
77.34 - 210.08	58.00 - 131.48	> 34.80	< 5.0	< 88.94

CALCULATION OF CHOLESTEROL IN BOTH UNITS [1]

In the USA, Europe and in some Asian countries, cholesterols are reported in mg/dL whereas in Canada, UK, Australia, New Zealand, South Africa and some other countries, they are reported in mmol/L. So a diabetic person, when in another country and having a blood test done, should be able convert the values from one system of units to the other in order to understand the normal range.

Notation: mg = milligram (1 gram = 1000 milligrams); dL = deciliter (1 liter = 10 deciliters); mmol = millimole (1 mole = 1000 millimoles); L = liter

Sample Calculation

Suppose total cholesterol is reported by a laboratory in Canada as 4.2 mmol/L. Convert the total cholesterol value to mg/dL as expressed in the USA.

Molecular Formula of Cholesterol is: $C_{27} H_{46} O$
Molecular Weight of Cholesterol is: 386.66 mg/mmol

To convert from mmol/L to mg/L, multiply by molecular weight.
To convert from mg/L to mg/dL, divide by 10 (1 liter is equal to 10 deciliters).

$$4.2 \text{ mmol/L} = (4.2 \text{ mmol/L}) (386.66 \text{ mg/mmol}) / (10 \text{ dL/L})$$
$$= 162.40 \text{ mg/dL}$$

Or, simply multiply with the conversion factor 38.67.
$$4.2 \text{ mmol/L} = (4.2 \text{ mmol/L}) \times (38.67) \text{ (mg/dL)} / \text{(mmol/L)} = 162.40 \text{ mg/dL}$$

Conversion Factor $= (386.66 \text{ mg/mmol}) / (10 \text{ dL/L})$
$$= 38.67 \text{ (mg/mmol)} / \text{(dL/L)} = 38.67 \text{ (mg/dL)} / \text{(mmol/L)}$$

To convert mmol/L of cholesterol to mg/dL, simply multiply the value by 38.67.
To convert mg/dL of cholesterol to mmol/L, simply divide the value by 38.67.

CAUSES OF HIGH CHOLESTEROL IN PEOPLE WITH DIABETES [1, 3]

● Heredity plays an important role as some people inherit gene deficiency from their parents. If there is a family history of high cholesterol or heart disease, the chances are some of the children pick up the disorders. It is always better to be aware of such genetic cause and be prepared to face and treat such condition, disease or disorder.

● A study at Kansas State University showed that extra insulin drawn into the bloodstream from the pancreas lowers HDL (good cholesterol) in the blood. Lowering HDL means more and more LDL (bad cholesterol) is deposited in the blood. The liver and muscles are the only places where extra glucose can be stored. Exercise uses the already stored glucose in the muscles allowing the newly flooded glucose from digested food into the muscles for storage and future usage. If the muscles are fully stored due to lack of exercise, then the glucose from digested food enters the bloodstream, raising glucose levels. People who are at high risk for diabetes exhibit higher levels of blood glucose. Increased glucose levels not only draw extra insulin and contribute to insulin resistance, but in addition lower HDL level and increase fat in the belly. This is why diabetic people tend to have higher levels of LDL and lower levels of HDL.

● Dr. Alan Rubin reported that poorly controlled high blood pressure increased total cholesterol by about 50 to 100 mg/dL (1.3 to 2.59 mmol/L).

● Excess weight is a contributing factor to increase of LDL.

● Stress and anxiety are the psychological factors that raise cholesterol levels. Research showed that people under pressure or experiencing depression overeat and console themselves by eating fatty foods. The saturated fat and cholesterol contribute to high LDL levels.

The symptoms and side effects of very high cholesterol are sensed and more or less recognizable as the person feels discomfort and heaviness in the chest when cholesterol levels go beyond normal. When it is more intense, the pain could lead to angina and coronary artery disease (CAD). CAD is developed due to the blockage of blood vessels which supply the heart with blood. Cholesterol, along with saturated fats and other greasy substances, forms a kind of plaque that can contribute to the narrowing of the coronary arteries. Heart attack occurs when one or more arteries are filled and blocked by plaque formation. The American Heart Association reports that Coronary Heart Disease (CHD) is the number one killer in America and almost 99.5 million Americans have high cholesterol levels. So a diabetic person must check his/her cholesterol levels on a routine basis once every 3 months, and should prepare for the appropriate treatment if the test shows abnormal cholesterol levels. Your main focus should be on LDL level.

HOW TO PREVENT HIGH CHOLESTEROL (LDL) & HEART DISEASE? [1, 2, 4]

(i) LOW-FAT & LOW-CHOLESTEROL DIET WITH DAILY EXERCISE
● A simple way of treating high total cholesterol and high LDL cholesterol is to consume a low-fat diet with daily exercise as is simultaneously applied to diabetes. You can control both diabetes and high cholesterols at the same time. Eating habits have to be carefully planned by looking into the cholesterol tables of all foods being consumed. Whatever plan is being used, low-fat diet works effectively only when the excess body weight is melted away.
● By eating whole foods only (no processed foods and no refined foods), with daily exercise, you can lose weight until your body mass index (BMI) or body fat percentage drops to perfectly normal. With consistent efforts and determination, you can do it.

- By minimizing the fat consumption, you lose weight easily. Eat egg-white omelet with a variety of vegetables so that your body gets enough protein. Do not eat meat-based products.
- The cholesterol level in the blood is the only way of establishing the risk for coronary heart disease. Saturated fat is responsible for the rise in cholesterol level. The amount of saturated fat from food being consumed raises bad cholesterol (LDL) level which in turn lead to thickening or clogging of arteries. The end result is the build-up of plaque in the arteries leading to coronary heart disease, arteriosclerosis and atherosclerosis. Arteriosclerosis is the stiffening or hardening of the artery walls, whereas atherosclerosis is the narrowing of the artery because of plaque build-up.

(ii) ALWAYS EAT PLANT-BASED FOODS: Foods such as whole grains, vegetables, beans, fruits, tofu, soymilk, etc. do not have cholesterol. Vegetable oils such as olive oil, canola oil, peanut oil, soybean oil, coconut oil, palm oil, etc. do not have cholesterol but some of these oils have saturated fats so avoid them. Coconut oil and palm oil are called "artery cloggers" as they can turn into bad fats through hydrogenation. Do not consume them.

(iii) DO NOT EAT (NEVER EAT) ORGAN MEATS: Organ meats such as liver, kidney and brain are extremely high in cholesterol and should not be consumed. The following table lists the organ foods and other animal products with high cholesterol content. Most commonly used food "Egg Yolk" is very high in cholesterol while "Egg White" has no cholesterol. Also "Egg White" is one 100% protein so consume it plenty to boost your protein intake.

Table 7.2 Cholesterol content of organ foods and other animal products.

Food Item	Serving SIZE	Cholesterol (mg)	Food Item	Serving SIZE	Cholesterol (mg)
Pig Brain	100 gm	2530	Duck Egg	100 gm	619
Cow Brain	100 gm	2054	Chicken Egg Yolk	1 Egg	266
Beef Kidney	100 gm	804	Chicken Egg White	1 Egg	0
Pig Kidney	100 gm	480			
Cow Kidney	100 gm	387	Shrimp	100 gm	154
Pig Liver	100 gm	368	Lobster (cooked)	100 gm	85
Beef Liver	100 gm	307			
			Butter	100 gm	260
Beef	100 gm	96	Cream	100 gm	140
Chicken (with skin)	100 gm	195	Cheese	100 gm	100
Chicken (skinless)	100 gm	79	Milk (whole)	250 gm	35
Fish (Salmon)	100 gm	35			

(iv) PRESCRIPTION DRUGS: Take prescription drugs (mostly statin drugs) if you do not experience any side effects. You should take liver test routinely when on statin drugs.
(v) SUPPLEMENTS: Take natural products or supplements (that contain Niacin, Red Yeast Rice, Psyllium, Blond Psyllium, Fenugreek, Garlic, Oat Bran, Artichoke, Barley, Sitostanol, Beta-itosterol, others).

The American Heart Association suggested that daily cholesterol intake through food consumption should be less than 300 mg. This suggestion is based on general public. The people with diabetes and heart disease should keep the cholesterol intake as low as possible. Dr. Dean Ornish in his prevention diet , and in his book "Program for Reversing Heart Disease" recommended a cholesterol intake of only 5 mg per day. [2]

CHOLESTEROL-LOWERING DRUGS [1]

The New England Journal of Medicine, September 1998 Issue, stated that prescription drugs showed powerful effects on many patients with heart disease and the cholesterol levels were significantly reduced after the consumption of the following cholesterol-lowering drugs.

FDA Approved Statin Drugs: The 6 statin drugs are Mevacor (lovastatin), Lescol (fluvastatin), Pravachol (pravastatin), Zocor (simvastatin), Baycol (cervastatin), and Lipitor (atorvastatin).

Caution: Baycol (cervastatin), a well-known statin drug, has been withdrawn from the market worldwide except in Japan after it was linked to 31 deaths in the USA and over 9 in other countries because Baycol destroyed muscle cells, which were then released into the bloodstream. There have also been reports that the situation with two more drugs, rhabdomyolysis and gemfibrozil, is also life threatening. Muscle pain is the common side effect of these drugs. The Wall Street Health Journal on 1st Feb 2002 raised side-effect concerns reported by doctors and patients that statin drugs cause memory loss, personality changes and irritability.

LISTEN TO THE EXPERTS

Dr. S. SWEENY'S EXPERIMENTS [1]
Dr. Sweeny conducted experiments in 1927 with young healthy medical students as volunteers. In the first experiment, he fed the students with high fat diet consisting of olive oil, butter, mayonnaise made from egg yolks, and 20% cream for 2 consecutive days. Then a glucose tolerance test was taken for 2 hours, monitoring glucose levels every 30 minutes. The results showed that the blood glucose levels of healthy non-diabetic students after 2 hours remained at or over 11 mmol/L (200 mg/dL), indicating that those students suffered **temporary diabetes**.

After the bodies had recovered from the high fat diet, the experiment was repeated with the same volunteers but this time with a high carbohydrate diet consisting of sugar, candy, pastry, white bread, baked potatoes, syrup, bananas, rice and oat meal for 2 consecutive days. Then a glucose tolerance test was taken again. The results of this experiment showed that the blood glucose levels of healthy non-diabetic students after 2 hours reached normal values under 7 mmol/L (126 mg/dL), indicating no symptoms of diabetes.

Dr. Sweeny then interpreted that high fat food such as fats and oils block the insulin flow towards the cells, and raise the glucose level in the bloodstream. If you live with higher glucose levels, insulin resistance develops, and over time Type 2 diabetes.

Dr. T.J. MOORE'S REPORT ON CHOLESTEROL CONTROL (Probably Very True!) [1]
Dr. T.J. Moore concluded after many years of research that "lowering your cholesterol is next to impossible with diet, and often dangerous with drugs and it won't make you live any longer."

In his paper The Cholesterol Myth, Dr. T.J. Moore wrote: "Since cholesterol compounds are synthesized within the body, its link with diet would seem to be tenuous and indirect. Perhaps only one person in seven could achieve over ten percent cholesterol reduction through diet."

Dr. GABE MIRKIN'S REPORT [1]

Darwin's theorem meant that when people who have inherited sickening genes give birth to children, then children usually die early and the genes disappear. But the genes of diabetics have been around for millions of years.

When there is plenty of food around, a lot of diabetics eat plenty and even prepare to die from heart attacks, heart disease, stroke, kidney failure, etc. On the other hand when there is not enough food around, diabetics eat less and live longer because those who store fat best burn fewest calories. For example, Pima Indians in the deserts of Arizona and New Mexico used to be "thin warriors" and were survived on only 700 kilocalories per day compared to the average European who needs more than double that, 2000 kilocalories per day. When Pima Indians were fed western fat food, almost all of them became obese and more than 70% of them became diabetic.

REFERENCES
1. Permanent Diabetes Control (Book), Subtitle: The Complete Guide to Living Like A Normal Person Forever, Authored by Rao Konduru, MS, PhD, Reviewed and Endorsed by Dr. Marshal Dahl, MD, PhD., Endocrinologist, Faculty of Medicine, University of British Columbia, Vancouver, British Columbia, Canada, First Published in 2003. www.mydiabetescontrol.com

2. Dean Ornish, MD, Program for Reversing Heart Disease, Ivy Books, Published by Ballantine Books, New York, 1996.

3. Alan L. Rubin, MD, Diabetes for Dummies, IDG Books Worldwide Inc., Foster City, CA, USA, 1999.

4. Andrew Weil, MD, Eating Well For Optimum Health, Borzoi Books, Published by Alfred A. Knopf, New York.

CHAPTER 8 EAT WHOLE FOODS ONLY
Avoid Processed Foods and Refined Foods

A Person With Diabetes Must Not Eat:
a. Processed Foods
b. Refined Foods
This Chapter Is Designed to Help You Understand All About It!

TABLE OF CONTENTS

EAT WHOLE FOODS ONLY [2]
Avoid Processed Foods and Refined Foods

WHOLE FOODS

Whole foods are natural raw foods possessing all the nutrients nature bestowed upon them when they were grown and produced in orchards, gardens, or greenhouses. Whole foods are foods that have not been processed, modified or refined by any means by adding preservatives, colors and/or other additives in order to improve their taste and/or to store them for extended periods for the future consumption.

Whole foods are the healthiest foods for the human body. They are authentically flavorful, have vibrant colors and rich textures. Whole foods are loaded with carbohydrates, proteins, micronutrient vitamins, minerals, antioxidants, phytonutrients, fiber, and do not contain unhealthy fats.

Examples of Whole Foods

All raw foods, unprocessed, unrefined and unpolished whole grains, coarse grains (cracked, not powdered), beans, peas, vegetables, legumes, fruits, all unprocessed animal products (still in their whole form without any modification) such as whole chicken, whole turkey, whole beef, whole fish, whole eggs and all dairy products in their original form. Rotisserie chicken falls under the whole foods category but Kentucky Fried Chicken or any kind of deep-fried and breaded chicken is considered as processed food. See a complete list of "vegetables and greens" at the end of this chapter.

PROCESSED FOODS [2]

Processed foods are foods manufactured from whole foods or foods in a food factory, by adding preservatives, artificial colors and flavors including salt (sodium), MSG (monosodium glutamate), hydrogenated oils, fillers, sugars and sweeteners in order to package, transport and preserve them for sale in supermarkets.

Being modified, processed foods lose the nutritional value that the whole foods originally possessed. They also get contaminated with artificial colors, flavors and other additives making them harmful and unhealthy if consumed with ignorance.

Processed meats are manufactured in meat factories by adding a coloring agent called "sodium nitrite" to make them look fresh and attractive to consumers. Some processed meats contain monosodium glutamate (MSG), an even more harmful agent. People with unhealthy lifestyle habits choose processed meats, and they all pay a big price down the road. Research suggests that processed meats are directly linked to chronic health diseases and even cancer. Processed meat contains several chemical compounds that are not naturally present in fresh meat. Many of these chemical compounds are harmful to health. All processed foods are "JUNK FOODS".

JUNK FOODS are strategically manufactured from both processed foods and refined foods, adding large quantities of sugar, salt, oil, fat and several other chemicals including artificial colors and flavors to boost our cravings. This makes us buy more and eat more. Junk foods sabotage our weight-loss efforts. People consume here and there junk foods such as pizza slices, chicken donair in middle eastern places, pita bread, whole wheat bread, deep-fried samosas and spring rolls, Oh HENRY bars, chocolate chewy candies, dipped cone ice creams, cashew clusters, etc. **World Cancer Research International** established that there is a link between processed foods and cancer.

Examples of Processed Foods [2]

- Processed meat, red meat, processed pork, all meats that have been smoked, salted, cured, dried and canned, corned beef, beef jerky, bacon, ham, meat loaf, hot dogs, frozen pizza with processed meat, kid's meal containing red meat, ravioli and meat pasta foods, meat balls with spaghetti, fried chicken, breaded chicken, fish and beef, salami, pepperoni, sausages (chicken, turkey, beef), sausage rolls, kebabs, spring rolls, deep-fried samosas stuffed with potatoes, chicken and beef, deep-fried pakoras, nuggets of all types, and many other forms of breaded meat being sold in supermarkets.
- All bakery items, all kinds of breads made from refined flour, all kinds of pita breads, middle-eastern breads, naan, roti and so on.
- Ready-to-eat meals in packages and from fast-food restaurants.
- Soy milk, almond milk, all kinds of fruit juices and soft drinks.
- All kinds of soups and soup mixes being sold in supermarkets.
- Breakfast cereals of all kinds, being sold in supermarkets.
- All products made from whole milk such as cheese, whey, tofu from soy.
- Canned and frozen vegetables and fruits.
- All kinds of chips and snacks being sold in supermarkets and convenience stores.
- Processed peanuts, almonds, cashews with added salt being sold in plastic bags as snacks.
  Note: Dry-roasted raw peanuts, raw almonds, raw walnuts, raw cashews are whole foods.
- All kinds of sauces & dressings being served in restaurants or sold in supermarkets.
- Countless other items being sold in the stores everywhere.

REFINED FOODS [2]

Refined foods are not whole foods but processed foods that do not contain the original nutrients given by nature. Refined foods have been transformed and/or ground to their refined form from whole foods, and transported to supermarkets for distribution and direct consumption by customers. A refined food doesn't entirely contain its original nutrients in the whole food form, but is mixed with preservatives and/or artificial colors and flavors. **The altered texture and flavor make the body crave more of it. That is why your body wants more and more processed foods and refined foods.**

The human body does not process refined foods in the same way as whole foods, partially due to the decreased fiber content in refined foods. Refined foods are also generally many times higher in calories than whole foods. So your daily calorie consumption is a lot higher if you eat refined foods.

Examples of Refined Foods

A typical example is the STARCHY WHITE FLOUR OR ALL-PURPOSE WHITE FLOUR made from grains (mostly wheat, rice or both) by crushing them in a grinding machine. Refined foods lose fiber content after they are processed. Pizza dough, muffins, chips, Doritos, all bakery items such as pastries, cookies, donuts, cakes, ice cream cones, all kinds of breads, pita breads that are made from refined flour.

REASONS WHY YOU HAVE FAT IN THE BELLY [2]

◌ You are tempted to overconsume flour-based foods because they look attractive to the eyes, are easier to chew in your mouth and are very tasty while chewing.

◌ When whole-kernel grains are crushed with machinery and refined to produce starch, 80 percent of the fiber is lost, and therefore the gut health suffers.

◌ When you overconsume processed and refined foods, many heath hazards develop: food cravings, spiked blood sugar levels, metabolic slowdown, food allergies, acid-alkaline imbalances, inflammation, gastrointestinal-disorders or GI disorders such as acid reflux, heartburn, dyspepsia/indigestion, nausea and vomiting, peptic ulcer disease, abdominal pain syndrome, belching, bloating, flatulence, biliary tract disorders, gallbladder disorders and gallstone pancreatitis, and others.

◌ Refined flours or foods made using refined flours act like sugars in the body, triggering weight gain and high blood sugar. People like to consume fancy food items made from refined flour because they taste better than whole foods and are easier to consume. Foods made from refined flour digest faster than whole foods, causing blood sugar spikes, which in turn demands an immediate spike in insulin levels in order to maintain normal blood sugar levels in the body. But when the pancreas fail to secrete enough insulin into the blood stream to transport the glucose, glucose gets accumulated in the blood stream resulting in type 2 diabetes. <u>When people eat foods made from refined flour, they feel hungry again within 2 hours and eat more with developed cravings, causing the liver to manufacture fat in the belly</u>. Obese and overweight people eventually develop type 2 diabetes. That is why if you eat whole foods, you would save your life and protect yourself from gaining weight and developing diabetes, sleep apnea, sleep disorders and other diseases.

Table 8.1 Good carbohydrates versus bad carbohydrates.

GOOD CARBOHYDRATES	BAD CARBOHYDRATES
● Complex carbs.	● Simple carbs.
● Digest slowly.	● Digest fast and raise blood sugar level.
● Prolonged energy.	● Short energy spike.
● High in fiber.	● Low in fiber.
● You feel full longer.	● You become hungry again.
● Natural sugar and low calories.	● Added sugar and more calories.
● Demand low levels of insulin.	● Demand higher insulin levels with spike in blood sugar.
● Used directly for the energy.	● Some are converted into fat cells.
● Low glycemic index.	● High glycemic index.
● Help with weight loss.	● Cause uncontrollable weight gain.

NUTRIENTS ARE NEEDED FOR THE HUMAN BODY SURVIVAL [2]

In order to function properly, the human body must possess sufficient nutrients. A nutrient is a chemical or substance that an organism needs to survive and grow, or a nutrient is a substance taken from the environment and used in an organism's metabolism. The nutrients that are essential for the survival of human beings are: proteins, carbohydrates, fiber, fats, oils, vitamins, minerals and water. Nutrients are directly used to build and repair tissues, regulate the body's processes throughout the day. Nutrients are further converted into and used as energy for the living human body. The living human body needs nutrients for energy, to grow, and to repair itself. In addition, the human body needs water and fiber as well. You must consume the following seven types of nutrients every single day to be able to survive:

1. Water: About 70% of the human body is water. Water is required for the digestion, transport of nutrients in and out of your body's cells, lubrication, temperature regulation, etc.
2. Carbohydrates: Carbohydrates are the main source of energy.
3. Fats: Fats are a source of energy, and are used to repair cell parts.
4. Protein: Proteins are the building blocks making up body tissues, muscles, skin, and organs.
5. Vitamins: Vitamins enable chemical reactions in the body.
6. Minerals: Minerals aid enzyme function, and are utilized for the bone structure.
7. Fiber: Fiber is not digested by your body. Instead, it passes relatively intact through your stomach, small intestine and colon and moves out of your body. Fiber helps maintain bowel health, normalizes your bowel movement, helps control blood sugar levels, lowers cholesterol levels and aids achieving healthy weight and prevents colorectal cancer. Whole foods contain a lot of fiber whereas the refined and processed foods have already lost a lot of fiber content while being processed in manufacturing factories.

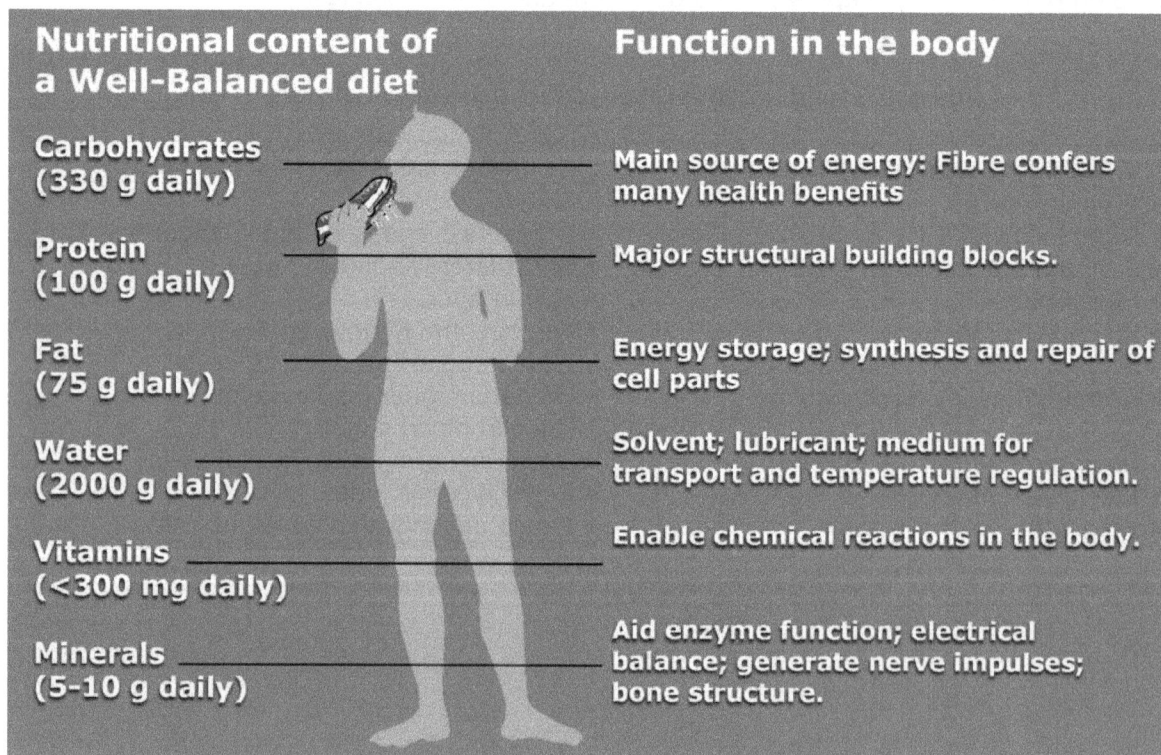

Nutritional content of a Well-Balanced diet	Function in the body
Carbohydrates (330 g daily)	Main source of energy: Fibre confers many health benefits
Protein (100 g daily)	Major structural building blocks.
Fat (75 g daily)	Energy storage; synthesis and repair of cell parts
Water (2000 g daily)	Solvent; lubricant; medium for transport and temperature regulation.
Vitamins (<300 mg daily)	Enable chemical reactions in the body.
Minerals (5-10 g daily)	Aid enzyme function; electrical balance; generate nerve impulses; bone structure.

Figure 8.1 Different nutrients and their functions in the body.

SIMPLE CARBOHYDRATES Vs COMPLEX CARBOHYDRATES [2]

Carbohydrates are a major source of energy that your body requires. Almost all foods "except meats, chicken, fish, egg whites, spices, oils, and water" are loaded with carbohydrates. Carbohydrates are made up of sugar, starch and fiber.

There are two types of carbohydrates: a. Simple Carbohydrates
b. Complex Carbohydrates

Table 8.2 Simple carbohydrates versus complex carbohydrates.

SIMPLE CARBOHYDRATES	COMPLEX CARBOHYDRATES
Simple carbohydrates are sugary food items with little or no fiber that digest quickly and raise blood sugar levels. All processed foods and foods made from refined flour are simple carbohydrates, and demand a lot of insulin to transport glucose into the blood stream. If the pancreas fail to secrete insulin according to the demand, the glucose buildup in the blood stream could result in type 2 diabetes. High glucose levels are also a cause for fat in the belly. Examples: raw sugar, brown sugar, all bakery items made by adding tons of sugar, refined flour and butter such as cookies, biscuits, muffins, cakes, candies, white bread, pie, pizza dough, breakfast sugary cereals, sodas, fruit juices, etc. ◦ You should deliberately identify and avoid simple carbohydrates in your diet, and consume only complex carbohydrates.	Complex carbohydrates are non-sugary food items with a lot of fiber along with vitamins & minerals that digest slower without any glucose spikes. All raw foods that are unprocessed and unrefined, contain complex carbohydrates. There are two types of complex carbohydrates: (i) Fibrous Foods (ii) Starchy Foods Fiber is essential for bowel movement, and lowers cholesterol levels. **Examples of Fibrous Foods:** whole grains, vegetables, raw fruits, beans, nuts & seeds. **Examples of Starchy Foods:** potatoes, legumes, whole wheat bread, raw cereal, oats, kidney beans, chick peas, rice, wheat, quinoa, etc. ◦ You should wisely include complex carbohydrates in your diet. All Whole Foods contain complex carbohydrates.

LIST OF VEGETABLES & GREENS (WHOLE FOODS) FOR EVERY DAY EATING [2]

Consume a variety of healthy vegetables and greens so that your body would get enough vitamins, minerals and fiber. Change the combination of vegetables and greens every day. You should prepare your egg-white omelet every day with different vegetables and greens. Some of these greens such as Kale, Spinach, Mustard Green, Chard should be added directly into the vegetables while making egg-white omelet. And some of the other greens such as Microgreens, Romaine, Iceberg, Alfalfa Sprouts and Beets can be eaten outside the plate to add nutritional value to your meal. It is important that you should watch the calories being consumed, and limit the quantity of vegetables and greens being consumed in every meal so that you meet the requirements of the weight-loss plan. In other words, do not overconsume these food items. Purchase and eat only "organic vegetables and greens" and wash them thoroughly before cooking and eating. And more importantly do not store these vegetables and greens for more than a week at home. If you do store them for more than a week, they could lose nutritional value. Make sure that you have eaten by covering most of these vegetables and greens, listed below, at least once every single week. Given below is the list of vegetables.

Table 8.3 List of vegetables & greens (whole foods) for every-day eating. [2]

LIST OF VEGETABLES AND GREENS (PREFERABLY ORGANIC)	
1. Kale, Chard, Collard Greens	31. Tomatoes (all kinds)
2. Fennel, Leeks, Broccoli Rabe (Rapini)	32. Lemons & Limes
3. Spinach, Curry Leaves	
	33. Parsley, Cilantro
4. Broccoli, Romanesco	34. Microgreens
5. Cauliflower	(nutrient levels are 6 times higher)
6. Mushrooms (all kinds)	35. Basil Herb
7. Egg Plant (all kinds)	36. Arugula
8. Onions (Yellow, Red & White)	37. Dandelion Green
9. Green Onions	38. Mustard Green, Mint Leaves
10. Scallions	39. Alfalfa Sprouts & Other Sprouts
11. Bell Peppers (Green, Red & Yellow)	40. Head Lettuce
12. Cucumber and Zucchini	41. Green Leaf Lettuce
13. Long English Cukes	42. Red Leaf Lettuce
14. Bok Choy & Goi Lan (Chinese)	43. Romaine Lettuce
	44. Butter Lettuce
15. Brussels Sprouts	45. Boston Butterhead
16. Asparagus	46. Iceberg Lettuce
17. Okra	47. Watercress, Dill
18. Green Long Beans/Yardlong Beans	
19. Peas	48. Sweet Corn (limited quantity)
20. Radishes	49. Russet Potatoes (limited quantity)
21. Cabbage (Green & Red)	50. White Potatoes (limited quantity)
22. Carrots	51. Red Potatoes (limited quantity)
23. Celery	52. Little Potatoes (limited quantity)
24. Butternut Squash	53. Sweet Potatoes (limited quantity)
25. Acorn Squash, Squash Carnival	54. Yams (limited quantity)
26. Kabocha	
27. Pumpkins	55. Beets (fresh, soft & juicy)
	56. Purple Top Turnips (limited quantity)
28. Garlic	57. Rutabagas, Daikon (limited quantity)
29. Ginger	58. Parsnips (limited quantity)
30. Horse Raddish	59. Artichokes (limited quantity)
	60. Celery roots (limited quantity)

REFERENCES

1. Permanent Diabetes Control (Book), Subtitle: The Complete Guide to Living Like A Normal Person Forever, Authored by Rao Konduru, MS, PhD, Reviewed and Endorsed by Dr. Marshal Dahl, MD, PhD., Endocrinologist, Faculty of Medicine, University of British Columbia, Vancouver, British Columbia, Canada, First Published in 2003. www.mydiabetescontrol.com

2. Reversing Obesity (Book), Self-Discovered Weight-Loss Method Illustrated, Authored by Rao Konduru, PhD, Published in 2018, Available on Amazon.com and other Amazon marketplaces, ASIN # B07BQYPC8C, ISBN # 9780973112030.

CHAPTER 9 DIABETES MEDICATIONS

Type 1 Diabetes
▶ **People With Type 1 Diabetes Inject Insulin Shots.**
Type 2 Diabetes
▶ **People With Type 2 Diabetes Take Oral Medications.**
▶ **Some People With Moderate Or Severe Type 2 Diabetes Inject Insulin Shots (As Oral Medications Do Not Work).**
▶ **This Chapter Is Designed to Help You Understand All About It!**

TABLE OF CONTENTS

WHO CAN USE ORAL MEDICATIONS & WHO CAN USE INSULIN SHOTS?
[1, 2, 3]

The International Diabetes Federation (IDF) reported in 2017 that there are approximately 425 million adults worldwide (ranging 20-79 years of age) living with diabetes. About 5 to 10% of these people suffer from type 1 diabetes, and the remaining 90 to 95% suffer from to type 2 diabetes. [3]

Type 1 Diabetes: Type 1 diabetes mellitus or insulin-dependent diabetes mellitus or adult diabetes, also called juvenile diabetes, is developed when the pancreas produces little or no insulin because the beta cells of the pancreas may have been totally damaged or destroyed. Type 1 diabetes is developed mostly in infants, children and young adults under the age 30 years. Insulin shots are certainly required to treat type 1 diabetes. As explained above, in order to optimize the insulin dose and insulin action, type 1 diabetics also need to exercise after every major meal consumption in order to slash the after-meal spikes and to tightly control diabetes.

Type 2 Diabetes: Nearly 40% of the adults in USA alone suffer from prediabetes or borderline diabetes, and at least some of them would soon be diagnosed with type 2 diabetes. The people with type 2 diabetes around the world can be categorized into 3 groups based on the severity of the disease: (i) mild, (ii) moderate and (iii) severe.

● For those people with prediabetes or borderline diabetes, or mild type 2 diabetes, diabetes can be controlled without any oral medication or insulin, but with healthy lifestyle (dietary changes) and regular exercise or physical activity. However high self-discipline is required to maintain healthy lifestyle.

● For some people with moderate type 2 diabetes, diabetes can be controlled with healthy lifestyle (dietary changes), and oral medication (s) along with regular exercise or physical activity. However high self-discipline is required to maintain healthy lifestyle.

● For those people with severe type 2 diabetes, and for some people with moderate type 2 diabetes, oral medications do not work effectively, and it would be difficult to achieve normal hemoglobin A1c. And so this group of diabetic people are advised to switch to insulin shots (both long-acting insulin and rapid-acting) along with after-meal exercise. Those diabetics who use insulin shots need after-meal exercise because insulin dose needs to be optimized. Injecting too much insulin without exercise has adverse side effects, and therefore insulin dose should be cut in half by incorporating an appropriate after-meal exercise plan.

● Some diabetic people with expert knowledge go easy on the dietary guidelines and still manage to control diabetes with insulin shots, keep their A1c perfectly normal, and live like a normal person. These people with expert knowledge know how to inject the right amount of rapid-acting insulin, by trial and error and exercise, and lower after-meal blood glucose spike quickly to normal, and know how to achieve normal A1c.

▶ Insulin is the best medicine to treat diabetes, and insulin shots always work for any kind of diabetes (either type 1 diabetes or type 2 diabetes). That is why, many doctors recommend their patients to switch to insulin shots.

LIST OF ORAL MEDICATIONS FOR TYPE 2 DIABETES [4, 5]

Table 9.1 The list of oral medications to treat type 2 diabetes.

ORAL MEDICATION	COMMENTS
1. Metformin or Biguanides. Examples include Glucophage & Glumetza. Most commonly prescribed oral medication to treat type 2 diabetes by many doctors. Depending on the progress, a doctor may also prescribe a 2nd medication in combination such as (i) Metformin-alogliptin (Kazano), and (ii) Metformin-canagliflozin (Invokamet).	It works by lowering glucose production in the liver and improving your body's sensitivity to insulin so that your body uses insulin more effectively. Side effects may include nausea and diarrhea. If there no significant progress, or if your after-meal glucose levels do not drop to normal within 2 hours consistently, you should switch to insulin shots.
2. Sulfonylureas. An alternative to Metformin medication. Examples include: (i) Glyburide (DiaBeta, Glynase), (ii) Glipizide (Glucotrol) and (iii) Glimepiride (Amaryl).	These medications stimulate the beta cells of the pancreas, and help your body secrete more insulin. Possible side effects include low blood sugar and weight gain.
3. Meglitinides (short or rapid-acting). Examples include: (i) Repaglinide (Prandin) and (ii) Nateglinide (Starlix). These medications work very similar to Sulfonylureas.	These medications also stimulate the beta cells of the pancreas, and help your body secrete more insulin much faster than sulfonylureas. Possible side effects include frequent low blood sugar and weight gain.
4. Thiazolidinediones. Examples include (i) Rosiglitazone (Avandia), and (ii) Pioglitazone (Actos) These medications work similar to Metformin.	These medications make the body's tissues more sensitive to insulin so that your body absorbs insulin faster. They have serious side effects are such as an increased risk of heart failure and anemia. Many people complained about Actos.
5. Sodium-Glucose Transporter Inhibitors. Examples include (i) Dapagliflozin (Farxiga), and (ii) Dapagliflozin-metformin (Xigduo XR).	These medications help get rid of the glucose through your urine. When heart disease, heart failure, or chronic kidney disease predominate, these medications also help treat the disease.
6. Alpha-Glucosidase Inhibitors. Examples are (i) Acarbose (Precose) (ii) Miglitol (Glyset)	These medications help your body break down starchy foods and table sugar. This effect lowers your blood sugar levels. For the best results, you should take these drugs before meals.
7. Dopamine Agonist. Bromocriptine (Cycloset) is an example.	This drug may affect rhythms in your body and may prevent insulin resistance.

⚫ Diabetes is a condition or disease that leads to unusually higher blood glucose levels in the bloodstream of your body. This happens when your body can't make or use insulin effectively. Insulin is a substance that helps transport glucose from the food to your body's trillions of cells. When the pancreas does not produce enough natural insulin, you need to inject artificial insulin.

INSULIN THERAPY

DISCOVERY OF ARTIFICIAL INSULIN [1]

Insulin is a miracle drug. Insulin was first discovered during 1921-22 by two Canadian doctors, Nobel Prize Winners, Dr. Frederick Banting and his student Dr. Charles Best at the University of Toronto, Toronto, Ontario, Canada (10b, 30). They were able to extract and purify insulin from the pancreases of several dogs that have anti-diabetic characteristics. Thereafter they successfully tested the extract on diabetic dogs. They reported that the action of the extracted insulin on diabetic dogs was outstanding. Immediately after that, they treated some diabetic people and brought the glucose levels to normal by injecting appropriate amounts of animal insulin extracted from cows and pigs. The whole medical community marveled at the miraculous effect of insulin, recognized as one of the most sensational medical breakthroughs ever, in bringing the rather starved and comatose diabetic people back to normal life.

Insulin is a hormone and therefore a protein that contains 51 amino acids, made from the pancreas gland. Insulin was the first hormone ever identified in 1921. The human body uses insulin to drive glucose from digested food. This fuel is used in turn by the cells to make energy. The beta cells of the pancreas produce insulin. Glucagon is another protein hormone produced by alpha cells of the pancreas. Glucagon stimulates the liver, kidneys and muscles to break down stored glucogen and releases glucose. Glucogen is stored in the liver and muscles for future use whenever there is excess glucose from digested food.

If the person is non-diabetic, there is always a counter-balance between the actions of insulin and glucagon so that the blood glucose levels remain normal at all times. When the beta cells of the pancreas of the human body do not function properly, then diabetes develops. Diabetics therefore need artificial insulin to be injected into their body's tissue.

COMMERCIAL OR SYNTHETIC INSULIN

In 1921, insulin was first manufactured from the pancreases of cows and pigs. It was available in the form of pure pork and mixed beef/pork insulin. In 1922, researchers first tested the insulin with a young patient. In 1939, insulin was first approved by FDA. In the 1980's advanced technology allowed the manufacture of human insulin. Research findings, through the development of recombinant DNA technique, revealed the fact that all humans have exactly the same insulin, and so there would not be any compatibility problem because injected insulin could not constitute a foreign protein to any person. Eventually the human gene, which codes for the insulin hormone (protein), was cloned and was captured inside of bacteria. After several modifications and manipulations performed on this gene, the bacteria were able to produce insulin constantly. Huge vats of bacteria nowadays make tons of a variety of human insulins. The most important among them are Humulin-U, Humulin-N, and Humulin-R. The fastest acting insulin available now is Humalog manufactured and sold by Eli Lilly.

Humalog was found to be the most effective insulin for any given food to quickly lower after-meal glucose levels close to normal with an appropriate combination of exercise. Refer to Chapter 4 for the practical results of the "Real-Life Case Study."

TYPES OF COMMERCIAL OR SYNTHETIC INSULIN [1, 6]

There are over 20 types of insulin available in USA today. There are 4 major types of insulin commercially available based on the promptness of action, duration and intensity of the insulin action upon injection into human body tissue. The following table shows the different types of insulin and their times of action. The times of action vary significantly from one individual to the other.

Table: 9.2 Commercially available insulins to treat diabetes.

Insulin Type	Action Begins	Peak	Duration
Rapid Acting Insulin			
a. Humalog (Lispro)	5 to 15 min	30 to 60 min	3 to 4 hours
b. Novo Rapid (Aspart)	5 to 15 min	1 to 2 hours	3 to 6 hours
or NovoRapid			
Short Acting Insulin			
a. Humulin-R (Toronto)	30 to 45 min	2 to 4 hours	6 to 8 hours
Intermediate Acting Insulin			
a. Humulin-N (NPH)	2 to 4 hours	6 to 12 hours	18 to 24 hours
b. Novolin	1 to 3 hours	5 to 8 hours	Up to 18 hours
b. Lente	2 to 4 hours	4 to 8 hours	10 to 16 hours
Long Acting Insulin			
a. Humulin-U(Ultralente)	3 to 5 hours	8 to 12 hours	18 to 24 hours
b. Lantus (Glargine)	1.5 hours	No Peak	24 hours
c. Toujeo	Up to 6 hours	No Peak	Up to 30 hours

ACTION PROFILE CURVES OF VARIOUS TYPES OF INSULIN [6a]
HOW FAST THE INSULIN WORKS AND HOW LONG THE INSULIN LASTS?

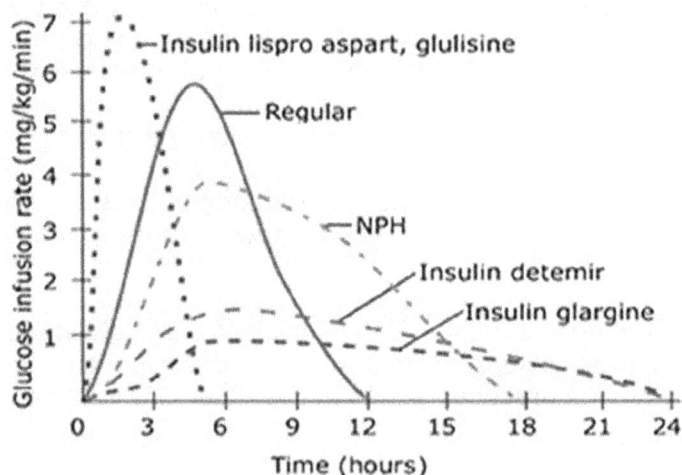

Figure 9.1 Action Profile Curves of various types of insulin.

HANDLING & STORAGE OF INSULIN [1]

The insulin should not be taken through mouth because it will be broken down in the stomach and does not help to normalize blood glucose levels. The insulin should be taken as a shot.

The insulin manufacturer usually provides instructions along with the insulin vial or pen. As soon as the insulin is purchased, the diabetic person should read the instructions on handling and storage, should check the expiration date and should never use the same insulin vial or pen loaded with a cartridge for more than 28 days. Some insulin pens such as Humulin-N, Humalog Mix 75/25 and Humulin Mix 70/30 are good for 10 days only.

A diabetic person, however, should attend a session at the nearest diabetic center to learn the handling and storage instructions from a nurse or healthcare professional in person, and should not depend on just reading material with instructions.

Caution: Any mishandled and/or improperly stored insulin could lead to erroneous results. There is no guarantee that the insulin being injected will act accordingly and lower glucose levels. Therefore after every insulin shot, the blood glucose level should be monitored in one or two hours to make certain that the injected insulin is acting accordingly and blood glucose levels are lowered.

Eli Lilly Company provided the following handling and storage precautions:
(i) Never roughly shake the insulin vial or pen loaded with a cartridge, but mix it very gently.
(ii) Avoid keeping insulin close to places that are too hot or too cold.
(iii) Never freeze insulin.
(iv) Any insulin vial or pen is considered "open" if the stopper or seal has been loosened.

Insulin Vial: Should be refrigerated if the vial is new and unopened.
After the vial is opened, it can be either refrigerated, kept in a cool place, or be left at room temperature outside the refrigerator.
Room temperature means 59 to 86 degrees Fahrenheit (°F)
Or 15 to 30 degrees Celsius (°C).
Insulin Pen: Should be refrigerated if the pen is new and unopened. After the pen is open, refrigeration is not required. After the pen is open, it can be left at room temperature.

Rotate Injection Sites, Or Face Lipohypertrophy! [2]
When injecting insulin, it is important to rotate the injection sites. Please do not inject repeatedly on the same area of your belly, and please do not re-use the syringes (never!). If you do so, you will develop lipohypertrophy. Lipohypertrophy is a medical term, meaning a lump under the skin, caused by the accumulation of extra fat at the site of many subcutaneous injections of insulin.

Longer Needles, Or Shorter Needles? [6b]
In the past, diabetics have been using 12.7 mm needles to inject insulin. Most recently, research proved that a needle depth of 5 mm works fine for all people, including children. With shorter needles (4 to 5 mm), inject at a 90-degree angle with no pinching of the skin. If longer needles are used, pinch up the skin to avoid injecting into intramuscular tissue. Also, hold the needle in the skin for 5 to 10 seconds after you give the insulin (even longer with higher doses) so the medication doesn't leak from the site. For very lean people, pinching the skin and injecting at an angle are recommended even with shorter needles.

INSULIN STRENGTH AND SYRINGE SIZE [1]

Insulin is sold in 3 different containers: (i). vials, (ii) cartridges, and (iii) pre-filled syringes. Vials require syringes and cartridges are used with pens.

When purchasing insulin and syringes, a diabetic person should note carefully the strength of insulin marked on the container and purchase appropriate syringes with a thorough concept. Any kind of misconception could lead to erroneous results or dangerous consequences. In North America, insulin is supplied at a strength of U-100. In Europe and in Latin America, insulin is supplied at a strength of U-40. U-100 insulin is 2.5 times stronger than U-40 insulin.

Table 9.3 Understanding Insulin Strength and Syringe Size

INSULIN STRENGTH	SYRINGE SIZE
A vial marked "U-100 or 100 u/mL" means	"Insulin U-100 1 cc" means
100 units of insulin substance are dissolved	1 cc is divided into 100 units.
in 1 mL of liquid	
A vial marked "10 mL U-100" has 1000 units of insulin.	"Insulin U-100 1/2 cc" means
A cartridge marked "3 mL 100 u/mL" has 300 units.	1/2 cc is divided into 50 units.
A vial marked "U-40 or 40 u/mL" means	"Insulin U-40 1 cc" means
40 units of insulin are dissolved in 1 mL of liquid.	1 cc is divided into 40 units.
A vial marked "10 mL U-40" has 400 units of insulin.	"Insulin U-100 1/3 cc" means
A cartridge marked "3 mL 40 U/mL" has 120 units.	1 cc is divided into 100 units
	but only 30 units are marked.

Proper attention should be paid while using the syringes. To avoid any confusion, U-100 insulin should be used with a U-100 syringe (1 cubic centimeter or 1 cc divided into 100 units or ½ cc divided into 50 units). U-40 insulin should be used with a U-40 syringe (1 cc divided into 40 units or ½ cc divided into 20 units). Sometimes, if the right syringe is not available, it is necessary to know how to calculate the correct amount of insulin for a particular syringe being used.

The following examples clearly illustrate the understanding of insulin strength. [1]

Example 1
John, a Type 1 diabetic person from Canada, traveled to Europe with his U-100 insulin. He usually takes 25 units of Humulin-N in the morning. He did not carry his U-100 syringes with him. He therefore purchased a U-40 syringe in a pharmacy in Europe. He calculated his insulin dose for U-40 syringe as follows:

25 units with U-100 syringe = 25 /2.5 = 10 units with U-40 syringe

He injected 10 units of Humulin-N with the U-40 syringe.
The conversion factor here is 2.5 (100 divided by 40 is 2.5).
Caution: If John had taken 25 units with the U-40 syringe, he would have had a severe insulin reaction or hypoglycemia.

Example 2

Mary, a Type 2 diabetic person from Europe, traveled to Canada with her U-40 insulin. She usually takes 12 unit of Humulin-N in the morning. She did not carry her U-40 syringes with her. She therefore purchases a box of U-100 syringes in a pharmacy in Canada. She calculated insulin dose for U-100 syringe.

12 units with U-40 syringe = 12 x 2.5 = 30 units with U-100 syringe

She injected 30 units of Humulin-N with the U-100 syringe.

Example 3

Paul, a Type 1 diabetic person from Canada, traveled to Europe. He is currently taking 25 units of Humulin-N from a U-100 vial with a U-100 syringe every morning. While traveling he lost his whole bag of insulin and syringes. He therefore purchased Humulin-N of U-40 vial and U-40 syringes from a pharmacy in Europe. He then made the following calculations.

25 units from U-100 vial = 25 x 2.5 = 62.5 units from U-40 vial.

If he had his U-100 syringe, he could have filled his syringe with 62.5 units.

But he does not have U-100 syringe, so he must use a U-40 syringe.

62.5 units with U-100 syringe = 62.5 / 2.5 = 25 units with U-40 syringe.

He injected 25 units of Humulin-N from the U-40 vial with a U-40 syringe. When he travels to Europe, he does not have to panic; he can purchase local insulin of U-40 strength and local syringes of U-40, and inject the same dose as in Canada. The dose is unchanged in this case.

Example 4

Edna, a Type 2 diabetic person from Europe traveled to Canada. She is currently taking 12 units of Humulin-N of U-40 vial with a U-40 syringe every morning. While traveling she lost her whole bag of insulin and syringes. She therefore purchased Humulin-N of U-100 vial and U-100 syringes in a pharmacy located in Canada. She then made the following calculations.

12 units from U-40 vial = 12 / 2.5 = 4.8 units from U-100 vial.
If she had her U-40 syringe, she could have filled her syringe with 4.8 units.
But she does not have U-40 syringe, so she must use a U-100 syringe.
4.8 units with U-40 syringe = 4.8 x 2.5 = 12 units with U-100 syringe.
She injected 12 units of Humulin-N from U-100 vial with U-100 syringe. When she traveled to Canada, she does not have to panic, she can purchase local insulin of U-100 strength and local syringes of U-100, and inject the same dose as in Europe. The dose is unchanged again in this case.

HOW TO PREPARE INSULIN INJECTION [1]

Procedure 1

Ravi takes 5 units of Humalog insulin with his lunch at noontime every day. The procedure is illustrated in the figure below:

Ravi measures 5 units of air into a "30-units 3/10 cc syringe" by pulling the plunger (Picture 1). He then pumps 5 units of air into the vial of Humalog through the rubber seal (Picture 2). Thus the vial is pressurized and is ready to deliver 5 units of insulin. He turns the vial of Humalog upside down with the syringe upright so that the tip of the needle is in the insulin (Picture 3). By keeping the syringe upright, he withdraws precisely 5 units of Humalog insulin into the syringe (Picture 4). He gets rid of the air bubbles, if any, with an up and down action of the plunger when syringe is half-filled. He then pulls out the needle from the vial of Humalog. The syringe is filled with 5 units of Humalog (Picture 5).
He injects 5 units of Humalog into the fatty tissue of his abdomen.

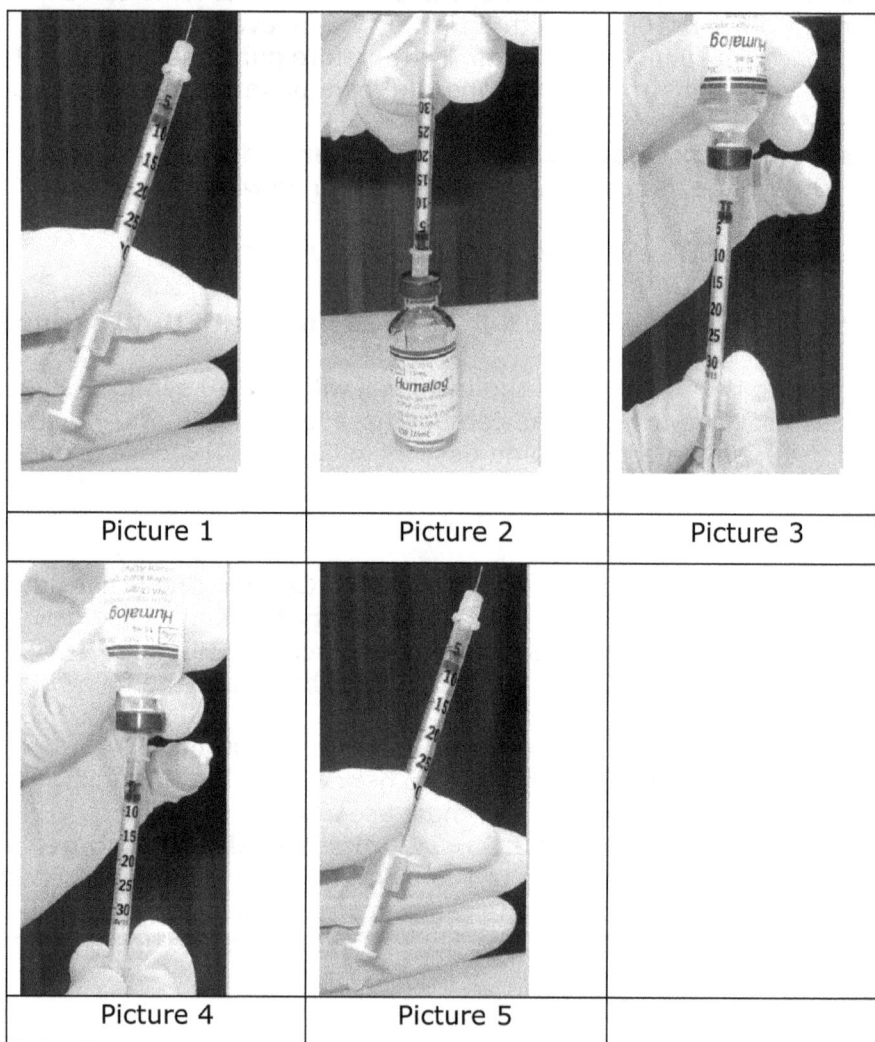

Picture 1	Picture 2	Picture 3
Picture 4	Picture 5	

Figure 9.2 Illustration of insulin injection.

HOW TO PREPARE MIXED DOSE OF INSULIN [1]

The following example demonstrates how to mix 2 different types of insulin:

Procedure 2

David being a Type 2 diabetic has been talking insulin shots for the last 2 years. He takes a mixed dose of insulin (15 units of Humulin-N and 5 units of Humalog) every morning before breakfast. To prepare the mixed dose he uses only one syringe.

15 units of Humulin-N + 5 units of Humalog = 20 units of mixed insulin

The sequence of steps is illustrated below in Figure 2.3.

David uses a "30-units 3/10 cc syringe" for his insulin injections. David measures 15 units of air into the syringe by pulling the plunger (Picture 6).

He inserts syringe through the rubber seal into the vial of Humulin-N (Picture 7).

He pumps 15 units of air into the vial of Humulin-N (Picture 8). Thus the vial is pressurized and is ready to deliver 15 units of insulin into the syringe.

He pulls out the needle from the vial of Humulin-N without filling the syringe with insulin. He then measures 5 units of air again into the same syringe by pulling the plunger (Picture 9).

He now pumps 5 units of air into the vial of Humalog through the rubber seal (Picture 10).

He turns the vial of Humalog upside down with syringe the upright so that the tip of the needle is in the insulin (Picture 11).

By keeping the syringe upright, he withdraws precisely 5 units of Humalog insulin into the syringe (Picture 12). He gets rid of the air bubbles, if any, with an up and down action of the plunger when the syringe is half-filled. He then pulls out the needle from the vial of Humalog with 5 units of Humalog.

He re-inserts the same syringe through the rubber seal into the vial of Humulin-N that was previously pressurized with 15 units of air. By turning the vial of Humulin-N upside down and by holding the syringe upright, he withdraws precisely 15 units of Humulin-N which makes up the total insulin reading of 20 units on the syringe (Picture 13).

The syringe is now filled with 20 units of mixed dose of insulin (15 units of Humulin-N and 5 units of Humalog). See Picture 14. He injects 20 units of the prepared mixed dose of insulin into the fatty tissue of his abdomen area.

Because he has been doing this every day, he prepares the mixed dose and injects into his fatty tissue in 30 to 40 seconds. It is possible with practice.

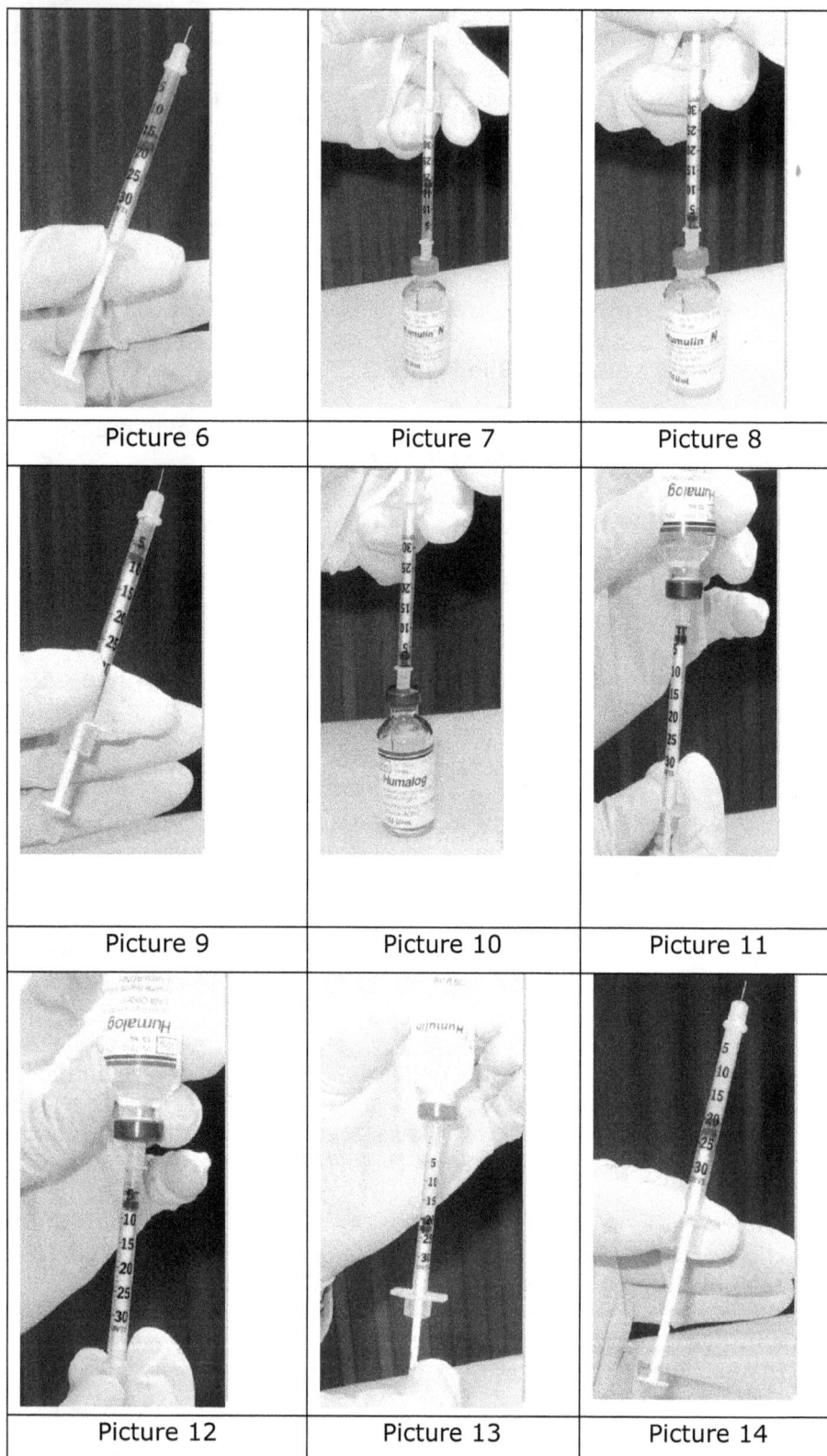

Figure 9.3 Illustration of injection of mixed dose of insulin.

INSULIN INJECTION SITES [1, 6a]

Insulin should be injected as a shot into the subcutaneous fatty tissue (under the skin) or directly into a vein. Insulin cannot be consumed as a pill because stomach acid would destroy the insulin before it can enter the bloodstream. Depending on the type of insulin and its corresponding action rate, the injected insulin is stored in the fat tissue, travels slowly and later passes into the bloodstream. Insulin can be injected to the fat tissue usually available in the upper arm, thigh, hip and abdomen of the human body. The standard depth of needle is 12.7 mm for an ordinary syringe and 8 mm when using a pen. Needles shorter than 8 mm are used for diabetic children but not recommended for adults. The ultra-fine syringes are highly recommended. Insulin is absorbed at different rates from different parts of the skin. An excellent spot would be the abdomen area (tummy) because the insulin is best absorbed there and passes into the bloodstream quickly. While using the abdomen area, the syringe should not be injected within a distance of 2 inches from navel (belly button). After the injection apply pressure gently over the site, and do not rub. After each injection, the site should be cleaned with soap, and the distance between current injection site and the next injection site should be 0.5 inch or 1.3 cm; otherwise fat tissue could be altered or get infected. The picture below shows the injection sites recommended by Eli Lilly and Co. (Reproduced with permission).

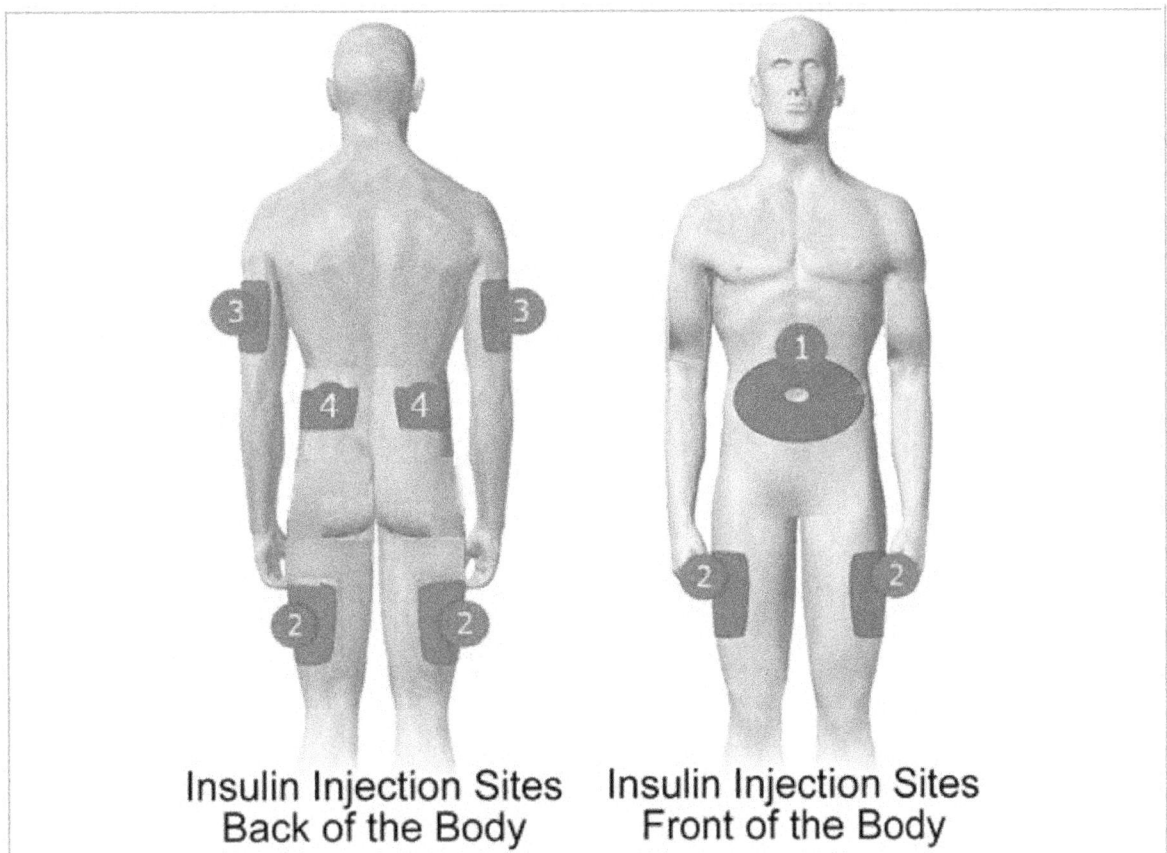

Insulin Injection Sites
Back of the Body

Insulin Injection Sites
Front of the Body

Courtesy of C. S. MOTT Children's Hospital, Michigan Medicine.
Figure 9.4 Insulin injection sites (Insulin works the best if injected on the belly).

SELF-BLOOD GLUCOSE TESTS AND FINGER-POKING [1]

Diabetic people should monitor blood glucose levels as many times as possible to control diabetes. When you do "Diabetic Research" on your own body, you may have to poke your finger 10 times or even more than 10 times a day in order to collect data, analyse and interpret the results. Frequent monitoring is also extremely important because only in that way you can take action, and inject insulin if needed, and achieve normal hemoglobin A1c and perfect diabetes control. Remember the pancreas monitors 500 times a day and automatically adjusts insulin secretion! A systematic procedure therefore is crucial to protect the fingers from getting ragged. The following picture shows how to do this carefully.

Finger-poking should be done with proper care by poking one finger a day, remembering it, and switching to next finger in the following day in the order so that you would not repeat poking on the same finger over and over again. For example it is necessary to poke 4 times a day. As marked in the picture, there are 12 poking sites on each finger and so each finger can be used for 3 days. Remembering each site poked, one can continuously poke all twelve sites in 3 days. Poke the first finger for 3 days beginning on the 1st of the month, then poke the second finger for the next 3 days, and so on, with the aid of a calendar. There are 10 fingers, and it would take 30 days (1 month) to finish poking the 10th finger. In this way each finger has 27 days per month to heal and restore. **Precautions:** Wash your poked finger with soap and clean it each time with a cloth, and always use only ultra-fine lancets with a high-quality lancing device.

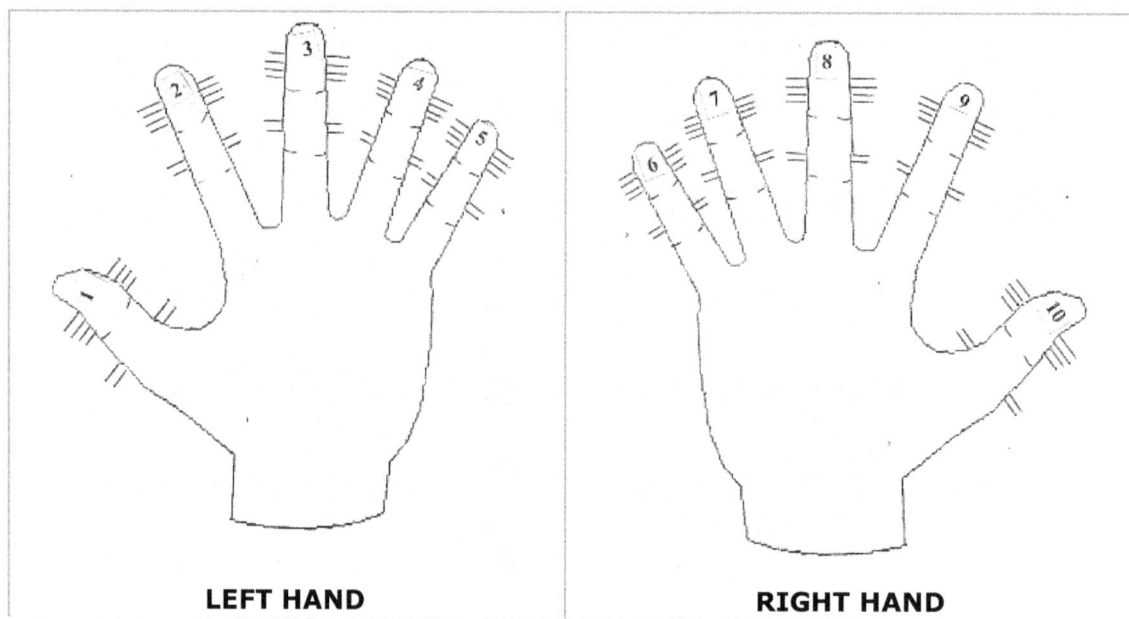

	LEFT HAND				RIGHT HAND	

2019 DECEMBER

SUN	MON	TUE	WED	THU	FRI	SAT
1	2	3	4	5	6	7
8	9	10	11	12	13	14
15	16	17	18	19	20	21
22	23	24	25	26	27	28
29	30	31				

Figure 9.5 Finger-poking should be done with proper care one finger a day.

INSULIN PUMPS [1]

Insulin pumps mimic pancreatic function. An insulin pump is a mini-device of about the same size as a pager in which most commonly a rapid-acting insulin such as Humalog is stored. The pump is able to deliver minute quantities of insulin ranging from one hundredth to one tenth of a unit. A needle is inserted under the subcutaneous fat tissue so that pre-determined doses of insulin are pumped at pre-determined intervals similar to the function of the pancreas. The device is automatic and there is no manual involvement.

The pancreas of a non-diabetic person stores about 200 units of insulin. The average basal rate is two units per hour. When food is consumed, the rise in glucose levels stimulates the pancreas and the secretion of insulin increases to four to six units per hour.

The amount of insulin to be delivered by the insulin pump in short intervals is programmable by the person using the pump. As a result, the effective action of the insulin becomes much smoother in controlling blood glucose levels.

This pump is usually designed to deliver insulin with two types of rates: (i) **basal rate** and (ii) **bolus rate**. The basal rate is a constant low flow of insulin similar to the secretion of insulin from the pancreas. The bolus rate is used to deliver extra insulin needed instantaneously depending on the amount of carbohydrate consumed. The basal rate is a substitute for intermediate or slow acting insulin and the bolus rate is a substitute for rapid-acting insulin. Whenever the diabetic person eats extra food, he/she can program the pump to increase the bolus rate to an extended period of time. The manufacturer usually provides the necessary training on self-programming skills.

When you are planning to use an insulin pump, you just talk to a major manufacturing company. They will arrange a free session with a sales representative at the comfort of your home or in location near you, and that representative would train you on everything about using the insulin pump. In addition, you can talk to the manufacturer over the phone and get all your question answered.

Caution:

a. Every diabetic person using any such insulin pump should bear in mind that the pump is not always guaranteed to work. Like any other instrument it may break down or stop working. That is why one should monitor glucose levels on a regular basis with a glucose meter to confirm the results and to make sure that the pump is working and blood glucose levels are controlled to the desired level.

b. Once every 3 months, a hemoglobin A1c test should be done to make certain that the diabetes is controlled. The pump itself does not take care of diabetes.

c. Companies that market insulin pumps may encourage the diabetic person to eat more or less any food whenever he/she wants because the insulin pump takes care of glucose levels. Even though these pumps can keep the diabetes under tight control, when a diabetic person eats food without appropriate care, he/she can gain weight, the cholesterol levels rise and over time the individual could face heart attack and/or heart disease. Hence, a diabetic person should always maintain keen attention to the food being consumed.

MEDTRONIC INSULIN PUMPS (MINIMED™ 670G & MINIMED™ 630G) [7]

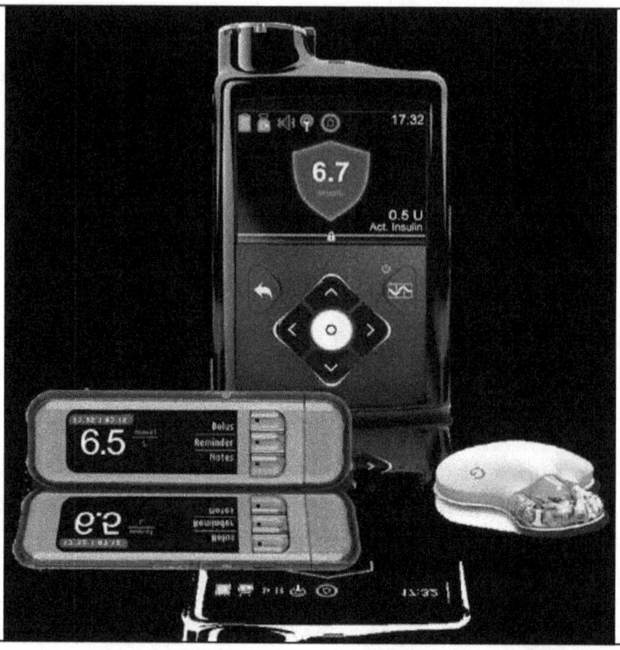

The website of Medtronic company claims that The MiniMed 670G system's revolutionary technology automatically works to keep your glucose levels in range, day and night.

The MiniMed™ 670G system with SmartGuard Auto Mode gives you freedom to think less about managing your diabetes. It focuses on you, so you can focus more on whatever the day brings.

https://www.medtronic.com

Courtesy of Medtronics

Figure 9.6 Insulin Pump MEDTRINIC MINIMED™ 670G.

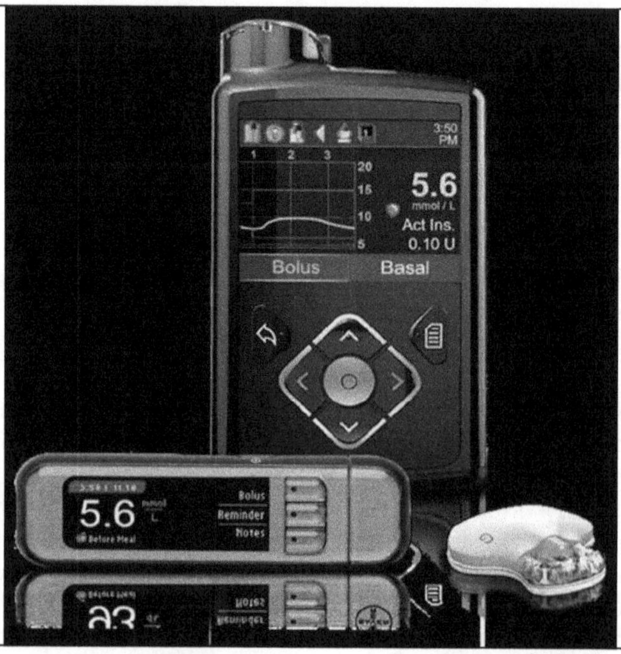

The website of Medtronic company claims that The MiniMed™ 630G with SmartGuard™ technology can help you get there. This insulin pump and sensor system steps in when you need it; with convenient options and features, it makes it easy to enjoy a day that revolves around you.

https://www.medtronic.com

Courtesy of Medtronics

Figure 9.7 Insulin Pump MEDTRONIC MINIMED™ 630G.

TANDEM INSULIN PUMP: t:slim X2 [8]

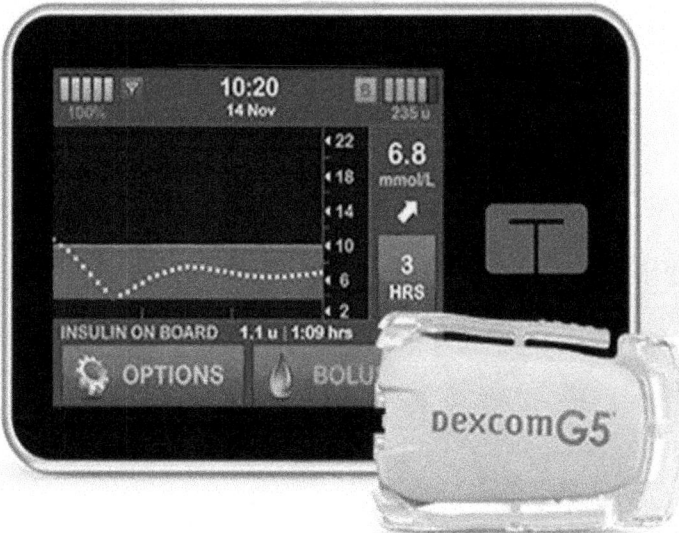

https://www.tandemdiabetes.com/

The website of Tandem Insulin Pump company claims that this is the only pump available with Dexcom G5® Mobile CGM integration. The t:slim X2™ insulin pump is approved to let you make treatment decisions without pricking your finger.

If your glucose alerts and readings do not match your symptoms or expectations, or you are taking medications containing acetaminophen, you should perform a fingerstick blood glucose test to confirm your blood glucose level.

Courtesy of Tandem Insulin Pump Company

Figure 9.8 Insulin pump Tandem.

OMNIPOD INSULIN PUMP [9]

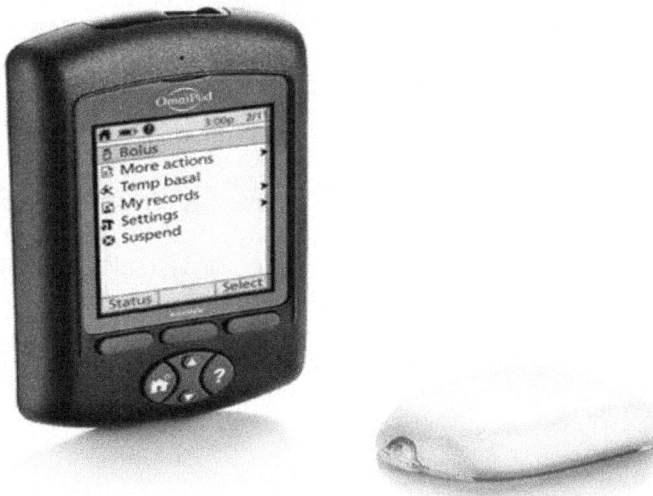

https://www.omnipod.com/

The website of OmniPod pump company claims that Our tubeless, waterproof Pod provides up to 3 days of insulin for people with diabetes. Omnipod® Insulin Management System lets you manage insulin delivery simply and discreetly. More convenient than daily insulin injections and more comfortable than traditional tubed pumps, the Omnipod® System enables you to live life more freely. Omnipod® Systems innovative design has been engineered for ease-of-use, and to manage insulin delivery simply and discreetly. It is more convenient than daily insulin injections and more comfortable and discreet than traditional tubed pumps.

Courtesy of OmniPod

Figure 9.9 Insulin pump OmniPod.

YpsoPump (Insulin Pump) [10]

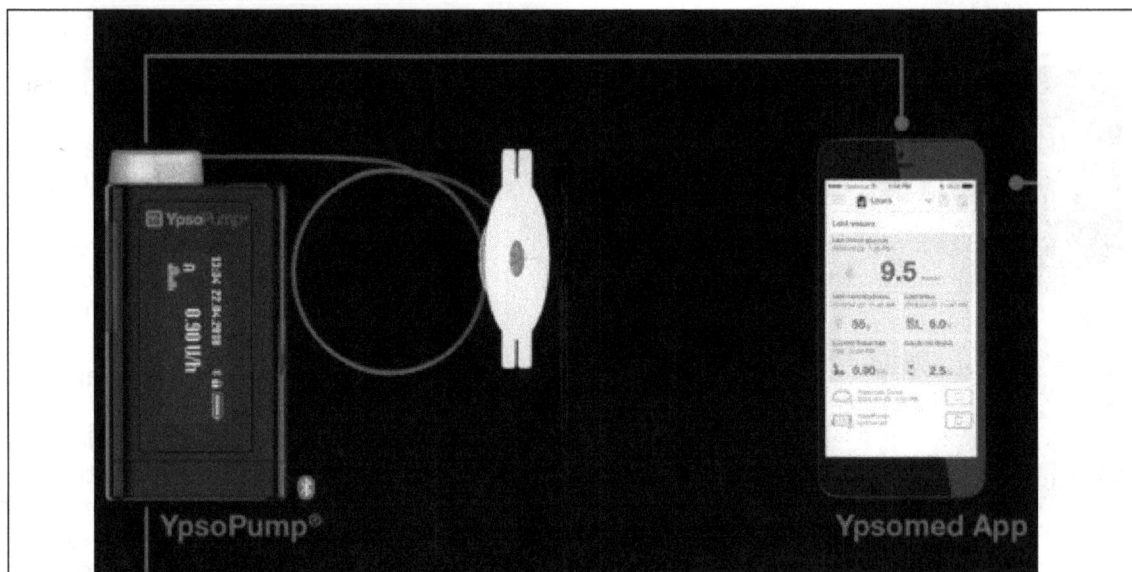

The website of YpsoPump company claims that: YpsoPump is the intuitive insulin pump system, the small insulin pump with a touchscreen, comprehensive data at your fingertips, and self-filled YpsoPump Reservoir for the insulin of choice. YpsoPump Orbit infusion set is for more freedom of movement. Orbit Inserter is designed for quick and safe insertion of the infusion set. And Ypsomed Software has the therapy management made easy.

https://www.ypsomed-diabetescare.com/

Courtesy of YpsoPump Company

Figure 9.10 Insulin pump YpsoPump.

Insulin Inhalers, Patches and Capsules [1]

Insulin inhalers, patches and capsules are under development. Compressed air is used to convert a dose of dry or dissolved rapid-acting insulin such as Humalog into particles that can be inhaled. It is called aerosolization. However they are not yet commercially available nor have they been safety-tested to control diabetes. Scientific research is underway to develop devices which can deliver insulin through nasal spray, skin patches, or oral capsules.

INSULIN-FREE WORLD [1]

The future holds strong hope for the permanent cure of Type 1 diabetes. The web site of "Insulin-Free World" discusses up-to-date advances in diabetes care.
        http://www.insulinfree.org/articmch.htm
The current news and scientific breakthroughs are as follows:

a. Artificial Pancreas: Medtronic, a MiniMed subsidiary, believes that Medtronic could bring an "artificial pancreas" to the market in the future.

b. Injected Stem Cells Reversed Type 1 Diabetes in Mice

Some university researchers in Spain developed a special gene therapy that restores islets without any cell transplants. They gave multiple shots of a drug that induces Type 1 diabetes in genetically engineered mice. They used a substance, insulin like growth factor (IGF-I), which promotes the growth and development of pancreatic tissue. After the therapy, they found that the glucose levels at first rose and over time returned to normal level, and the mice experienced a rebound in beta cells. Thus they successfully reversed Type 1 diabetes in genetically engineered mice. However the research failed when they tried to duplicate this gene therapy to actual mice because the actual mice died when they tried. They still believe that in the near future, gene therapy will permanently cure Type 1 diabetes.

c. Pancreas Transplantation: Some 14,000 pancreas transplantations have already been performed worldwide.

d. Simultaneous Transplantation of Kidney and Pancreas:

Simultaneous Transplantation of Kidney and Pancreas is becoming increasingly popular for diabetic people who suffer serious kidney disease. Upon successful transplantation the body begins producing proper hormones again eliminating the need for daily insulin injections.

e. Islet Transplantation – Edmonton Protocol

In 1999, at the University of Alberta, Edmonton, Alberta, Canada, Type 1 diabetic people were completely freed from insulin injections through a new treatment of islet transplantation called the Edmonton Protocol. After that the clinic was funded to continue research by extending the islet transplantation treatment plan to 40 more Type 1 diabetics around the world. Further information about this islet transplantation program can be found on the following web site:

Islet Transplantation Procedure

A typical transplantation requires about one million islets collected from two deceased donors. Specialized enzymes are used to remove islets from the pancreas of donors. A catheter is placed through the upper abdomen into the liver. The islets are then injected into the large vein in the liver via the catheter. If this attempt is successful, the islets of Langerhans should attach to the blood vessels. After a while, the islets of Langerhans begin producing insulin from beta cells. Blood glucose levels are continuously monitored and artificial insulin is also injected at the beginning of transplantation to lower glucose levels whenever needed. The transplantation is continued through the infusion of islets until the insulin produced by the islets lowers blood glucose levels to normal without any artificial insulin. It takes less than an hour to complete the transplantation.

The major obstacle in this islet transplantation is that the immune system could reject the functioning of transplanted islets. To prevent any such rejection, anti-rejection drugs are prescribed. These drugs may have to be taken forever to keep the transplanted islets functioning without any rejection problems.

REFERENCES

1. Permanent Diabetes Control (Book), Subtitle: The Complete Guide to Living Like A Normal Person Forever, Authored by Rao Konduru, MS, PhD, Reviewed and Endorsed by Dr. Marshal Dahl, MD, PhD., Endocrinologist, Faculty of Medicine, University of British Columbia, Vancouver, British Columbia, Canada, First Published in 2003. www.mydiabetescontrol.com

2. The Secret to Controlling Type 2 Diabetes, Subtitle: Addendum to Permanent Diabetes Control, Authored by Rao Konduru, Published in 2019, ISBN # 9780973112054, Available on Amazon.com, www.mydiabetescontrol.com

3. Diabetes Facts & Figures (Statistics) by International Diabetes Federation (IDF) https://www.idf.org/aboutdiabetes/what-is-diabetes/facts-figures.html

4. Type 2 Diabetes by Mayo Clinic, Diabetes Medications and Insulin Therapy, 2019 https://www.mayoclinic.org/diseases-conditions/type-2-diabetes/diagnosis-treatment/drc-20351199

5. The Complete List of Diabetes Medications by Healthline. https://www.healthline.com/health/diabetes/medications-list

6. Insulin Types by Healthlink BC, https://www.healthlinkbc.ca/health-topics/aa122570

6a. Insulin Action Profiles Different Types of Insulin http://www.partone.lifeinthefastlane.com/insulins.html#id

6b. Do I Need a Longer Insulin Needle? This question was answered by Christy L. Parkin, MSN, RN, CDE, Diabetes Forecast, The Healthy Living Magazine, 2019. http://www.diabetesforecast.org/2013/dec/do-i-need-a-longer-insulin.html

7. Medtronic Insulin Pumps by Medtronic, 2019 https://www.medtronic.com/ca-en/index.html https://www.medtronic.com/ca-en/diabetes/home.html Insulin Pumps https://www.medtronic.com/ca-en/diabetes/home/products/insulin-pumps/minimed-670g.html

8. Insulin Pump Tandem, Tandem Diabetes Care, 2019. https://www.tandemdiabetes.com/en-ca/home https://www.tandemdiabetes.com/en-ca/products/t-slim-x2-insulin-pump

9. Omnipod Insulin Pump by Insulet Corporation, 2018. https://www.myomnipod.com/en-ca/home https://na.myomnipod.com/become-a-podder-ca-demokit?

10. YpsoPump (Insulin Pump) by Ypsomed Canada Inc. https://www.ypsomed-diabetescare.com/en-CA/products/infusion-systems/ypsopump-insulin-pump.html

CHAPTER 10 EXERCISE WITH DIABETES

TABLE OF CONTENTS

INTRODUCTION [1]

"Exercise is the best medicine," said Hippocrates (a Greek physician, known as the Father of Medicine, who lived from 460 BC to 377 BC). But mankind disregarded this. Priority was given to liberty, and the daily use of head, pen and paper instead of both feet. Consequently, the belly has become ugly, contributing to obesity, hypertension, high cholesterol and eventually diabetes.

Exercise can change the diabetic person's life forever as long as he/she implements it **after every major meal** in a strictly disciplined manner. As discussed in previous chapters, glucose from digested food is transported to each and every cell of the human body as the source of energy. On each cell, there are receptor-sites referred to as "little doors". When the person is obese, most of these little doors remain closed, not effectively utilizing the glucose that is already present in the bloodstream as the source of energy. With exercise the little doors are opened more frequently than they are without exercise so that glucose molecules can be effectively attached to the trillions of cells of the human body. Any deficiency regarding the opening of the little doors contributes to become obese and to lack energy, and lead a person to Type 2 diabetes.

Dr. Sweeney's experiments concluded that fats and oils interfere with the insulin flow on the body's cells while transporting glucose molecules. The cells of the body become unable to respond to the natural insulin produced by the pancreas and also to artificially injected insulin. As a result, the person is diagnosed with insulin resistance which in a later stage turns into Type 2 diabetes. These findings indicated that burning fat on a regular basis is of paramount importance for a diabetic person.

The liver and muscles are the only place where extra glucose is stored. While exercising, active muscles use glucose for energy. When the stored glucose is used up, additional glucose flows from the liver into the bloodstream. If the muscles use more glucose than is being supplied from the liver, then the blood glucose level falls. Because the blood glucose level does not rise during exercise, for a non-diabetic person or for a Type 2 diabetic person, there is no demand for insulin flow from the pancreas. For a Type 1 diabetic person or a diabetic person who uses insulin shots, the injected dose is the source of insulin. However the action of insulin during exercise maximizes and lowers blood glucose levels much more quickly than it does for a non-diabetic person. That is why preparing to face and treat insulin reaction (hypoglycemia) during exercise is very important. Adjustment of insulin dose to avoid any hypoglycemia should be learned through experience and proper care.

ADVANTAGES OF EXERCISE [1]

♦ Exercise is called "the invisible insulin" for diabetic people.
♦ Exercise lowers glucose level by speeding the transport of glucose into cells.
  Lower glucose level means lower insulin need & lower demand on pancreas.
♦ Exercise also improves the flow of artificial insulin injected, and cuts its dosage up to 60%.
♦ Exercise improves muscle stimulation, reduces stress, and improves sleep at night.
♦ Exercise increases the efficiency of heart and lungs, and keeps the body alert.
♦ Exercise improves quality of sleep, gives freshness and improves self-image.
♦ Exercise on a regular basis also lowers total cholesterol & LDL cholesterol levels.
♦ Exercise helps you lose weight, keeps your body weight normal and toned, and also improves your overall health.
♦ Did you know many people reversed type 2 diabetes by losing weight?

Burning calories can be accomplished through a variety of exercises and sports such as Walking, Running, Treadmill, Swimming, Aerobics, Bicycling, Bowling, Skiing, Skating, Stretching, Dancing, Playing Tennis and other Sports.

HOW TO EXERCISE?

a. You can go out and walk on the road for an hour.
b. You can go to a large shopping mall and walk for an hour if the mall allows.
c. You can go to a local gym every day and exercise for 1 hour or more.

While any type of exercise would do the job, for a diabetic person, "Walking, Treadmill, Biking and Swimming" are most suitable and comfortable to burn calories.

Walking is the most comfortable and easily manageable exercise for everybody. Walking at a normal pace of about 3 miles per hour burns approximately 250 to 300 calories per hour depending on the weight of the person. Walking does not hurt the body like other exercises do. A diabetic person should walk an hour after every major meal to lower glucose levels.

Treadmill being an indoor exercise is suitable for young diabetics. In cold weather, when climate is not suitable for walking, running on treadmill is an excellent option. The person can monitor calories burned and heart rate by inputting the body's weight, duration and speed. Vigorous treadmill exercise burns fat quickly and efficiently. One can see a significant loss in weight by monitoring it before and after a vigorous extended treadmill exercise.

Biking is as good as treadmill with its advantage being an indoor exercise.

Swimming is strongly recommended for improving freshness and self-image. Exercise can be continued as long as the energy lasts, and more importantly until the blood glucose level is at or above 4 mmol/L or 72 mg/dL.

ENERGY EXPENDITURE IN EXERCISE [1]

Metabolism is the process by which a food substance is handled in the body and in which a source of energy such as food is converted into energy or heat to be used or absorbed by the body's cells. Metabolism is a two-part process. The first part is **catabolism** in which the body uses food for energy. The second part is **anabolism** in which the body uses food to build or mend cells. Insulin is necessary for the metabolism of foods. Metabolism is also defined as the mechanism inside the body that is responsible for burning the calories ingested through food substances.

When people exercise calories are lost. Metabolism varies from person to person as each individual body's cells absorb the food energy differently. Metabolism is faster/slower than the normal rate. Any confusion regarding calories should be clarified. Calories, either food calories listed on labels or books and calories burned being displayed on exercise machines always refer to **kilocalories**.

Energy expenditure means the calories burned either with or without physical activity or exercise. MET (Metabolic Equivalent) is a standard term developed by health fitness experts. MET has been defined as the energy expenditure per one kilogram of body weight per hour of sitting quietly. It was confirmed that an average adult spends about 1 kilocalorie per hour per 1 kilogram of his/her body weight by sitting quietly or lying down without doing any exercise.

Example 1
a. A person weighing 40 Kg (89 lb) loses 40 Kcal in 1 hour, 80 Kcal in 2 hours, and so on without any physical activity.
b. A person weighing 70 Kg (156 lb) loses 70 Kcal in 1 hour, 140 Kcal in 2 hours, and so on without any physical activity.

The energy expenditure for each type of physical activity is different because one activity requires more or less energy than another. To determine the energy expenditure for a given physical activity, the MET value has to be multiplied by the weight of the individual in kilograms and by the time spent in physical activity in hours. Heath fitness experts have already determined and tabulated the MET values for a variety of physical activities. Listed below, in Table 6.1, are MET values for a few physical activities. Using these MET values, we can calculate the calories burned in 1 hour or more time.

Example 2
A person weighing 130 lb (58.5 Kg) is walking at 2.0 mph.
From Table 6.1, the MET value = 2.5
Calories burned in 1 hour = 58.5 x 2.5 x 1 = 146 Kcal

Example 3
A person's weighing 130 lb (58.5 Kg) is walking at a normal pace at 3 mph.
From Table 6.1, the MET value = 3.5
Calories burned in 1 hour = 58.5 x 3.5 x1 = 204.8 Kcal
Similarly, using MET values, the calories burned for a person weighing 155 lb (69.75 Kg) and 190 lb (85.5 Kg) for different activities are calculated and tabulated as shown in Table 5.1.

Table 10.1 MET Values and Calories Burned (Kcal).

		Calories Burned in 1 Hour (Calculated from MET values)		
		130 lb	155 lb	190 lb
	MET	58.5 Kg	69.75 Kg	85.5 Kg
Resting (no activity)	1.0			
Walking at 2.0 mph	2.5	146.0	174.4	213.8
Walking at 2.5 mph	3.0	175.5	209.3	256.5
Walking at 3.0 mph	3.5	204.8	244.0	299.3
Walking at 4.0 mph	4.0	234.0	279.0	342.0
Bicycling at 10.0 mph	6.0	351.0	418.5	513.0
Swimming (light)	8.0	468.0	558.0	684.0
Running at 6.0 mph	10.0	585.0	697.5	855.0

This is what exactly the exercise machines do. Exercise equipment such as treadmills is designed and built to display calories being burned per hour and exact calories lost during a workout, indicating the total energy expenditure. Exercise machines are developed with electronic controllers and sensors that read the body weight and the intensity of the exercise and calculate and display the calories burned in a given period of exercise. These machines have incorporated the MET values in their database and have been calibrated properly, tested at a variety of intensity levels and for long periods before they are marketed. Whenever we use an exercise machine either in a gym or in a private location, each machine asks questions such as body weight, chosen program, intensity level, and the duration of exercise. Based on the intensity of the program, the machine calculates and displays calories burned for a particular workout.

A treadmill stores the MET values as a function of body weight, kind of program such as Fat Burn, Hill, Random, Manual, Cardio, Fit Test, etc., and intensity of the exercise such as speed and inclination. When the person performs an exercise for a given period of time, the machine calculates and displays the calories burned.

HEART RATE [1]

The pulse rate, or the heartbeat, can be sensed and counted by touching some areas such as the wrist, neck or the top of the foot where the artery passes closest to the skin. The pulse rate is counted by placing the index finger over and middle finger under the wrist, and by pressing firmly until the pulse is sensed.

The acceleration and deceleration of blood and vibration of the heart cause the sound of heartbeat. The adult average heartbeat is 72 times per minute. The normal heart rate while resting is as follows:

Table 10.2 Normal Heart Rate Ranges.

Type of People	Beats Per Minute
Infants	100 to 160 beats per minute
Children (1 to 10 years)	70 to 120 beats per minute
Children (over 10 years)	60 to 100 beats per minute
Adults of all ages	60 to 100 beats per minute
Trained Athletes	40 to 60 beats per minute

If the pulse rate is not within the normal range as indicated above, something is wrong, and the person should consult a healthcare professional.

The maximum heart rate and target heart rate can be calculated:
Maximum Heart Rate = 220 bpm (beats per minute) – Age
Target Heart Rate = 60 to 70% of Maximum Heart Rate

Example 4
A 50-year-old person is weighing 70 Kg.
Maximum Heart Rate = 220 – 50 = 170 bpm
70% of Maximum Heart Rate = 0.70 x 170 = 119 bpm
60% of Maximum Heart Rate = 0.60 x 170 = 102 bpm
His target heart rate should be between 102 bpm and 119 bpm—which is safe for this person at any level of intensity of a particular activity.

TOTAL FOOD ENERGY REQUIREMENT [1]

Basal Metabolic Rate (BMR) is the total calorie intake a normal human body needs for survival including heart beat, breathing, maintaining human digestive system, body temperature, etc.

The very approximate short-cut rule is to multiply the body weight in pounds by 10 to obtain the basic energy in kilocalories, and then correct this basic energy value taking physical activity into account. This also depends on many factors such as age, gender, size and body composition.

Example 5: A 52-year-old person weighing 155 lb (69.75 Kg) and 5' 6" (168 cm) tall would need 1550 Kcal per day for survival. If this person plans a daily exercise of walking for 1 hour at normal pace (3 mph.), he/she would need an extra 244 Kcal. The total calories required = 1550 + 244 = 1794 Kcal.

More Accurate Method to Calculate Basal Metabolic Rate (BMR)
Harris Benedict Formula
BMR for Men = 66 + (13.7 x Weight in Kg) + (5 x Height in cm) – (6.8 x Age in yr)
BMR for Women = 655 + (9.6 x Weight in Kg) + (1.8 x Height in cm) – (4.7 x Age in yr)

If we use Harris Benedict formula in Example 5, BMR would be 1508 Kcal.

WEIGHT LOSS [1]

HOW TO EXPLAIN 3500 Calories = One Pound?

Most health fitness experts very commonly state that one pound of body mass contains 3500 calories. That is to say in order to lose one pound of body weight, one has to burn 3500 calories. The following is the probable explanation:

> 1 gram of fat contains 9 kilocalories.
> 1 lb = 0.45 Kg = 450 grams ⇨ 450 x 9 = 4050 Kilocalories.
> But human body fat contains up to 20% water.
> Supposing a water composition of 13.58% (remaining 86.42% body fat),
> 4050 kilocalories is corrected to obtain 4050 x 0.8642 = 3500 Kilocalories.

Therefore, theoretically, 1 lb of body fat is equivalent to 3500 Kilocalories. If a person is planning to lose 1 lb of weight, he/she should lose 3500 Kcal. This can be accomplished in a week/month depending on one's abilities and fitness skills.

By burning 500 Kcal per day through exercise, or by eating 500 Kcal less food per day, it would take 1 week (7 days) to lose 1 pound of body weight. To lose 10 pounds, it may take 10 weeks and so on.

By losing 250 Kcal per day through exercise, or by eating 250 Kcal less food per day, it would take 2 weeks (14 days) to lose one pound of body weight. To lose 10 pounds, in this case, it may take 20 weeks and so on.

OPERATION OF TREADMILL [1]

Refer to the next page to see a picture of the treadmill. To operate the LifeFitness treadmill (9100 HR or 9500HR), the following instructions are used:

Digital Instruction	What Person Should Do (An example)
Press START to begin	Press START button
Enter Weight (Lbs)	Enter 162, Press START button
Select Program	Press "Manual" key
Choose Program Goal	Enter 1, Press START button
Enter Time (Minutes)	Enter 15, Press START button
Select Your Speed (mph)	Enter 4.0, Press START button

Greeting: "HAVE A GOOD WORKOUT."

After the treadmill starts, speed can be adjusted, either increased or decreased using up-down arrow keys. After 15 to 30 minutes or more of exercise, the treadmill runs 1 minute more to cover the cooling period. While running on the treadmill to get the heart rate, wipe hands and hold the sensors located on the front rod firmly for 1 minute. The machine displays heart rate in bpm (beeps per minute). To discontinue anytime, press STOP.

The following results are then displayed on the digital display (in this example of chosen weight, type of program and intensity of exercise).

Time: 15.00 min	Speed: 4.0 mph
Cool down Period: 1.00 min	Last minute: 4.5 mph
Calories/hr: 334	Inclination: 0.5
Total Calories: 89	Distance: 1.07 miles

Interpretation: Lost 89 kilocalories by running on the treadmill at 4 miles per hour for 15 minutes.

There are several programs available such as Fat Burn, Hill, Random, Manual, Cardio, Fit Test, etc. Each option represents a different level of intensity of exercise. The intensity of exercise can also be adjusted with the up-down arrows.

The total energy expenditure in Kcal/hr can be controlled by choosing the appropriate speed. For example for a body weight of 160 lb, the machine showed the following values:

Table 10.3 Speed Versus Calories Burned (Weight = 160 lb)

Speed (mph)	Inclination	Kcal/hr	Speed (mph)	Inclination	Kcal/hr
3.0	0	254	4	0	314
3.0	0.5	269	4	0.5	334
3.0	1.0	285	4	1.0	355
3.5	0	284	5	0	674
3.5	0.5	302	5	0.5	686
3.5	1.0	320	5	1.0	700

From the above table the person can choose the appropriate speed and can plan ahead the desired calories to be lost. One should not try high speed if it causes pain in the legs.

Life Fitness World Headquarters
10601 W. Belmont Ave
Franklin Park, IL 60131
Toll Free: 1-800-634-8637
Tel: 1-847-288-3300
www.Lifefitness.com

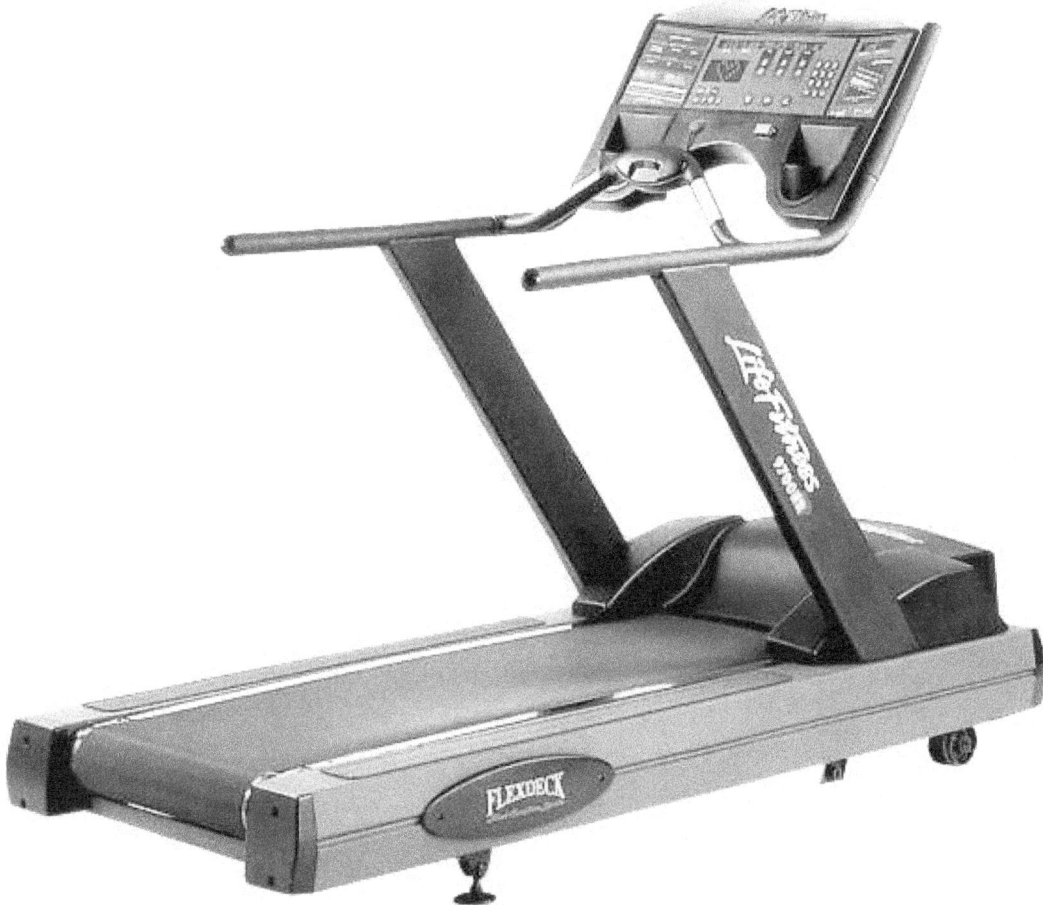

Courtesy of LifeFitness

Figure 10.1 LifeFitness Treadmill (Reproduced with permission).

BODY MASS INDEX (BMI) [1]

When diets do not work, and when the diabetic person is fed up with muscle pain and other side effects of prescriptions and other products, the alternative available is to bring the Body Mass Index (BMI) to normal somehow by losing weight through exercising or by eating only limited calories of food. As long as the Body Mass Index (BMI) is between 19 and 22, the cholesterols should remain normal or close to normal. People with BMI over 22 tend to have high cholesterols.

Body Mass Index (BMI) is calculated by the following formula:

Body Mass Index = Weight (Kg) / [Height (m)]^2

If the weight is known in pounds, convert to Kg.
If the height is known in feet and inches, convert to meters.

1 Kg = 2.2222 Pounds; 1 Pound = 0.45 Kg;
1 Meter = 39.37 Inches = 3.281 Feet; 1 Inch = 0.0254 Meters

National Heart, Lung and Blood Institute (NHLBI) and National Institute of Diabetes and Digestive and Kidney Diseases (NIDDK) released United States Federal guidelines defining "OVERWEIGHT" as a body mass index (BMI) value between 25 and 29.9, and "OBESITY" as a body mass index (BMI) value greater than or equal to 30. A value of BMI below 25 is considered normal.

Sample Calculation

Bill is 5′ 6″ tall and currently weighs 190 pounds (lb). How many pounds should Bill lose to bring his body mass index (BMI) to normal?

Height = 5′ 6″ → 66 Inches → (66)(0.0254) → 1.68 m
Weight = 190 lb → (190/2.2222) = 85.50 Kg
BMI = (85.50)/(1.68)^2 = 30.29

Similarly, Bill's body mass index (BMI) is calculated at several weights as shown in the table below until the BMI drops to 24. That means Bill's correct weight should be 150 lb to reach normal body mass index (BMI). Bill should lose 40 lb to reach normal body weight.

Table 10.4 Body Mass Index (BMI) is calculated at several weights, and normal body weight is determined by trial and error.

Weight (Lb)	Weight (Kg)	Height (m)	BMI	Assessment
190	85.50	1.68	30.29	Obese
180	81.00	1.68	28.70	Overweight
170	76.50	1.68	27.10	Overweight
160	72.00	1.68	25.51	Above Normal
150	**67.50**	**1.68**	**23.92**	**Normal**

P.S.: A value of BMI below 25 is considered normal.

EXERCISE AND SWEATING (PERSPIRATION) [1]

Body Temperature Rises During Exercise because more than 70% of the energy that powers the muscles is lost as heat. This is why people say, "calories are lost or burned" . Heat that is expressed in calories is lost through every type of physical activity. The normal temperature of a healthy human body is 98.6º F or 37º C. To keep the body temperature from rising too high, the heart beats rapidly, and pumps blood via blood vessels to supply oxygen to the muscles. Heat from the muscles is then transferred to the blood, and the blood gets heated. The heart then upon the brain's order pumps heated blood from the muscles to the skin surface where the water content of the blood gets evaporated, dissipating its heat into the environment. The cooled blood then is re-circulated to the bloodstream. Immediately after exercising, the heart slows down lowering the amount of blood being pumped to the skin surface, thereby increasing the body temperature and therefore people sweat even more.

Excess Body Heat generated during exercise can escape from the body by three forms of heat transfer phenomena: conduction, convection and radiation. Conduction takes place while excess heat is being transferred to sweat (blood) that is evaporated on the skin. Convection takes place while excess heat is being transferred to the air surrounding the body. Radiation takes place while excess heat is being transferred by means of the electromagnetic emission of rays to nearby cooler objects.

Drink 8 Cups of Purified Water Per Day (1 glass = 1 cup = 8 ounces = 250 mL)
Sweating or perspiration is the result of exercise and the body's water can be lost either by exercise or by an increase in the ambient temperature. Before and during exercise it is recommended to drink plenty of water. A normal adult should drink sufficient water, distributing it properly to each meal being consumed, to maintain the fluid balance, normal body temperature and good health. Much water is required to keep the contents of the digestion process in liquid state. Insufficient water consumption can cause constipation problems.

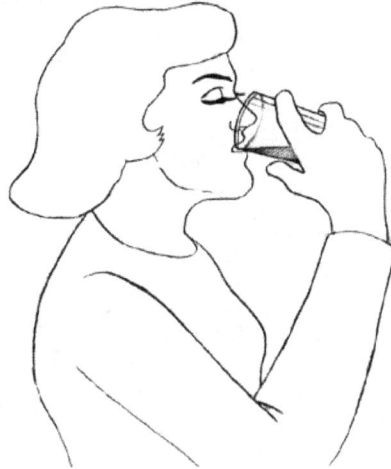

Figure 10.2 Drink 8 cups of purified water (RO water or distilled water) per day.

What Kind of Water Should A Diabetic Person Drink? Please do not drink tap water, well water, or bottled water. Please always drink purified water that is either neutralized or slightly alkalized, and remineralized up to a TDS (Total Dissolved Solids) level of 200 ppm.
Please refer to the book "Drinking Water Guide", authored by Rao Konduru, PhD.
www.drinkingwaterguide.com

PRECAUTIONS WHEN EXERCISING WITH DIABETES [1]

a. **Hypoglycemia (Low Blood Sugars Due to Insulin Reaction)** may occur while exercising. While exercising with insulin dose injected, appropriate steps should be taken to avoid or treat any adverse effect. It is well known that too much insulin drops blood glucose level suddenly, which could develop into a dangerous situation such as a sudden collapse. Refer to Chapter 7 where the calculation of insulin dose is explained. Exercise stimulates insulin action and the action of a rapid-acting insulin such as Humalog is so powerful and abrupt that the blood glucose level falls quickly. Arrangements should be made to make certain that a friend, coach or teammate is around who understands the symptoms of hypoglycemia. Those people who are trying a rapid-acting insulin for the first time must take serious care in identifying and treating the hypoglycemia until the body is accustomed to the combined action of insulin and exercise.

- **The symptoms of hypoglycemia are**: Nervousness, lack of energy, sweating, excessive hunger, poor coordination, blurred vision, drowsiness and dizziness.

Immediate consumption of sugar, glucose cubes, candy, orange juice or Coke helps recovering from hypoglycemia.

b. **Do not Exercise When Your Blood Glucose Level Is Beyond 13 mmol/L or 234 mg/dL**: It is strongly advised not to exercise if your blood glucose level is over 13 mmol/L or 234 mg/dL. At high glucose levels, whenever there is lack of insulin in the body, ketones accumulate. Ketones can poison and even kill the body's cells if allowed for a long time in the bloodstream. So diabetic people must take appropriate insulin dose before meals, monitor and make sure that the after-meal glucose level is under 13 mmol/L (234 mg/dL) before starting an exercise.

c. **Hypoglycemia Later in the Night** may attack during sleep. For some insulin dependent diabetic people, exercise can lower blood glucose levels several hours after the exercise is performed, even during sleep. Different people react differently to exercise and/or insulin. Depending on the body's response to exercise, a pattern of unusual effects of exercise is possible. The individual of this type should record these effects through monitoring blood glucose levels as frequently as possible, study them carefully, understand the probable cause and implement a method through adjusting insulin dose, the amount of food being consumed and the duration and intensity of exercise. This kind of self-healing approach could not only lower after-meal glucose levels and control diabetes but in addition safeguard the diabetic person from any upcoming danger.

An insulin-dependent diabetic (either type 1 or type 2) should study the combined influence of a rapid-acting insulin and after-meal exercise through consuming a variety of heavy meals. In a few months, he/she can research and control diabetes.

A Type-2 diabetic who depends on oral medications, but do not inject insulin shots, can also use the same technique of lowering after-meal blood glucose level thorough after-meal exercise. If the after-meal glucose level does not drop through a medication, then a type-2 diabetic should switch to insulin shots.

REFERENCE

1. Permanent Diabetes Control (Book), Subtitle: The Complete Guide to Living Like A Normal Person Forever, Authored by Rao Konduru, MS, PhD, Reviewed and Endorsed by Dr. Marshal Dahl, MD, PhD., Endocrinologist, Faculty of Medicine, University of British Columbia, Vancouver, British Columbia, Canada, First Published in 2003. www.mydiabetescontrol.com

CHAPTER 11 HEART DISEASE AND DIABETES

TABLE OF CONTENTS

CHAPTER 11 HEART DISEASE AND DIABETES [1]

INTRODUCTION[1]

Believe it or not, the following staggering information is true:

♦ The World Health Organization (WHO), the International Society and Federation of Cardiology (ISFC) and the United Nations Educational, Scientific and Cultural Organization (UNESCO) jointly reported in a press release in 1997 that cardiovascular diseases kill more than any other disease around the world. Every year, an estimated 15 million deaths are reported, which is about 30% of total deaths around the world, and many more millions of people are disabled due to heart and blood vessel diseases.

♦ More than 80 percent of people with diabetes die from some form of heart or blood vessel disease.

♦ Cardiovascular disease has been the number one killer in the USA since 1900. Heart disease is found to be the first leading cause of death, and stroke is found to be the 3rd leading cause of death.

♦ About 61 million Americans (about one-fourth of the population) live with the complications of heart disease and stroke. In 2001, the cost for all cardiovascular diseases in the USA alone was $300 billion.

♦ Every 33 seconds, a person dies from cardiovascular disease in the USA alone.
♦ Every 34 seconds, a person dies from a form of heart disease in the USA alone.
♦ Every day, more than 2500 Americans die from heart disease.
♦ Every year, more than 250,000 people die of heart attack in the USA before they reach a nearby hospital.
♦ In 1991, 923,000 Americans died from heart and blood vessel diseases.

♦ Also, in countries like Russia, Romania, Bulgaria, Hungary, Bulgaria, Czechoslovakia and Poland, heart disease contributes to the highest number of deaths. The lowest death rates of heart disease were in Japan, France, Spain, Switzerland and Canada.

CARDIOVASCULAR DISEASE [1]

Cardiovascular disease is categorized into two major parts, heart disease and stroke. The majority of the cases fall into heart disease.

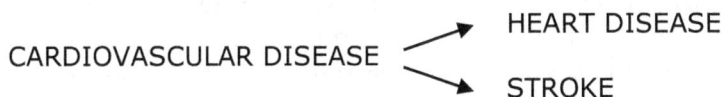

CARDIOVASCULAR DISEASE → HEART DISEASE
→ STROKE

The causes of heart disease are heredity, diabetes, high cholesterol, tobacco smoking, high blood pressure, stress, obesity, lack of exercise, male sex, age over 65, high blood homocysteine, etc. The causes of stroke are all the above plus blood clots and sudden occlusion of an oxygen-supplying artery to the brain.

FUNCTION OF THE HEART [1]

The human heart is an amazing machine designed to provide energy to all parts of the human body and without which a human being cannot survive. The heart is the never-ceasing pump that supplies blood throughout the body. In order to move the blood, the heart pulls in blood by dilating (opening wider) and pushes it out by contracting (squeezing). Arteries carry oxygen-rich blood away from the heart. Veins carry waste or impure blue blood back to the heart in order to be purified. Capillaries connect arteries to veins. The body's cells draw fuel in the form of chemicals and oxygen from the blood and convert it into energy to work.

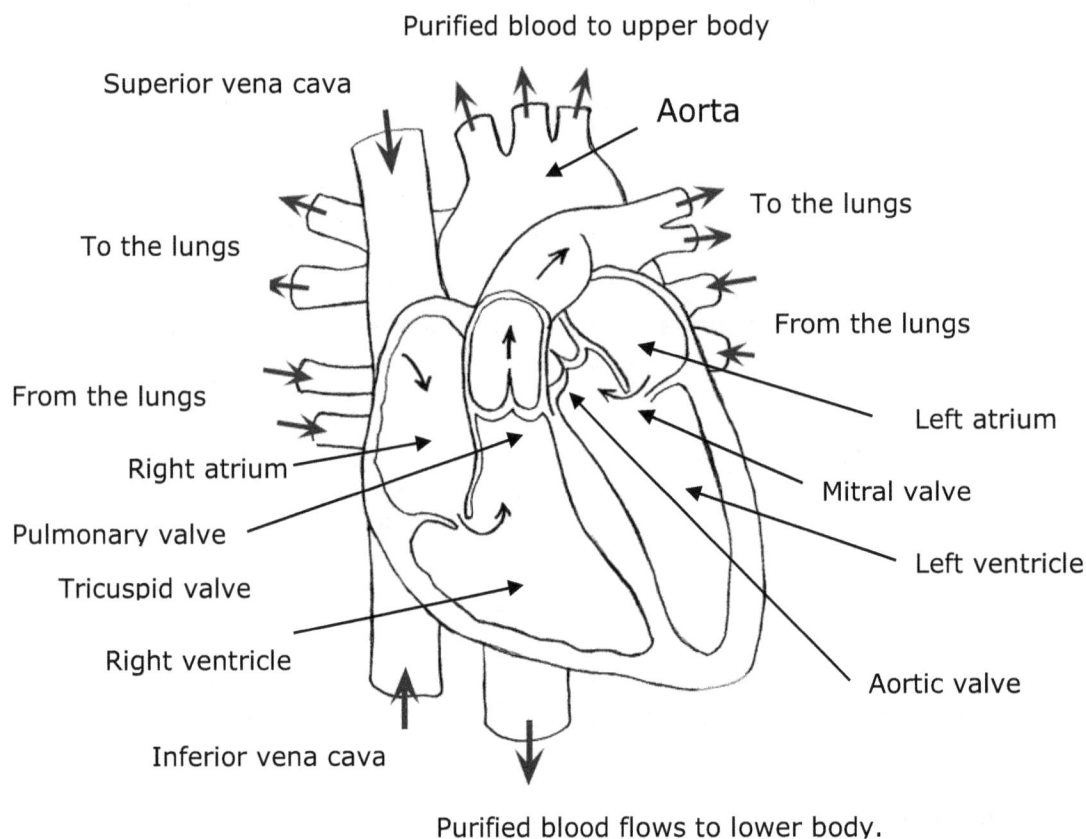

Purified blood to upper body

Superior vena cava

Aorta

To the lungs

To the lungs

From the lungs

From the lungs

Right atrium

Left atrium

Mitral valve

Pulmonary valve

Tricuspid valve

Left ventricle

Right ventricle

Aortic valve

Inferior vena cava

Purified blood flows to lower body.

Figure 11.1 The components of the heart and its four valves.

The human heart as shown in the figure above is a hollow organ, roughly the size of a clenched fist, shaped like an upside-down pear. An adult heart weighs between 9 and 11 ounces (between 255 and 311 grams). The heart is made up of muscle and this muscle is divided into four chambers—two atriums and two ventricles. There are four one-way valves that connect the chambers and the main artery, the aorta. The upper chambers are called the left atrium and right atrium. The lower chambers are called the left ventricle and right ventricle. Veins from all over the body carry and bring waste-rich blue blood to the superior vena cava from the upper part of the body and to the inferior vena cava from the lower part of the body, and then the blood enters the right atrium. The atrium is like a storage room. When the right atrium is filled with waste-rich blood, it contracts, pushing blood into the right ventricle through a one-way valve (tricuspid valve).

The ventricle, unlike the atrium, is a very powerful pump. The waste-rich blood from the right ventricle is pushed through another one-way valve (pulmonary valve) into a narrow tunnel called the pulmonary artery, which leads to the lungs. There are two lungs that cover the heart and are structured with bellows. When we breathe, air enters the lungs (air contains 21% of oxygen) and the chest moves up and down or in and out. When the impure blue blood enters the lungs, amazingly the blood gets purified in the lung capillaries, carbon dioxide is removed from the impure blood, and the blood is enriched with oxygen and leaves the lungs as pure bright red blood. The purified oxygen-rich blood then enters the pulmonary veins which carry the blood into the left atrium. From the left atrium, the purified blood is pushed again through another one-way valve (mitral valve) into the left ventricle, which is the strongest and most powerful chamber of the heart. This highly pressurized chamber supplies the oxygen-rich blood throughout the body. The left ventricle contracts and the purified blood first enters via another one-way valve (the aortic valve) into the aorta which is the largest and strongest artery in the entire body. From the aorta, the blood travels through arteries towards all the muscles and organs. The blood is further cleaned when it passes through the liver and kidneys. The blood picks up nutrients from the small intestine walls and supplies it to the trillions of the body's little cells. This process is called the systemic circulation. When blood is carried from the heart to the lungs where it gets purified and returned to the heart, it is called pulmonary circulation.

To summarize: When the heart contracts, the blood is pushed out of the left ventricle and when it dilates (expands), the blood comes back into the right atrium. When the heart contracts again, the blood moves into the right ventricle and then into the lungs. When the heart dilates again, the blood returns to fill the left atrium, and so on. We can use a stethoscope to hear pulmonary circulation. Two sounds we hear, "lub" and "dub," are the ventricles contracting and the valves closing. The adult heart dilates and contracts about 72 times per minute. In an average lifetime, the human heart beats about two and half billion times without ever pausing to rest, thus giving life to human body.

HEART VALVES AND VALVE DISEASE [1]

When the blood passes from one chamber to another, the action of the one-way valves is of paramount importance in order to avoid any backward flow and the exchange of oxygen and carbon dioxide. There are four one-way valves inside the heart:

- ♦ **Tricuspid valve** is between the right atrium and the right ventricle
- ♦ **Pulmonary valve** is between the right ventricle and the pulmonary artery
- ♦ **Mitral valve** is between the left atrium and the left ventricle
- ♦ **Aortic valve** is between the left ventricle and the aorta

When the valves fail to function properly, they make a sound called a **murmur** and valve disease develops. There are two types of malfunctions: the first being regurgitation, in which the valve does not close completely allowing the blood to flow backwards; and the second being a stenosis, in which the valve opening becomes narrowed, restricting the blood flow. When a murmur problem or valve discomfort develops, the cardiologist orders several detection tests, recommends either some medications or valve surgery to repair the valves.

ATHEROSCLEROSIS AND ARTERIOSCLEROSIS [1]

Atherosclerosis is a disease process, in which the arteries are clogged due to a buildup of cholesterol and other fatty substances, called plaque, within the walls of the arteries, developed over a period of many years. It is the major form of heart disease in Western countries. Atherosclerosis develops in large and medium sized arteries in the body especially in the heart. The commonly affected areas are the aorta, the coronary arteries and the cerebral arteries (which supply blood to the brain). It also affects the arteries in the legs and abdomen. This disease process is depicted in the figure below.

Arteriosclerosis is another type of disease process, in which the arteries are hardened and lose elasticity. The symptoms of atherosclerosis/arteriosclerosis are shortness of breath, discomfort in the chest and angina. When the artery is fully blocked, the blood supply to the heart muscle is reduced, oxygen supply will be interrupted, and then a heart attack occurs. If the blood supply to the brain is cut off, then a stroke occurs.

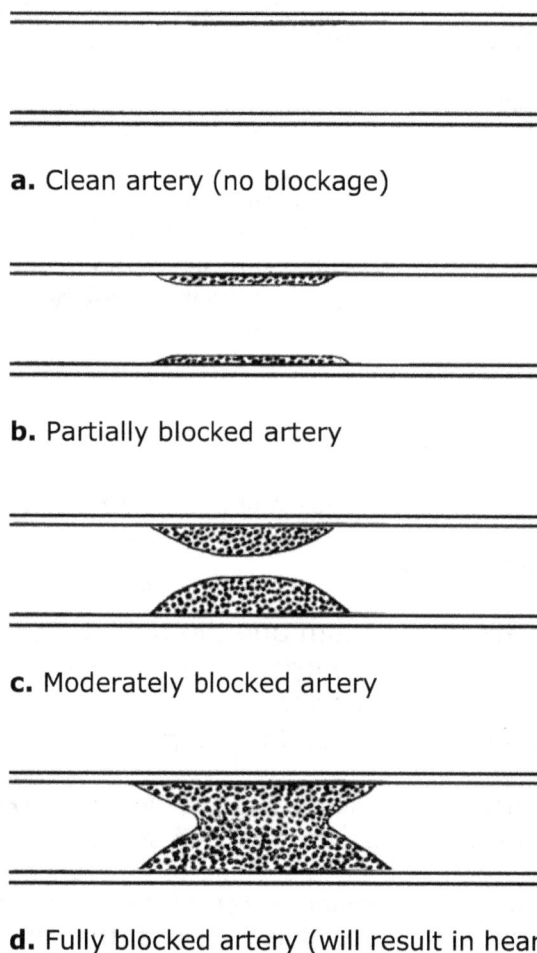

a. Clean artery (no blockage)

b. Partially blocked artery

c. Moderately blocked artery

d. Fully blocked artery (will result in heart attack)

Figure 11.2   Development of atherosclerosis in an artery.

BLOOD PRESSURE [1]

Blood pressure is defined as the force with which the blood flows against the walls of blood vessels or arteries. This pressure is expressed in millimeters of mercury (mm Hg) or pounds per square inch (psi). The blood pressure of a person is measured and expressed in two different readings, systolic pressure and diastolic pressure. Systolic pressure is the highest pressure in the artery when the heart is pumping blood to the body. Diastolic pressure is the lowest pressure in the artery when the heart relaxes between heartbeats.

Illustration

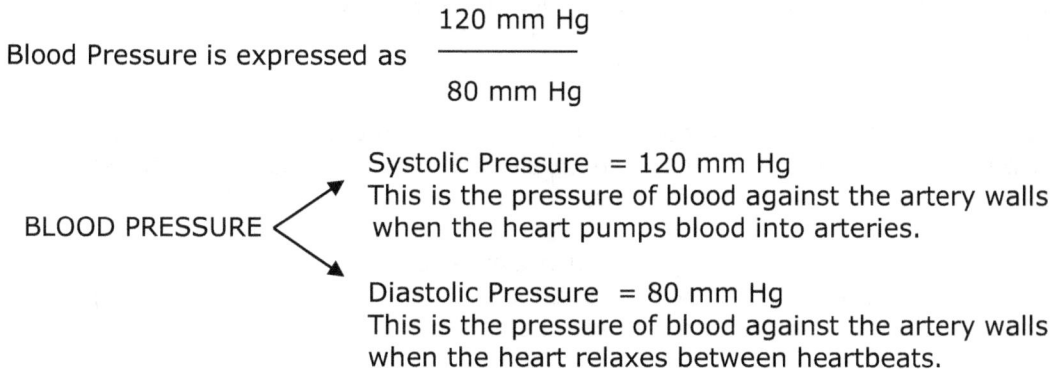

Blood Pressure is expressed as

$$\frac{120 \text{ mm Hg}}{80 \text{ mm Hg}}$$

BLOOD PRESSURE

Systolic Pressure = 120 mm Hg
This is the pressure of blood against the artery walls when the heart pumps blood into arteries.

Diastolic Pressure = 80 mm Hg
This is the pressure of blood against the artery walls when the heart relaxes between heartbeats.

According to the National Heart, Lung and Blood Institute, a division of the US Federal Government's National Institute of Health, the following table shows the normal ranges of blood pressure.

Table 11.1 Normal blood pressure Levels.

	BLOOD PRESSURE (mm Hg)		
	Normal	High Normal	High Blood Pressure
Systolic	< 130	130 to 139	> 140
Diastolic	< 85	85 to 89	> 90
With Diabetes and Kidney Disease			
Systolic	< 120	< 130	> 130
Diastolic	< 79	< 80	> 80

Symbols: < means less than; > means greater than

Blood pressure equal to or below 120/80 mm Hg is considered optimal (the perfect normal). Blood pressure above and beyond 140/90 mm Hg is considered high blood pressure and immediate action is required to lower and control it.

LOW BLOOD PRESSURE
If the blood pressure is below 80/60 mm Hg, then the person is said to have low blood pressure. With low blood pressure, which is rare, a person feels dizziness, tiredness and lack of energy.

HIGH BLOOD PRESSURE OR HYPERTENSION [1]

When the blood pressure is above 140/90 mm Hg, the person is said to have hypertension or high blood pressure.

60 to 65% of diabetics suffer from high blood pressure. More than 50 million Americans have high blood pressure, which is the leading contributor to heart disease. 35% of them do not know that they have high blood pressure.

When the pressure in the blood vessels increases, the heart needs to work harder than usual, and as a result the heart gets strained and tends to enlarge, causing heart attack and/or stroke. High blood pressure contributes to an increase in cholesterol level for diabetic people.

When the high blood pressure is detected, doctors usually prescribe medications such as diuretics and beta blockers which are capable to eliminate the excess fluids and salt from the body—thereby lowering the blood pressure.

Consuming less salt helps lower the high blood pressure or hypertension. Getting enough calcium, potassium and magnesium, and through eating a low-fat diet with a variety of vegetables, fruits, legumes, soymilk and tofu also helps lower the high blood pressure.

Some doctors recommend heart patients a daily mega dose of vitamin-C (500 mg to 1000 mg), vitamin-E (300 IU) and multi-vitamins, and a daily low dose of coated aspirin (81 mg) as they improve the vascular function in arteries, avoid blood clots and protect a person from suffering a heart attack.

However, diabetics can treat and control high blood pressure with after-meal exercise and a well-planned meal of known nutritional composition with minimal fat content (Refer to chapter 3 to calculate nutritional composition of any meal and to minimize fat content). As a matter of fact, controlling diabetes (keeping the hemoglobin A1c always normal or close to normal) would minimize many heath risk factors including high blood pressure, and rejuvenates the person.

BLOOD PRESSURE MONITORS [1]

There are two types of blood pressure monitors available in the market today:

    a. Aneroid Monitors and
    b. Digital Monitors

In aneroid monitors, the cuff is inflated manually by squeezing a rubber bulb. The blood pressure is read on a dial gauge. Aneroid monitors come with a built-in stethoscope and they are easily portable. Digital monitors on the other hand have automatic cuff, are more accurate and easier to use, and blood pressure is displayed digitally. Digital monitors are available in many drug stores for home use. Some pharmacies (Safeway, Shoppers Drug Mart, and others) have already installed blood pressure monitors on their premises as a courtesy to their customers, and anybody can monitor blood pressure free of cost.

HEART ATTACK: SYMPTOMS AND TREATMENT [1]

Call 911 and request an emergency ambulance or ask a friend or relative to drive you to an emergency hospital (do not drive yourself, and leave your door unlocked and lights on) if any of the following symptoms are predominant:

- Sudden chest pain or discomfort in the heart
  (because one or more arteries may have been fully blocked).
- Sudden shortness of breath.
- Back pain, neck pain, pain in one or both arms, jaw or stomach.
- Sudden vomiting, nausea, cold sweat and lightheadedness.

A heart attack occurs when part of the heart muscle is damaged or dead because it is not receiving enough or any oxygen. If any artery is blocked, the heart muscle will no longer receive enough oxygen. A heart attack can also occur due to a blood clot in a narrowed artery that goes to the heart. All the above could result in from atherosclerosis, in which the arteries are clogged by a kind of plaque made from cholesterol and other fatty substances.

As soon as the person experiencing a heart attack reaches the emergency unit, the medical staff will first spray nitro (nitrolingual 0.4 mg), under the tongue, which prevents angina and gives quick relief. They also quickly install an intravenous line in the arm, and inject clot busters (a medication that opens the blocked artery immediately). A person who has suffered a heart attack in most circumstances is treated with an angioplasty or a bypass surgery immediately.

STROKE: SYMPTOMS AND TREATMENT [1]

Call 911 and request an emergency ambulance or ask a friend or relative to drive you to an emergency hospital (do not drive yourself, and leave your door unlocked and lights on) if any of the following symptoms are predominant:

- Sudden numbness in the face, arm or leg mostly on one side of the body.
- Sudden loss of vision for a short time, sudden dizziness or imbalance.
- Sudden difficulty in walking and loss of consciousness.
- Sudden vomiting, nausea or fever not caused by viral illness.
- Sudden severe headache for unknown reasons.

Hospital intensive care, rehabilitation and prescription drugs are the primary treatments for stroke. If the stroke is severe, for example, if the neck artery is clogged due to a blood clot, surgery is used to remove the plaque.

A stroke can be treated in the long run by properly understanding, treating and minimizing several persisting risk factors such as diabetes, heart disease, high blood pressure and cigarette smoking.

Diabetics should control **insulin dose, food intake and after-meal exercise** until the hemoglobin A1c drops to its normal range, as suggested in this book, in order to wipe out the total risk associated with heart disease and stroke. The diabetes treatment plan presented in this book (Chapter 3 & Chapter 4) is the simplest, easiest and efficient self-healing treatment.

MEDICAL CHECK-UP AND DETECTION [1]

When a patient approaches a cardiologist with discomfort in the chest or shortness of breath, either while resting or while walking, the cardiologist organizes a series of tests to detect a heart disease: [92]

Chest X-Ray

X-rays pierce the skin and muscle but are blocked by bones and a few organs such as the heart, which cast a shadow in the x-ray output. The shadow is invisible to the human eye but can be recorded and the results can be interpreted after creating a special film. The shadow of the heart formed in the x-ray output reveals to the specially trained x-ray technician information about the heart, its size, its shape and its enlargement if any. From the x-ray report, the cardiologist detects tentatively if the patient has any heart disease or not. The output also shows the lungs and blood vessels. However, this chest x-ray test alone will not be the final answer.

Echocardiogram or Ultrasound Study

The ultrasound with its high frequency is capable of penetrating the human skin and muscle but reflects when it hits an organ such as the heart. By studying the reflected ultrasound waves, the specially trained technician, nurse or doctor creates a picture of the heart. The patient is asked to lie on a couch and some jelly is applied on the chest. The jelly helps to transmit the ultrasound waves from the machine to the body. On the echocardiogram, it is possible to see different parts of the heart (the chambers, the valves, the aorta, and the pulmonary artery). By viewing this picture on a video screen, it is possible to detect any heart disease such as holes in the walls between chambers, any blockage or leaks in the valves and the direction of the blood flow.

Electrocardiogram

The electrocardiogram, also called EKG or ECC, is a graph recording the electrical activity of the heart. While pumping blood throughout the body, the heart contracts, and creates a weak electric current. From this point onwards, the current flows through a well-defined path through the rest of the heart. The flow of the current can be detected and recorded by electrodes, which are simply metal plates placed on the chest, wrists and ankles. The recorder draws a graph. Jelly applied to the chest, wrists and ankles helps better conduct the current and communicate with the instrument to record the current. The test takes only a few minutes. From the EKG graph, the cardiologist or doctor understands if there is any unusual pattern of electrical activity across the heart. The graph also indicates whether or not any chamber of the heart is enlarged or thick-walled.

Cardiac Catheterization

Chest x-ray, ultrasound and electrocardiogram are noninvasive tests (which means there in no insertion of any sort of tube or needle into the chest or other parts of the body). But catheterization is an invasive test in which a thin plastic tube called a catheter is threaded into the groin or the forearm after a needlestick. The catheter is then guided into the heart, and a dye is injected into the heart. As the dye is opaque to the x-rays, it does not allow x-rays to pass through. The shadow thus obtained in the x-ray output has the shape of the heart. The pressure in the four different chambers and the concentration of oxygen in the blood are also measured during this test. By analyzing the x-ray, the doctor can draw conclusions about the shape of the heart and its defects if any. This test is also called an angiogram.

There are some other tests such as a CT Scan (Computerized Tomography Scan), PET Scan (Position Emission Tomography Scan), RI Scan (Radio Isotope Scan) and MRI (Magnetic Resonance Imaging). Each of these tests is performed to obtain specific information concerning a heart disease. Usually it is a combination of several tests that detects whether or not the person is experiencing any heart disease in given case.

Stress Test

Most cardiologists equip their clinics with a treadmill hooked to instruments to monitor heart rate and blood pressure and to an electrocardiogram. The person is asked to run on a treadmill and the speed and inclination of the treadmill are increased. If the heart patient has any clogging in arteries, he/she will feel instant chest pain, and become tired, and may not continue to the end point— confirming clogging of the arteries. Healthy people continue the test till the end point with normal blood pressure, heart rate and electrocardiogram results.

HEART DISEASE [1]

Coronary heart disease (CHD) or coronary artery disease (CAD), and arteriosclerotic heart disease (AHD) are the alternative names used to describe human heart disease. Coronary is a Latin word, meaning crown (a model of the coronary arteries and its branches, when seen in isolation, resembles a crown). Heart disease, if not resolved with medications, can be treated by angioplasty or bypass surgery.

ANGIOPLASTY

The percutaneous transluminal coronary angioplasty (PCTA), balloon angioplasty or simply angioplasty is widely used to treat a coronary artery disease (CAD). In angioplasty, the clogged heart arteries are opened and the blood flow restored in the heart. The first balloon angioplasty was performed in 1977 by a Swiss physician, Dr. Andreas Gruentzig.

There are 3 angioplasty procedures most commonly used:
   ♦ Balloon angioplasty
   ♦ Stent Angioplasty
   ♦ Laser Angioplasty

Balloon angioplasty is performed by passing a balloon catheter through a guiding catheter into the artery where the deposited plaque is present. A guide wire inside the balloon catheter is then advanced into the artery until the tip is beyond the blockage. The balloon catheter is then moved over the guide wire until the balloon is in the exact position of the narrowing. The balloon is then inflated several times until the plaque is compressed and blood flow restored. The balloon is then deflated. The balloon catheter, guide wire and guiding catheter are then removed from the artery.

Stent Angioplasty is performed for some people, when the balloon angioplasty may not be the sufficient treatment to restore the blood flow in the artery. In that case, a coronary stenting procedure is accompanied by balloon angioplasty. A stent is a device made of expandable metal mesh that is placed and left at the narrowing of the artery to keep the artery open after the catheter is removed. This procedure prevents the buildup of the plaque again.

Laser Angioplasty is often used in combination with the balloon angioplasty when the blockage is hardened and difficult to remove. In laser angioplasty, a thin tube is advanced into a blocked artery, and then a laser emits short pulses of photons that cause the plaque to vaporize. The laser drills holes in the hardened plaque, and then the plaque is removed with balloon angioplasty.

ANGIOPLASTY PROCEDURE [1]

The angioplasty or cardiac catheterization procedure takes approximately 1 to 2 hours. During this invasive procedure, the patient is asked to lie on a special operating table or bed, and x-ray cameras are positioned above and below focusing on the chest area. A monitor shows a picture of the patient's heart.

A nurse inserts an intravenous line (Iv) into the patient's arm which allows injection of a calming medication (sedative), blood thinner (anticoagulant) or other medications during the procedure without sticking the patient with more needles. Other devices are attached to monitor blood pressure and heart rate during and after the angioplasty. A urinary catheter is also inserted.

The injection site is usually the groin (the area between the upper thigh and belly). Some surgeons choose to use the arm as the injection site, though a new technique uses the wrist. The site is shaved and cleaned to make sure no infection occurs. The surgeon injects the local anesthetic into the groin and the injection site is numbed. The surgeon then places a sheath on the area and inserts the catheter into the artery of the groin and then advanced into the heart by viewing the video monitor which guides the procedure. At that time the patient may feel some discomfort. Then an x-ray of the coronary artery is taken from which the surgeon is able to determine the size of the artery and of the narrowing of the blockage. Based on this information, the surgeon picks an appropriate noncompliant balloon, which expands to a pre-designated maximum diameter so that it will not expand to more than the diameter of the artery. For example, a surgeon might pick a 3 millimeter balloon to treat an artery of 3 millimeters diameter.

After the blockage of the artery is located, a balloon-tipped catheter is inserted into a guiding catheter. A guide wire inside the balloon catheter is then advanced through the artery until the tip is beyond the blockage. The balloon catheter is moved over the guide wire until the balloon perfectly fits the blocked area. The balloon is then inflated to push the deposited plaque further against the wall. Thus the blockage is cleared gradually in several attempts, by inflating and deflating the balloon, which takes up to several minutes. When the angioplasty procedure is completed, the guiding catheter and balloon catheter with balloon are removed from the artery. The procedure is depicted below in the figure below.

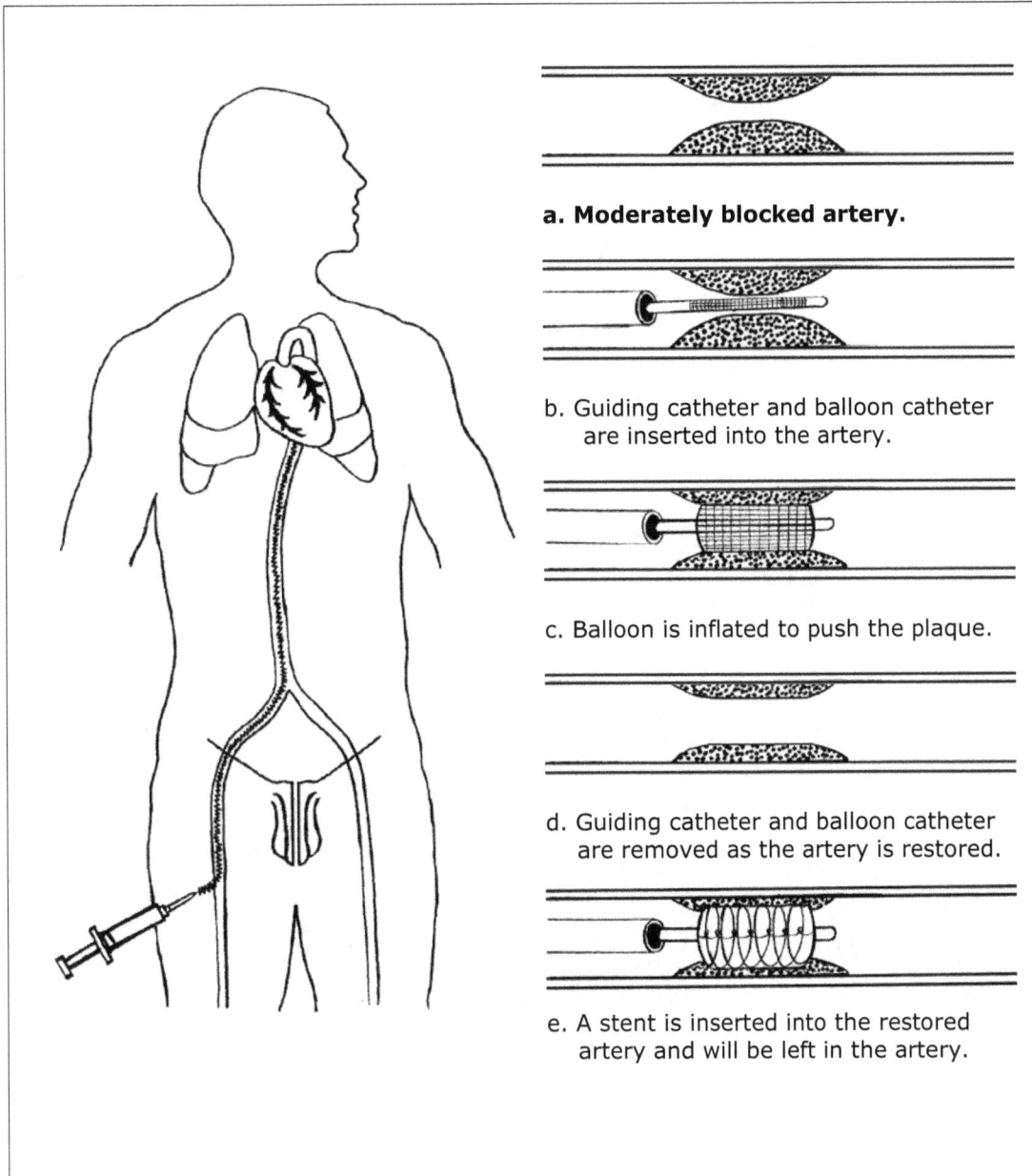

a. Moderately blocked artery.

b. Guiding catheter and balloon catheter are inserted into the artery.

c. Balloon is inflated to push the plaque.

d. Guiding catheter and balloon catheter are removed as the artery is restored.

e. A stent is inserted into the restored artery and will be left in the artery.

Figure 11.3 Angioplasty procedure.

Once the angioplasty is completed, the patient is transported to the rest room. The patient will be instructed to keep his/her leg straight so that the groin area will not be disturbed. The next step is to remove the sheath from the groin area. The action of the anticoagulant that was injected just before the procedure lasts from 4 to 6 hours. So after 6 hours, the surgeon who performed the angioplasty comes back and removes the sheath by applying pressure gently on the groin area. Then the groin area is cleaned and bandaged. There are also new methods available to remove the sheath, and to seal and stitch the area, immediately after the angioplasty. The next day, the patient is allowed to go home.

Angioplasty gives immediate relief from a heart attack or blockage of an artery. However, there is no certainty that angioplasty works for everyone. Many patients require repeat angioplasty, and keep themselves busy with ongoing visits to the cardiologist and eventually become candidates for bypass surgery.

BYPASS SURGERY [1]

Open heart bypass surgery, also called coronary artery bypass grafting (CABG), is one of the medical wonders of the 20th century, and saved hundreds of thousands of lives—without which many people would be dead or have had repeat heart attacks or could have suffered intractable and debilitating chest pains. Many heart patients have tremendously improved the quality and longevity through the bypass surgery.

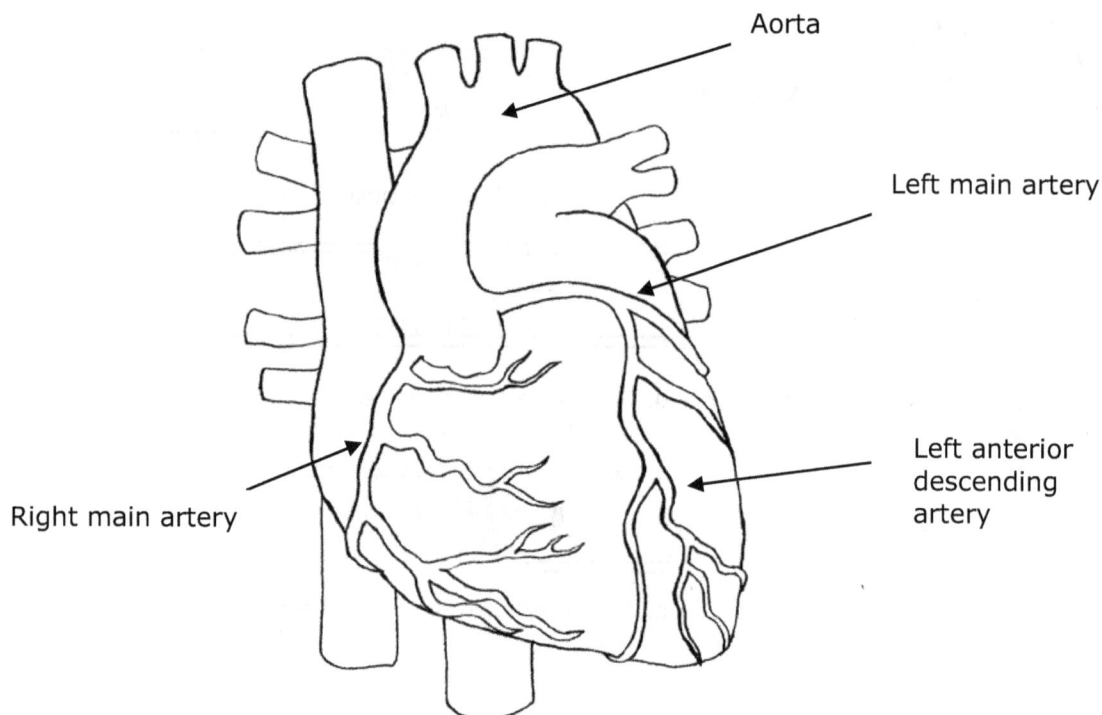

Figure 11.4 Heart with left and right arteries.

Figure 11.4 depicts the left main artery, right main artery, left anterior descending artery and the aorta (there are many more arteries not shown). The procedure of bypass surgery, as shown in Figure 11.5, is usually performed in sequence after an angiogram in which the surgeon detects the exact blockage of an artery or arteries so that the surgeon has a clear idea of which arteries are to be grafted. The patient is asked to lie on the operating bed or table, which is then transported from the rest room to the operating room. The x-ray cameras are carefully positioned above and below focusing on the chest area. A monitor shows a picture of the patient's heart. A nurse inserts an intravenous line (Iv) into the patient's arm. Other devices are attached to the patient's body that allow the surgeon to monitor blood pressure and heart rate during and after the surgery. The surgery requires general anesthesia to put the patient to sleep. An artificial breathing machine is required to give oxygen immediately after the anesthesia. The patient is also hooked to a special device called a heart-lung machine to keep the oxygen-rich blood circulating during the surgery. The surgeon then cuts and opens the chest area (Refer to Figure 11.5). The procedure involves the removal of a clean and unclogged small blood vessel or vein from a leg or from the chest. The vein is then sewn to the aorta and to a spot beyond the blockage on the artery to restore the blood flow through the clogged artery. This is called artery bypass grafting. This bypass grafting can be done for one, two, three or even four clogged arteries The single bypass, double bypass, triple bypass and quadruple bypass are depicted in Figures 11.6a and 11.6b.

After the completion of the surgery, the patient is disconnected from the heart-lung machine. The chest opening is then closed and stitched perfectly. The person will then be transported back to the rest room to recover from the surgery. The breathing machine is disconnected as soon as the patient is found awake. The person should stay in the hospital at least a couple of days or a week. Complete recovery may take up to two months. After the surgery, the patient will be given a series of prescription drugs to take on a daily basis.

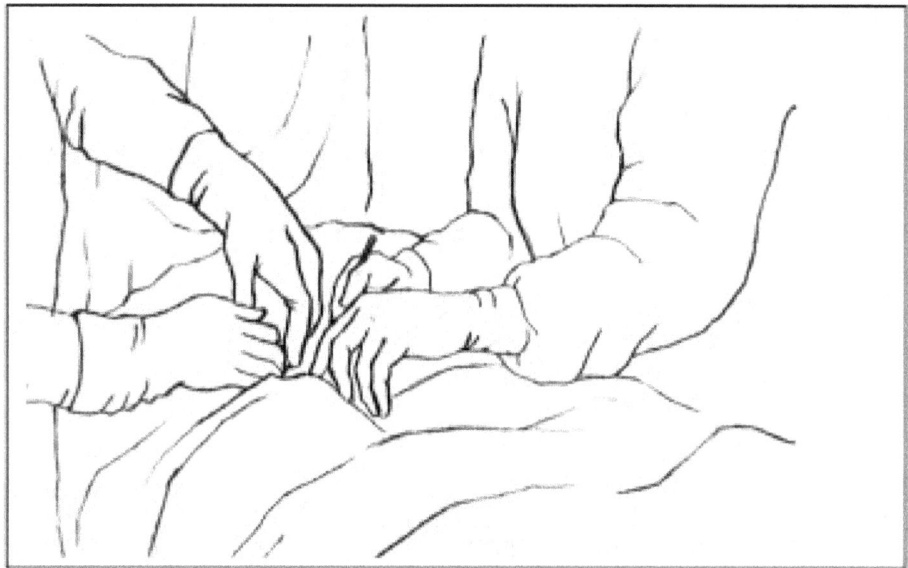

Figure 11.5 Surgeons performing open heart bypass surgery.

BEFORE BYPASS	AFTER BYPASS
a. Left artery blocked at one spot	a. Single bypass
b. Left artery blocked at two spots	b. Double bypass

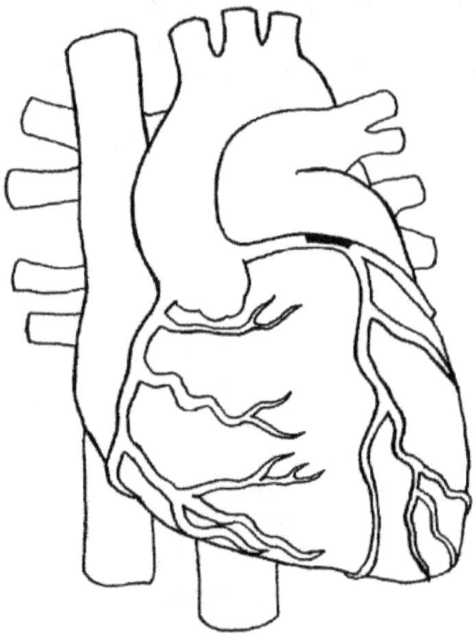

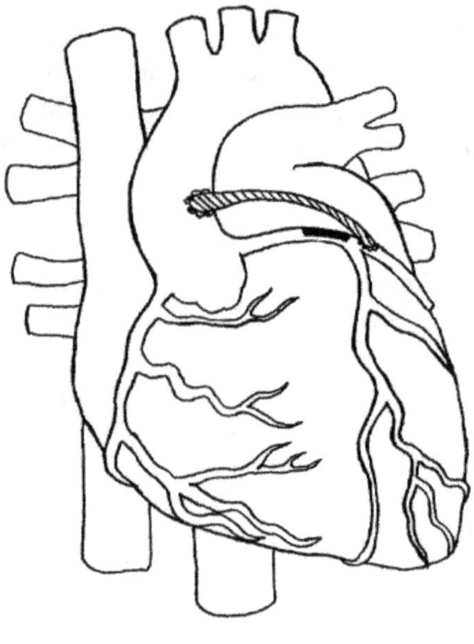

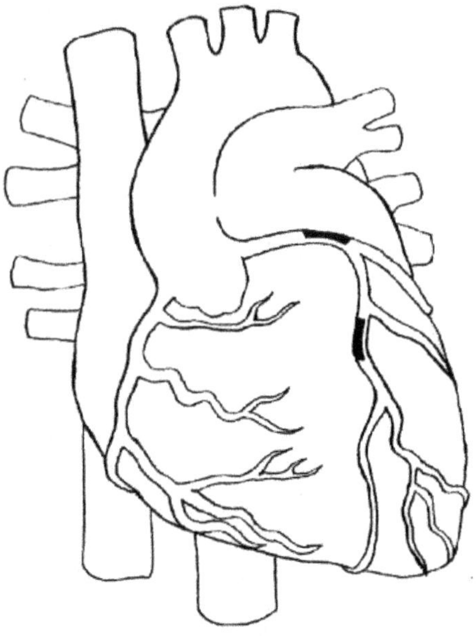

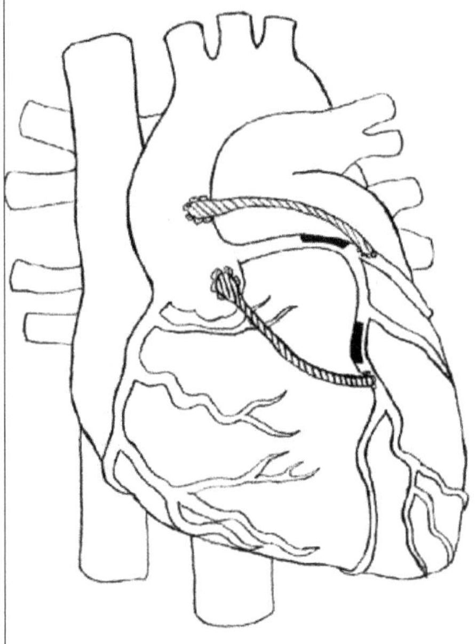

Figure 11.6a Bypass surgery (single, double, triple and quadruple).

BEFORE BYPASS	AFTER BYPASS
c. Arteries blocked at three spots	c. Triple bypass
d. Arteries blocked at four spots	d. Quadruple bypass

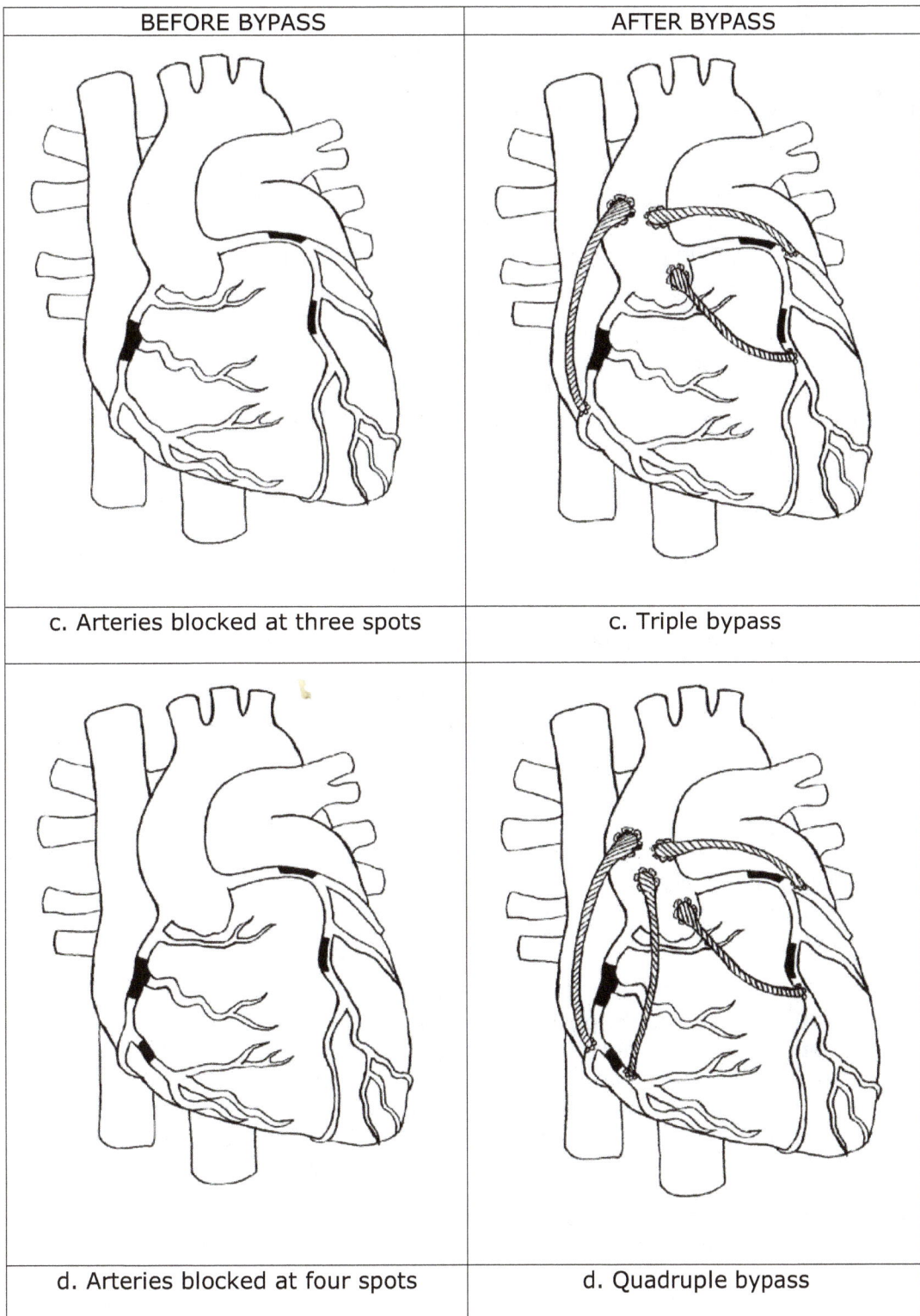

Figure 11.6b Bypass surgery (single, double, triple and quadruple).

DO DIABETICS HAVE TO GO THROUGH ALL THE ABOVE? [1]

A diabetic person should read through all the above, in detail, concerning heart disease and its possible remedies. Diabetic people tend to have higher cholesterols, which contributes to plaque buildup in the arteries. Only by mastering the details of this topic, heart disease, can one guide oneself to combat, control or permanently wipe out the heart disease. Simply taking some prescription drugs or going through surgical procedures will not completely wipe away the heart disease. One has to understand his/her diseased heart through a lot of reading, research, dedication and consistent efforts of self-discipline with good eating habits and after-meal exercise.

Diabetes causes high blood glucose levels. Living with elevated blood glucose levels is dangerous. At elevated blood glucose levels, glucose sticks to the surface of the body's cells for a long time and is then converted to a poison called sorbitol—which acts like an alcohol and punches holes in the cells, contributing largely to heart attack and heart disease. Controlling diabetes permanently through lowering hemoglobin A1c level to normal and keeping the total cholesterol, HDL, LDL and triglycerides levels consistently normal certainly helps reverse heart disease.

It is up to the individual to decide whether or not surgery is essential for him/her in the current circumstances. If the situation gets serious beyond the person's ability to take any decision, he/she would have no choice but to undergo surgery in the emergency care unit. Heart bypass surgery is undoubtedly helping many people and saving their lives temporarily. However, how long the bypass surgery lasts is still a puzzling question. Even after a successful bypass surgery, many people deal with numerous problems of further heart disease and other complications caused due to the side effects of prescription drugs.

THE AUTHOR SPEAKS OUT [1]

After having been diabetic for almost 20 years, I suffered a sudden heart attack. Until then, I never thought about diabetes and its control. I was just taking insulin shots and never did anything to control my diabetes.

When I had the heart attack, I called 911 and an ambulance carried me to Royal Columbian Hospital. Since then, my health problem has abruptly been linked to a devastating secondary problem, that is, the hospital environment and its way of treating patients such as myself. I had 2 angioplasties within a week, and I had to go through an enormous pain due to the way the nurses and the staff treated me. They did many humiliating things to me. I wished I had never lived in this world. I felt I was being treated like an animal so abrasively.

I was given some 10 different prescription drugs, and was asked to take them without fail. They spent hours in instructing me on how to take those drugs every day. They were more concerned about me taking those drugs on an ongoing basis than anything else. I was told convincingly that I had regained my health and that I could eat anything I wished. I started eating in restaurants as usual including hamburgers, cheeseburgers and French fries. After the angioplasty was performed, I had a bladder infection because the urinary catheter that was installed in my penis was not clean enough or not installed properly. After I came home, I had a very high fever and severe shakes and vibrations, and called the ambulance once again to go to the emergency unit. This time the treatment got even worse. I was placed in a tightly packed room of 4 or 5 elderly patients who were snoring all the time, yelling and murmuring. I found the nurses always jumping into that room arguing with them and demanding them to do this thing and that thing. I could not sleep well. My intravenous line (Iv) was dislocated from my arm and was hurting very badly and nobody showed up to fix it for a number of hours. A nurse did in fact came to see me and promised that she would come back in a short while to fix my Iv but did not show up. Somehow, I was discharged from the hospital after a terrible week. I was glad to be out of that hospital. It was a big relief.

Within a few months after having 2 angioplasties, I started feeling discomfort, shortness of breath and a severe pain in my chest whenever I took a short walk. I did not even know at that time that the pain that I was suffering from was called angina due to clogged arteries. I went to see my cardiologist on June 25, 1998, and he asked me to take a stress test. My stress test was not normal. I could not even complete my stress test on the treadmill. With severe pain in my chest, I discontinued the treadmill and almost collapsed. My cardiologist diagnosed severe heart disease and admitted me, on his special recommendation, into an intensive care unit in the Vancouver General Hospital where they performed an angiogram, and the results showed that **my left main artery was 75% blocked.** I was told that the 3-vessel tube on my left main artery was severely blocked with plaque and that the only way they could fix that problem was with a bypass surgery. The physician-in-charge came to see me the next morning and asked me to sign a paper (a disclaimer and my approval to undergo bypass surgery) so that I would be operated on by the next day. He said that he had seen my angiogram report, and he tried to convince me that it was extremely urgent that I should undergo bypass surgery immediately or I risk suffering a second heart attack or die. I did not have the courage to accept that offer. I hesitated a lot and refused to sign the paper. I now realize that I must have had a vision, deep in my heart, that bypass surgery was unnecessary. I was probably guided by that vision in the right direction. I immediately told the physician-in-charge that I needed some time to think about it and I promised that I would decide about it within a week. I was then discharged from the hospital. I came home. I never went back to that hospital or any other hospital again.

My cardiologist was found to be very much disappointed and upset and started treating me with anger and bad temper, as he did not like my refusal to go through bypass surgery. He prescribed nitro spray (Nitrolingual 0.4 mg) and nitro patches which gave immediate relief whenever I had angina. I started using nitro spray whenever I took a short walk. He also prescribed a beta blocker (Acebutalol) for my heart. During the month of September, 1998, I noticed a huge change in my sexual desire. I noticed that I lost my erections and potency. I called the manufacturer of the beta blocker and I was informed that the beta blocker that I had been taking could cause impotence. I immediately discontinued that beta blocker. The same cardiologist prescribed another drug similar to the beta blocker and warned me that I must take it. But I never took it.

I also began experiencing dental problems with serious gum disease and my dentist said many of my teeth might have to be taken out.

After a couple of months, I began experiencing prostate problems (frequent urination, burning in the urethra and no erection). I went to see an urologist a few times. I took the ultrasound exam, which was actually normal. After examining my urethra, the urologist recommended prostate surgery and made an immediate appointment to arrange my surgery¾which was later found to be 100% unnecessary. I learned from my family doctor that my ultrasound exam was normal and so no surgery would be necessary. It was totally incompetent and sloppy professional practice. But there was nothing I could do about it.

Had I gone through that prostate surgery, there was a great risk that I could have been totally disabled and/or could have become impotent for the rest of my life. After all these strange experiences, I decided to stay away from hospitals, drugs, and surgery.

I then became serious about my health. I started thinking sharply about alternative ways of healing my heart. I began researching books, contacting people in health food stores, reading alternative health magazines and newsletters, and contacting people who wrote articles in those magazines about how to heal heart disease. Someone on the phone recommended a book called "Program for Reversing Heart Disease" by Dr. Dean Ornish. I purchased that book and read it very anxiously. This is the kind of book that put me on the right track. I tried to do something very simple on my own. I called it a self-prevention diet. Through self-prevention diet and after-meal exercise, diligently on a daily basis, I brought down my cholesterols from very high (arteries clogged) to normal (arteries unclogged). I also controlled my diabetes and reversed my heart disease (Refer to Chapter 4, Permanent Diabetes Control). I no longer have angina, my heart is clear and better than ever, my natural erections came back, my prostate problem disappeared, my teeth got stronger and my gum disease is wiped out and my total heath in general is rejuvenated.

After my heart disease was reversed, I saw my cardiologist. He was very much surprised to find that my heart was perfectly normal and I was no longer using nitro spray nor was I taking any heart medications. He asked me to take a stress test. No problem at all, I ran on the treadmill like an athlete and passed the stress test. My cardiologist was convinced that my heart was normal and that a bypass surgery was unnecessary.

However my cardiologist and his medical secretary were continued to be very much disappointed, upset and started treating me with anger and bad temper, as they did not like my refusal to go through bypass surgery. They were found to be so uncomfortable to see me with normal heart. I never understood why my cardiologist was so eager, curious and obsessed to have me had a bypass surgery, and what kind of advantage he could attain from it.

++

NOTICE TO READERS & DISCLAIMER
The material presented specifically in this chapter is for educational purposes only. It is designed to help diabetics to understand what heart disease is and to have an idea about how angioplasty and bypass surgery are performed in the hospital so that they can take appropriate steps through a health care professional. The author does not assume any liability for any insufficient information or inaccuracies. This is not a professional medical guide on performing angioplasty and/or bypass surgery or to have them performed.

++

REFERENCE
1. Permanent Diabetes Control (Book), Subtitle: The Complete Guide to Living Like A Normal Person Forever, Authored by Rao Konduru, MS, PhD, Reviewed and Endorsed by Dr. Marshal Dahl, MD, PhD., Endocrinologist, Faculty of Medicine, University of British Columbia, Vancouver, British Columbia, Canada, First Published in 2003. www.mydiabetescontrol.com

++

CHAPTER 12 DIABETES GLOSSARY

ANGIOGRAM
A dye is injected into the heart through catheterization and x-ray taken which shows the shadow that has the shape of the heart. By analyzing the x-ray, the doctor detects the defects if any. The doctor also views the arteries on the monitor and detects if there is any blockage or narrowing.

ANGIOPLASTY
A non-surgical procedure in which a balloon catheter is inserted into the artery and the balloon inflated in order to spread away the plaque that was accumulated within the artery.

ANTICOAGULANT
A kind of medication, given to heart patients, that keeps the blood from clotting. It is also called blood thinner.

AORTA
The main artery that carries blood, through small arteries or blood vessels, away from the heart towards all the muscles and organs.

ARTERIOSCLEROSIS
A disease process in which the arteries are hardened and lose elasticity.

ARTERY
A blood vessel that carries oxygen-rich blood to all over the body.

ATHEROSCLEROSIS
A disease process in which fat, cholesterol and other greasy substances combine to form plaque on the artery walls, which can clog the arteries and restrict the blood flow.

BASAL METABOLIC RATE
The total calorie intake a normal human body needs for survival including heart beating, breathing, maintaining human digestive system, body temperature, etc.

CALORIE
The unit of heat necessary to raise the temperature of one gram of water one degree centigrade. A kilocalorie is the unit of heat necessary to raise the temperature of one kilogram of water one degree centigrade. All food labels represent kilocalories (not calories). Calories burned displayed by exercise machines are also kilocalories (not calories).

CHOLESTEROL
A biochemical, greasy or waxy fat-like substance called lipid found in the bloodstream and in all cells. LDL is bad cholesterol and HDL is good cholesterol.

DIABETES MELLITUS
Diabetes is a Greek word meaning "to siphon." Mellitus is a Latin word meaning "honey." Diabetes Mellitus means sweet urine being siphoned through the urinary system out of the body. Diabetes develops when the pancreas makes little or no insulin. Finely crushed and chewed meal is broken down into glucose, which is the body's main source of energy. Without insulin, glucose cannot reach the body's cells but remains in the bloodstream. When the pancreas produces no insulin at all, Type-1 diabetes develops. When the pancreas does not produce enough insulin or when the body does not make use of insulin properly because of metabolic disorder, Type-2 diabetes develops.

DOUBLE SHOT
A rapid-acting insulin injected twice in this case study: first shot just before the meal consumption and exercise and second shot after the exercise in order to keep up the blood glucose levels normal for an extended period of time (up to 6 hours).

EXERCISE
A physical activity, treadmill, regular walk, biking, swimming or other, by which the body burns calories, improves muscle stimulation by speeding the transport of glucose evenly to the cells. Exercise is also called "invisible insulin" for diabetic people because it lowers blood glucose levels.

FINGERSTICKING OR FINGER-POKING
In a fingerstick blood glucose test, a drop of blood is withdrawn from the finger by means of a lancing device and placed on a glucose meter strip to measure glucose of a diabetic person.

FOOD
Food is what we consume every day to live. Every food contains three major components, carbohydrate, protein and fat. Carbohydrate and protein contain 4 kilocalories per gram while fat contains 9 kilocalories per gram.

GESTATIONAL DIABETES
Is developed temporarily in women during pregnancy mainly during the last three months. If diagnosed with gestational diabetes, nearly 40% of women usually develop Type-2 diabetes within 15 years.

GLUCOSE
Food consumed, mostly the carbohydrate source, is broken down by digestive juices into simple sugars called glucose or blood sugar. Glucose, found in the bloodstream, is the main source of energy for the body's cells.

GLUCOSE TOLERANCE TEST

A test that determines whether or not a person is diagnosed with diabetes. The person is asked to consume 75 grams of concentrated glucose solution, and the glucose levels are then monitored at intervals of 15 or 30 minutes for a period of 2 to 3 hours. Unusually high glucose levels over long hours indicate diabetes.

GLYCOGEN

The long chains of glucose stored in the liver, muscles and kidneys for future use.

GLUCAGON

A hormone secreted by the alpha cells of the pancreas which stimulates the liver to break down already stored glycogen to glucose and to release it into the bloodstream. Commercial glucagon is also available as medication to be injected into the body to raise the glucose level.

GLUCOSE METER

A simple self-blood glucose-monitoring manual instrument that easily monitors blood glucose. Diabetic people use glucose meter every day to monitor and record their blood glucose levels.

GLUCOWATCH® BIOGRAPHER

A real time blood glucose-monitoring unit (FDA approved in 2001) marketed by Cygnus Inc. as of April 15, 2002. It monitors blood glucose level every 20 minutes for 12 consecutive hours and stores data. After shutting down for a 3-hour warm-up period, it resumes operation.

HEART

It is a never-ceasing pump that supplies blood throughout the body to provide energy.

HEART ATTACK

When the blood flow in an artery is fully blocked, a small or large portion of the heart muscle damages and heart attack occurs.

HEAVY MEAL

Any big meal over 800 kilocalories is considered a heavy meal in this case study. An insulin-dependent diabetic person must inject a rapid-acting insulin before a heavy meal and do exercise after a heavy meal to keep up normal glucose levels for long time (up to 6 hours). For a heavy meal a double-shot of rapid-acting insulin is required in this case study.

The meaning of heavy meal or major meal is the same in this case study.

HEMOGLOBIN A1c

A protein molecule that carries oxygen from the lungs to the body's cells. Red blood cells live in the body for 60 to 90 days during which time the glucose present in the bloodstream is bound to hemoglobin to form glycohemoglobin or glycosylated hemoglobin. There are three types of hemoglobin:

A1a, A1b and A1c. Measurement of hemoglobin A1c reflects the average blood glucose level and its control over the preceding 90 days.

HIGH BLOOD PRESSURE

When the blood pressure is above 140/90 mm Hg, the person is said to have high blood pressure or hypertension.

HYDROGENATED FATS

Unsaturated fats that are manufactured from unsaturated fatty acids in which the vacant carbon atoms are artificially bound with hydrogen to make the hydrocarbon chain saturated. In this process of hydrogenation, the liquid oil is solidified. An example is margarine.

HYPERGLYCEMIA

Occurs when blood glucose levels are elevated, and the person experiences extreme thirst, frequent urination and loss of appetite.

HYPOGLYCEMIA

Occurs when blood glucose levels are too low (below 4 mmol/L or 72 mg/dL), and the person experiences nervousness, sweating, hunger, blurred vision and imbalance. One should consume sugar, candy, juice or Coke to treat hypoglycemia.

INSULIN

A hormone made and secreted by the beta cells of the pancreas into the bloodstream to help deliver glucose to the body's cells. Without insulin, glucose cannot get into the body's cells. Commercial insulin is sold in many forms such as Humalog, NovoRapid or Novolog, Lantus, Humulin-N, Humulin-R.

INSULIN PUMP

An insulin pump is a painless insertion mini-device available for diabetic people in which most commonly a rapid-acting insulin such as Humalog is stored in order to deliver minute quantities of insulin ranging from one hundredth to one tenth of a unit according to the programmed instructions.

ISLETS OF LANGERHANS

The human pancreas is comprised of about one million cells in total. About 1 to 2% of these cells are endocrine or islets of Langerhans which produce both insulin and glucagon. The other 98%, exocrine cells, produce digestive juices.

KETONES

A kind of acids body produces and releases in the blood and urine when blood glucose levels are too high (over 13.mmol/L or 234 mg/dL).

LIGHT MEAL

Any meal under 800 kilocalories is considered a light meal in this case study. For a light meal, it was possible to keep up normal blood glucose levels for a long time with single shot of rapid-acting insulin and exercise.

MAJOR MEAL

Any big meal over 800 kilocalories is considered a major meal in this case study. An insulin-dependent diabetic person must inject a rapid-acting insulin before a major meal and do exercise after a major meal to keep up normal glucose levels for long time (up to 6 hours). For a major meal a double-shot of rapid-acting insulin is required in this case study. The meaning of major meal or heavy meal is the same in this case study.

METABOLISM

A process in the body in which a source of energy such as food is converted into energy or heat to be used or absorbed by the body's cells.

MELLITUS

It is derived from a Latin word meaning honey.

METABOLIC EQUIVALENT (MET)

The energy expenditure per kilogram of body weight per hour for sitting quietly. It was confirmed that an average adult spends about 1 kilocalorie per hour per 1 kilogram of his/her body weight for sitting quietly or lying down without any exercise.

MONOUNSATURATED FATS

Fats that are liquid at room temperature but begin to solidify when placed in a cooler or refrigerator. Examples are olive oil, canola oil, peanut oil, etc.

OMEGA-3 AND OMEGA-6 FATTY ACIDS

Polyunsaturated fatty acids where 3 and 6 refer to the first carbon double bond located in hydrocarbon chain. They are called "Essential Fatty Acids." The human body does not produce them. People should consume them.

OPEN HEART SURGERY

A bypass surgery made to operate on the heart by opening the chest, and grafting a new blood vessel between aorta and a spot beyond the blockage of the artery in order to restore the blood flow in the artery.

PANCREAS

A soft, pinkish-gray banana-shaped gland of about 15 to 25 cm long, connected to the upper part of the small intestine by means of a duct. The pancreas produces both insulin and glucagon to maintain normal glucose levels.

PREVENTION DIET

Any simple diet by eating which one can keep the total cholesterol under 150 mg/dL (3.88 mmol/L) and HDL Ratio under 3.0.

PROSTAGLANDIN

A hormone-like chemical produced in the human body under the influence of essential fatty acids such as omega-3 and omega-6. Prostaglandin type E1 plays an important role in male sexual function and this chemical is being used to treat erectile dysfunction.

POLYUNSATURATED FATS

Fats that are liquid at room temperature and also in a cooler or refrigerator but react quickly with oxygen and get rotten or sour. Examples are sunflower oil, sesame oil, soy oil, etc.

PULMONARY CIRCULATION

The circulation of the blood between the heart and lungs while the blood gets purified in the lungs and returned to the heart.

RED BLOOD CELLS

Saucer-shaped red cells in the blood plasma that carries oxygen to all the body's cells. Hemoglobin is present in the red blood cells.

SATURATED FATS

Fats that contain saturated fatty acids with a fully saturated hydrocarbon chain. Saturated fats are solid and stable at room temperature and do not react readily with oxygen at room temperature. A fat product is made up of fatty acids and glycerol.

SINGLE SHOT

Single dose of rapid-acting insulin Humalog injected just before a meal in this case study.

SORBITOL

Sorbitol occurs naturally in a wide variety of fruits and barriers and is used extensively in manufacturing sugar-free candies, frozen desserts and baked goods. It provides one-third fewer calories than sugar (2.6 calories per gram). The human intestinal tract does not allow sorbitol to be absorbed so when we eat sorbitol, it passes through the body and does not contribute any calories whatsoever. If consumed too much it could cause diarrhea. When sorbitol is formulated on the body's cells as a result of the elevated glucose levels over a long period of time, it acts as an alcohol and punches holes in the cells and becomes largely responsible in developing long term side effects of diabetes (heart attack, stroke, heart disease, kidney disease, eye disease, nerve damage and others).

STRESS TEST

To detect heart disease, a person is asked to run on a treadmill, speed is increased, heart rate, blood pressure are measured and electrocardiogram is taken. If the person feels pain in the chest during the test and/or if the electrocardiogram is not normal, the person will be diagnosed with heart disease.

STROKE

A sudden disruption of blood flow to the brain caused due to a blood clot, narrowed artery or a leak in the blood vessel.

TRANS FATS

Partially hydrogenated fats resulted by adding hydrogen atom mainly to vegetable oils and are used extensively in fast food restaurants and bakeries. Examples are cookies, cakes, French fries, chips, etc. They are not good for diabetic people as they could clog arteries.

TRIGLYCERIDES
Another form of fat, a small portion of which is found in the bloodstream and the large portion in the fat tissue. The body needs insulin to clean up this type of fat from the blood.

UNSATURATED FATS
Fats that contain unsaturated fatty acids in which not all carbon atoms are bound with hydrogen atoms but one or more positions are vacant. Unsaturated fats are usually liquid at room temperature. There are two types of unsaturated fats such as monounsaturated fats and polyunsaturated fats.

VEIN
A blood vessel that returns blood to the heart from the body or lungs.

WHITE BLOOD CELLS
Blood is made up of several kinds of tiny cells such as red blood cells, white blood cells and platelets. White blood cells fight off germs and protect the human body from getting sick. White blood cells do not contain hemoglobin.

Suggested References

1. Diabetes Glossary by Endocrineweb.
https://www.endocrineweb.com/conditions/diabetes/diabetes-glossary

2. Diabetes Glossary by Cleveland Clinic.
https://my.clevelandclinic.org/health/articles/9829-diabetes-glossary

3. Diabetes Glossary by Centers for Disease Control & Prevention (CDC).
https://www.cdc.gov/diabetes/library/glossary.html

4. Diabetes Glossary by Your Dictionary.
https://www.yourdictionary.com/diabetes

5. Diabetes Glossary by The Diabetes Council
https://www.thediabetescouncil.com/diabetes-dictionary-common-terms-to-know-for-diabetics/

About the Author

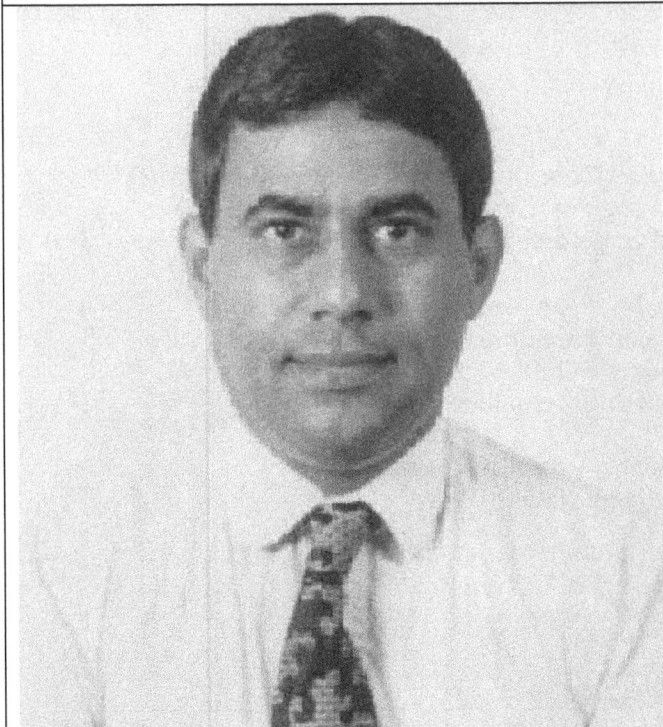

Dr. Rao M Konduru was a Chemical Engineer, and held two Master's degrees and two doctorates and two post-doctoral titles, all in chemical engineering. He published a book in 2003 titled "Permanent Diabetes Control," which earned immense respect and appreciation. Many people said it was a wonderful book. After suffering from a sudden heart attack in 1998, even though his left artery was 75% clogged with severe angina, he said "NO" to bypass surgery. He did what none of us would even think of doing. He simply relied on his natural self-prevention diet and exercise, and with it he reversed his critical diabetic heart disease in a matter of months, and developed a method to accomplish Permanent Diabetes Control. He also came up with a trial-and-error procedure to determine the optimal insulin dose that would tightly control diabetes, and would allow a diabetic person to live like a normal person for the rest of his/her life.

Dr. Rao M Konduru maintained his hemoglobin A1c level under 6.0% consistently. His personal best hemoglobin A1c level of 5.0% was an extraordinary result any diabetic person would hope to accomplish in a lifetime. Perhaps Dr. Rao M Konduru was the only diabetic person lived in this world with "Permanent Diabetes Control".

Once again, health demons such as uncontrollable weight gain, sleep apnea and chronic insomnia came his way. He did not give up, but persisted on discovering new, natural and effortless treatments of his own in reversing these most difficult disorders. His extensive scientific research experience and his powerful knowledge helped him battle and combat these life challenges. He figured out their root causes, and developed natural yet powerful techniques to cure these health disorders himself. After losing 40 pounds of weight and 12 inches around the waist, he successfully reversed his obesity, obstructive sleep apnea and chronic insomnia. He carefully created and published the following excellent guidebooks on Amazon so that others can benefit and be inspired to achieve similar results. His most recent book "Drinking Water Guide" is a 540-page book of wealth of information on drinking water for the rest of us.

1. Permanent Diabetes Control — www.mydiabetescontrol.com
2. The Secret to Controlling Type 2 Diabetes — www.mydiabetescontrol.com
3. Reversing Obesity — www.reversingsleepapnea.com/ebook2.html
4. Reversing Sleep Apnea — www.reversingsleepapnea.com
5. Reversing Insomnia — www.reversinginsomnia.com
6. Reversing Insomnia in 3 Days — www.reversinginsomnia.com
7. Drinking Water Guide — www.drinkingwaterguide.com
8. Drinking Water Guide-II — www.drinkingwaterguide.com
9. The Origin of the Earth's Water — www.drinkingwaterguide.com
10. Autobiography Of Dr. Rao M Konduru — www.mydiabetescontrol.com/Bio/

- Prime Publishing Co.

PLEASE WRITE A REVIEW ABOUT THIS BOOK

Now that you have read this book, please write a review about this book, and post your review on Amazon.

a. Please log into your Amazon account,
b. Search for this book "Permanent Diabetes Control (Author: Rao Konduru, PhD)", or by using ISBN # 9780973112009, and click on the book cover & scroll down,
c. Click on "Customer Reviews", click on "Write a customer review" button, and "Create Review" box pops up.
d. Kindly write your REVIEW in the Write-Your-Review box, type a Headline, and click on 5 stars overall rating (you can give up to 5 stars).
e. Click on "Submit" button, and your review will be registered on Amazon.
f. Amazon will acknowledge your review with an email confirmation!

Thanks for posting your review!
Your opinion counts!

YOUR OPINION
COUNTS!

Kindle eBook Is Available on Amazon

You can read this book on your computer, laptop, tablet, e-reader, iPhone, or any Kindle device by purchasing Kindle eBook. It is available on Amazon. Please log into your Amazon account, and search for "Permanent Diabetes Control, Kindle eBook" or by using ASIN # B07RDZR1QW.

The End Of The Book "Permanent Diabetes Control"!

BEST WISHES!

www.ingramcontent.com/pod-product-compliance
Lightning Source LLC
Chambersburg PA
CBHW061754210326
41518CB00036B/2329